Blueprints **Notes & Cases**
Pathophysiology:
Pulmonary, Gastrointestinal and Rheumatology

Blueprints Notes & Cases
Series Editor: Aaron B. Caughey MD, MPP, MPH

Blueprints *Notes & Cases—Microbiology and Immunology*
Monica Gandhi, Paul Baum, C. Bradley Hare, Aaron B. Caughey

Blueprints *Notes & Cases—Biochemistry, Genetics, and Embryology*
Juan E. Vargas, Aaron B. Caughey, Annie Tan, Jonathan Z. Li

Blueprints *Notes & Cases—Pharmacology*
Katherine Y. Yang, Larissa R. Graff, Aaron B. Caughey

Blueprints *Notes & Cases—Pathophysiology: Cardiovascular, Endocrine, and Reproduction*
Gordon Leung, Susan H. Tran, Tina O. Tan, Aaron B. Caughey

Blueprints *Notes & Cases—Pathophysiology: Pulmonary, Gastrointestinal, and Rheumatology*
Michael Filbin, Lisa M. Lee, Brian L. Shaffer, Aaron B. Caughey

Blueprints *Notes & Cases—Pathophysiology: Renal, Hematology, and Oncology*
Aaron B. Caughey, Christie del Castillo, Nancy Palmer, Karen Spizer, Dana N. Tuttle

Blueprints *Notes & Cases—Neuroscience*
Robert T. Wechsler, Alexander M. Morss, Courtney J. Wusthoff, Aaron B. Caughey

Blueprints *Notes & Cases—Behavioral Science and Epidemiology*
Judith Neugroschl, Jennifer Hoblyn, Christie del Castillo, Aaron B. Caughey

Blueprints Notes & Cases
Pathophysiology:
Pulmonary, Gastrointestinal and Rheumatology

Michael Filbin, MD
Clinical Instructor, Department of Emergency Medicine
Harvard Affiliated Emergency Medicine Residency
Massachusetts General Hospital
Boston, Massachusetts

Lisa M. Lee, MD
Resident, Obstetrics and Gynecology
University of California, San Francisco
San Francisco, California

Brian L. Shaffer, MD
Resident in Obstetrics, Gynecology, and Reproductive Sciences
University of California, San Francisco
San Francisco, California

Aaron B. Caughey, MD, MPP, MPH
Clinical Instructor, Division of Maternal-Fetal Medicine
Department of Obstetrics & Gynecology
University of California, San Francisco
San Francisco, California
Division of Health Services and Policy Analysis
University of California, Berkeley
Berkeley, California

Series Editor: Aaron B. Caughey, MD, MPP, MPH

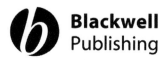
Blackwell
Publishing

© 2004 by Blackwell Publishing

Blackwell Publishing, Inc., 350 Main Street, Malden, Massachusetts 02148-5018, USA
Blackwell Publishing Ltd, 9600 Garsington Road, Oxford OX4 2DQ, UK
Blackwell Science Asia Pty Ltd, 550 Swanston Street, Carlton South, Victoria 3053, Australia

02 03 04 05 5 4 3 2 1

ISBN: 1–4051-0351–5

Library of Congress Cataloging-in-Publication Data

Filbin, Michael R.
    Pathophysiology. Pulmonary, gastrointestinal, and rheumatology / Michael Filbin, Lisa M. Lee, Brian L. Shaffer. — 1st ed.
      p. ; cm. — (Blueprints notes & cases)
    Includes index.
    ISBN 1-4051-0351-5 (pbk.)
    1. Respiratory organs—Pathophysiology—Case studies. 2. Gastrointestinal system—Pathophysiology—Case studies.
3. Joints—Pathophysiology—Case studies. I. Lee, Lisa M. II. Shaffer, Brian L. III. Title. IV. Title: Pulmonary, gastrointestinal,
and rheumatology. V. Series.
    [DNLM: 1. Respiratory Tract Diseases—physiopathology—Problems and Exercises. 2. Gastrointestinal Diseases—
physiopathology—Problems and Exercises. 3. Rheumatic Diseases——physiopathology—Problems and Exercises. WF 18.2
F479p 2003]
    RC711.F54 2003
    616.2'0047—dc21
                                   2003007077

A catalogue record for this title is available from the British Library

Acquisitions: Beverly Copland
Development: Selene Steneck
Production: Jennifer Kowalewski
Cover design: Hannus Design Associates
Interior design: Janet Bollow Associates
Typesetter: Peirce Graphic Services, in Stuart, Florida
Printed and bound by Courier Companies, in Westford, MA

For further information on Blackwell Publishing, visit our website: www.blackwellpublishing.com

Notice: The indications and dosages of all drugs in this book have been recommended in the
medical literature and conform to the practices of the general community. The medications
described do not necessarily have specific approval by the Food and Drug Administration for
use in the diseases and dosages for which they are recommended. The package insert for each
drug should be consulted for use and dosage as approved by the FDA. Because standards for
usage change, it is advisable to keep abreast of revised recommendations, particularly those
concerning new drugs.

Contents

Reviewers

Faunda Campbell
Class of 2004
Drexel School of Medicine
Philadelphia, Pennsylvania

Meena Nahata
Class of 2004
Nova Southeastern University College of Medical Sciences
Ft. Lauderdale, Florida

Christopher Teng
Class of 2004
SUNY Downstate College of Medicine
Brooklyn, New York

Val Tramonte II
Class of 2004
University of Nevada School of Medicine
Reno, Nevada

Leslie Van Schaack
Class of 2004
Medical College of Virginia
Richmond, Virginia

Preface

The first two years of medical school are a demanding time for medical students. Whether the school follows a traditional curriculum or one that is case-based, every student is expected to learn and be able to apply basic science information in a clinical situation.

Medical schools are increasingly using clinical presentations as the background to teach the basic sciences. Case-based learning has become more common at many medical schools as it offers a way to catalogue the multitude of symptoms, syndromes and diseases in medicine.

Blueprints **Notes & Cases** is a new series by Blackwell Publishing designed to provide students a textbook to study the basic science topics combined with clinical data. This method of learning is also the way to prepare for the clinical case format of USMLE questions. The eight books in this series will make the basic science topics not only more interesting, but also more meaningful and memorable. Students will be learning not only the why of a principle, but also how it might commonly be seen in practice.

The books in the *Blueprints* Notes & Cases series feature a comprehensive collection of cases which are designed to introduce one or more basic science topics. Through these cases, students gain an understanding of the coursework as they learn to:

- Think through the cases
- Look for classic presentations of most common diseases and syndromes
- Integrate the basic science content with clinical application
- Prepare for course exams and Step 1 USMLE
- Be prepared for clinical rotations

This series covers all the essential material needed in the basic science courses. Where possible, the books are organized in an organ-based system.

Clinical cases lead off and are the basis for discussion of the basic science content. A list of **"thought questions"** follows the case presentation. These questions are designed to challenge the reader to begin to think about how basic science topics apply to real-life clinical situations. The **answers to these questions** are integrated within the **basic science review and discussion** that follows. This offers a clinical framework from which to understand the basic content.

The discussion section is followed by a high-yield **Thumbnail table and Key Points box** which highlight and summarize the essential information presented in the discussion.

The cases also include two to four **multiple-choice questions** that allow readers to check their knowledge of that topic. Many of the answer explanations provide an opportunity for further discussion by delving into more depth in related areas. An **answer key** for these questions is at the end of the section for easy reference, and **full answer explanations** can be found at the end of the book.

This new series was designed to provide comprehensive content in a concise and templated format for ease in learning. A dedicated attempt was made to include sufficient art, tables, and clinical treatment, all while keeping the books from becoming too lengthy. We know you have much to read and that what you want is high-yield, vital facts.

The authors and series editor for these eight books, as well as everyone in editorial, production, sales and marketing at Blackwell Publishing, have worked long and hard to provide new textbooks to help you learn and be able to apply what you've learned. We engaged in multiple student email surveys and many focus groups to "hear what you needed" in new basic science level textbooks to meet the current curriculums, tests, and coursework. We know that you value this "student to student" approach, and sincerely hope you like what we have put together **just for you.**

Blackwell Publishing and the authors wish you success in your studies and your future medical career. Please feel free to offer us any comments or suggestions on these new books at blue@bos.blackwellpublishing.com.

Acknowledgments

To my family, friends, colleagues, and patients, all who provide inspiration for my work.
Mike

To Lishiana—my wife and best friend, for all of your patience, love, and support.
Brian

For my husband, Neal, and my parents, Dan and Barbara, who have always supported me in whatever endeavors I have chosen to pursue.
Lisa

Thanks to the staff at Blackwell Publishing, particularly Selene and Jen, for all of their hard work. Thanks to Mike, Brian, and Lisa for putting their talent and energy into this project. Special thanks to my family, Bill, Carol, Ethan, Samara, Jim, Wendy, Nicole, and my wife, Susan, for their continued support of my academic and clinical career.
Aaron

Abbreviations

A-a gradient	difference in partial pressure of oxygen between alveoli and arterial blood
abx	antibiotics
ACTH	adrenocorticotropic hormone
ADH	antidiuretic hormone
AFP	alphafetal protein
ALT	alanine aminotransferase
AMP	adenosine monophosphate (adenylic acid)
ANA	antinuclear antibody
ANCA	antineutrophil cytoplasmic antibody
ARDS	acute respiratory distress syndrome
AST	aspartate aminotransferase
ATN	acute tubular necrosis
BS	barium swallow
BUN	blood urea nitrogen
CA	cancer
CA	carbonic anhydrase
Cao_2	arterial oxygen content
CCK	cholecystokinin
CF	cystic fibrosis
CFTR	cystic fibrosis transmembrane regulator
Cl	chloride
CMV	cytomegalovirus
CNS	central nervous system
CO	carbon monoxide
CO_2	carbon dioxide
$[CO_2]$	concentration of dissolved CO_2 in serum measured by partial pressure P_{CO2}
COHb	carboxy-hemoglobin
COPD	chronic obstructive pulmonary disease
CREST syndrome	calcinosis, *Raynaud's phenomenon, esophageal disease, sclerodactyly, telangectasia*
CRF	chronic renal failure
CSF	cerebrospinal fluid
CT	computed tomography
CVAT	costovertebral angle tenderness
CX	dissolved gas

DIC	disseminated intravascular coagulation
DIP	distal interphalangeal
DLCO	diffusion capacity of gas across the alveolar capillary membrane
DVT	deep venous thrombosis
ECG	electrocardiogram
ELISA	enzyme-linked immunosorbent assay
EM	electron microscopy
ER	emergency room
ERCP	endoscopic retrograde cholangiopancreatography
ESR	erythrocyte sedimentation rate
EtOH	alcohol
FEV	forced expiratory volume
FEV_1	forced expiratory volume in 1 second
Fio_2	fractional percentage of oxygen in inspired air
FRC	functional residual capacity
FVC	functional vital capacity
GAS	group A streptococci
Gen	in general
GERD	gastroesophageal reflux disease
GGT	γ-glutamyl transferase
GI	gastrointestinal tract
GMP	guanylic acid
GU	genitourinary system
H_2HCO_3	carbonic acid
HAV	hepatitis A virus
HBsAb	hepatitis B surface antibody
HBcAb	hepatitis B core antibody
HBcAg	hepatitis B core antigen
HBeAb	hepatitis B envelope antibody
HBeAg	hepatitis B envelope antigen
HBsAg	hepatitis B surface antigen
HBV	hepatitis B virus
HCl	hydrochloric acid
HDV	hepatitis D virus
HEV	hepatitis E virus

HCV	hepatitis C virus
HCVAb	hepatitis C antibody
HCO_3^-	bicarbonate
$[HCO_3^-]$	concentration of serum HCO_3^-
H&E	hemotoxylin and eosin
Hgb	hemoglobin concentration
HGPRT	hypoxanthine-guanine phosphoribosyltransferase
HIV	human immunodeficiency virus
HRT	hormone replacement therapy
HSV	herpes simplex virus
Hx	history
IBD	inflammatory bowel disease
ICU	intensive care unit
IMP	inosinic acid
IPF	idiopathic pulmonary fibrosis OR interstitial pulmonary fibrosis
J receptors	juxtacapillary receptors
KD	Kawasaki's disease
LAD	left anterior descending coronary artery
LDL	low density lipoprotein
LES	lower esophageal sphincter
LM	light microscopy
LT	labile toxin
MHC	major histocompatibility complex (molecules; proteins)
mmHg	millimeters of mercury
MV	minute ventilation
Na	sodium
NAD^+	nicotine adenine dinucleotide, oxidized form
NADH	nicotine adenine dinucleotide, reduced form
NEC	necrotizing enterocolitis
NG	nasogastric (decompression)
NPPV	noninvasive positive-pressure ventilation
NSAID	nonsteroidal anti-inflammatory drug
N/V	nausea and vomiting
OCP	oral contraceptive pill
OTC	over the counter (over-the-counter drugs)
P_{50}	oxygen tension that produces 50% hemoglobin saturation
PA_{CO_2}	partial pressure of carbon dioxide in alveoli
Pa_{CO_2}	partial pressure of carbon dioxide in arterial blood
PA_{O_2}	partial pressure of oxygen in alveoli
Pa_{O_2}	partial pressure of oxygen in arterial blood
PAS	periodic acid Schiff
PBC	primary biliary cirrhosis
P_{CO_2}	partial pressure of carbon dioxide as measured by blood gas analysis
PDGF	platelet-derived growth factor
PEEP	positive end-expiratory pressure
PFT	pulmonary function test
P_i	interstitial hydrostatic pressure
π_ι	interstitial oncotic pressure
π_π	capillary oncotic pressure
PID	pelvic inflammatory disease
Pi_{O_2}	partial pressure of inhaled oxygen
PMN	polymorphonuclear (leukocyte)
P_{O_2}	partial pressure of oxygen as measured by blood gas analysis
P_p	capillary hydrostatic pressure
PPD	purified protein derivative
PRPD	5-phosphoribosyl-1-pyrophosphate
PSC	primary sclerosing cholangitis
PT	prothrombin time
PTH	parathyroid hormone
PTT	partial thromboplastin time
PUD	peptic ulcer disease
Pv_{O_2}	partial pressure of oxygen in venous blood
Px	partial pressure
Q	perfusion
RBBB	right bundle branch block
Re	Reynold's number
RNA	ribonucleic acid
RNP	ribonucleoprotein
RV	residual volume
Sa_{O_2}	arterial oxygen concentration
SIADH	syndrome of inappropriate antidiuretic hormone
SLE	systemic lupus erythematosus

ST	stable toxin	**V**	ventilation
SVC	superior vena cava	**V$_A$**	alveolar ventilation
TB	tuberculosis	**VC**	vital capacity
TLC	total lung capacity	**Vco$_2$**	carbon dioxide produced by peripheral tissue
TSS	toxic shock syndrome	**VEGF**	vascular endothelial growth factor
UC	ulcerative colitis	**VLDL**	very low density lipoprotein
UDC	uridine diphosphate	**V/Q ratio**	ventilation-perfusion ratio
UES	upper esophogeal sphincter	**VS**	vital signs
UGT	UDP-bilirubin glucuronosyltransferase	**WBC**	white blood cell (count)

Normal Ranges of Laboratory Values

BLOOD, PLASMA, SERUM

Alanine aminotransferase (ALT, GPT at 30 C)	8–20 U/L
Amylase, serum	25–125 U/L
Aspartate aminotransferase (AST, GOT at 30 C)	8–20 U/L
Bilirubin, serum (adult) Total // Direct	0.1–1.0 mg/dL // 0.0–0.3 mg/dL
Calcium, serum (Ca^{2+})	8.4–10.2 mg/dL
Cholesterol, serum	Rec: < 200 mg/dL
Cortisol, serum	0800 h: 5–23 μg/dL // 1600 h: 3–15 μg/dL
	2000 h: ≤ 50% of 0800 h
Creatine kinase, serum	Male: 25–90 U/L
	Female: 10–70 U/L
Creatinine, serum	0.6–1.2 mg/dL
Electrolytes, serum	
Sodium (Na^+)	136–145 mEq/L
Chloride (Cl^-)	95–105 mEq/L
Potassium (K^+)	3.5–5.0 mEq/L
Bicarbonate (HCO_3^-)	22–28 mEq/L
Magnesium (Mg^{2+})	1.5–2.0 mEq/L
Ferritin, serum	Male: 15–200 ng/mL
	Female: 12–150 ng/mL
Follicle-stimulating hormone, serum/plasma	Male: 4–25 mIU/mL
	Female: premenopause 4–30 mIU/mL
	midcycle peak 10–90 mIU/mL
	postmenopause 40–250 mIU/mL
Gases, arterial blood (room air)	
pH	7.35–7.45
P_{CO_2}	33–45 mm Hg
P_{O_2}	75–105 mm Hg
Glucose, serum	Fasting: 70–110 mg/dL
	2-h postprandial: < 120 mg/dL
Growth hormone—arginine stimulation	Fasting: < 5 ng/mL
	provocative stimuli: > 7 ng/mL
Iron	50–70 μg/dL
Lactate dehydrogenase, serum	45–90 U/L
Luteinizing hormone, serum/plasma	Male: 6–23 mIU/mL
	Female: follicular phase 5–30 mIU/mL
	midcycle 75–150 mIU/mL
	postmenopause 30–200 mIU/mL
Osmolality, serum	275–295 mOsmol/kg
Parathyroid hormone, serum, N-terminal	230–630 pg/mL
Phosphate (alkaline), serum (p-NPP at 30 C)	20–70 U/L
Phosphorus (inorganic), serum	3.0–4.5 mg/dL
Prolactin, serum (hPRL)	< 20 ng/mL
Proteins, serum	
Total (recumbent)	6.0–7.8 g/dL
Albumin	3.5–5.5 g/dL
Globulin	2.3–3.5 g/dL
Thyroid-stimulating hormone, serum or plasma	0.5–5.0 μU/mL
Thyroidal iodine (^{123}I) uptake	8–30% of administered dose/24 h
Thyroxine (T_4), serum	5–12 μg/dL
Triglycerides, serum	35–160 mg/dL
Triiodothyronine (T_3), serum (RIA)	115–190 ng/dL
Triiodothyronine (T_3), resin uptake	25–35%
Urea nitrogen, serum (BUN)	7–18 mg/dL
Uric acid, serum	3.0–8.2 mg/dL

CEREBROSPINAL FLUID

Cell count	0–5 cells/mm^3
Chloride	118–132 mEq/L
Gamma globulin	3–12% total proteins
Glucose	40–70 mg/dL
Pressure	70–180 mm H$_2$O
Proteins, total	< 40 mg/dL

HEMATOLOGIC

Bleeding time (template)	2–7 minutes
Erythrocyte count	Male: 4.3–5.9 million/mm^3
	Female: 3.5–5.5 million/mm^3
Erythrocyte sedimentation rate (Westergren)	Male: 0–15 mm/h
	Female: 0–20 mm/h
Hematocrit	Male: 41–53%
	Female: 36–46%
Hemoglobin A$_{1C}$	≤ 6%
Hemoglobin, blood	Male: 13.5–17.5 g/dL
	Female: 12.0–16.0 g/dL
Leukocyte count and differential	
Leukocyte count	4500–11,000/mm^3
Segmented neutrophils	54–62%
Bands	3–5%
Eosinophils	1–3%
Basophils	0–0.75%
Lymphocytes	25–33%
Monocytes	3–7%
Mean corpuscular hemoglobin	25.4–34.6 pg/cell
Mean corpuscular hemoglobin concentration	31–36% Hb/cell
Mean corpuscular volume	80–100 μm^3
Partial thromboplastin time (activated)	25–40 seconds
Platelet count	150,000–400,000/mm^3
Prothrombin time	11–15 seconds
Reticulocyte count	0.5–1.5% of red cells
Thrombin time < 2 seconds deviation from control	
Volume	
Plasma	Male: 25–43 mL/kg
	Female: 28–45 mL/kg
Red cell	Male: 20–36 mL/kg
	Female: 19–31 mL/kg

SWEAT

Chloride	0–35 mmol/L

URINE

Calcium	100–300 mg/24 h
Chloride	Varies with intake
Creatine clearance	Male: 97–137 mL/min
	Female: 88–128 mL/min
Osmolality	50–1400 mOsmol/kg
Oxalate	8–40 μg/mL
Potassium	Varies with diet
Proteins, total	< 150 mg/24 h
Sodium	Varies with diet
Uric acid	Varies with diet

Pulmonary

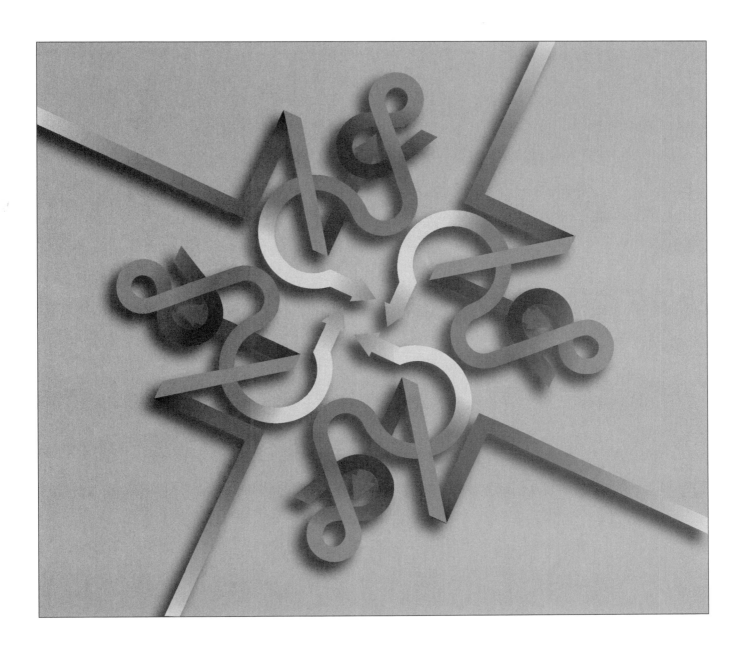

HPI: TS, a 22-year-old college wrestler, is preparing for his upcoming senior season as a heavyweight wrestler. Despite his heavyweight status, TS is in very good shape and likes to run stairs to get ready for the extreme cardiopulmonary demands of wrestling. He runs the 250-step aisle in the stands of his college stadium. It takes TS 2 minutes to run to the top and 3 minutes to walk back down. At maximal workload his total body oxygen consumption increases from about 0.5 liters per minute at rest to about 4.0 liters per minute at maximal exercise workload. To facilitate this increase in oxygen consumption his cardiac output increases from about 5 liters per minute to 25 liters per minute, and his ventilation increases from 15 liters per minute to 150 liters per minute. As TS arrives at the top the second time he is breathing at 40 times per minute, his heartbeat is 146 beats per minute, his chest is burning, he feels starved for oxygen, and his muscles begin to fatigue. He is now delivering the maximal amount of oxygen to his muscle tissue, but it is not enough to keep up with the current oxygen consumption rate. He begins to fatigue as anaerobic metabolism creates lactic acid.

Thought Questions

■ Which mechanisms allow oxygen transport from the outside world to enter end-organ tissues that utilize oxygen as fuel?

■ Which component of oxygen transport is the rate-limiting factor at maximal workload and oxygen utilization?

■ Which respiratory muscles are involved in inspiration and expiration and how does the mechanism of breathing change during exercise?

Basic Science Review and Discussion

Oxygen Transport There are five major mechanisms of oxygen transport from the outside world to its final destination in end-organ tissues that utilize oxygen for fuel:

1. *Ventilation* is the mechanical process of drawing air into the airways and alveoli via negative pressure created by active expansion of the chest wall.

2. *Alveolar diffusion* is the transfer of oxygen molecules across the alveolar cell membrane, interstitium, and pulmonary capillary membrane into the pulmonary circulation.

3. *Binding* is a function carried out by hemoglobin in red blood cells whereby four oxygen molecules are bound to a hemoglobin moiety.

4. *Circulation* refers to cardiac output that propels oxygenated blood to the peripheral capillary tissue beds.

5. *Peripheral diffusion* occurs in oxygen-utilizing tissues as oxygen molecules are off-loaded from saturated hemoglobin molecules across capillary membranes and interstitial tissue into cells that utilize oxygen.

There is a limit to oxygen utilization and thus a maximum workload achievable before oxygen utilization in peripheral tissues surpasses oxygen delivery. At this point anaerobic metabolism comes in to play and its by-product lactic acid

begins to accumulate in peripheral tissues. This is referred to as the anaerobic threshold and corresponds with maximal oxygen consumption. Of the five steps of oxygen transport, cardiac output is the rate-limiting factor that determines maximal oxygen consumption in a healthy person.

Mechanisms of Ventilation The diaphragm is the most important muscle for inspiration. It is attached to the lower portion of the rib cage and—when contracted—pushes the contents of the abdomen downward, which increases the vertical dimension of the thorax. The contraction of the diaphragm also pulls up on the naturally down-sloping rib cage that is hinged to the vertebrae in a bucket-handle fashion. Lifting the individual bucket handles acts to increase the anteroposterior dimension of the thorax (Figure 1-1). The increased volume of the thorax creates a negative intrathoracic pressure that draws air through the airways and into the alveoli. The diaphragm is innervated by the phrenic nerve that originates from the cervical levels C3–5. The diaphragm is unique in that it acts as both an involuntary and voluntary muscle. During sleep and rest,

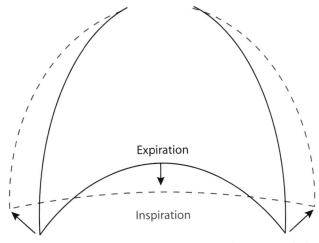

Expiration

Inspiration

Figure 1-1. Diaphragm depression and ribcage elevation results in increased thoracic volume during inspiration.

the diaphragm contracts involuntarily at a rate determined by respiratory centers in the medulla. This process can be overcome voluntarily by conscious breath holding, increased inspiratory excursion, or forceful exhaling.

Also important during inspiration are the external intercostal muscles that connect adjacent ribs. These are oriented in a forward down-sloping direction as they connect the top rib with the bottom rib. This contraction acts to lift the rib cage as a whole, increasing the anteroposterior dimension of the thorax. During exercise, the tidal volume can be increased by using accessory muscles of inspiration. These include the scalene muscles that lift the first two ribs and the sternocleidomastoids that elevate the sternum. During maximal exertion, the diaphragm can increase its excursion to 10 cm (usually 1 cm at rest); therefore, the diaphragm is still the most important muscle involved in increasing tidal volume during exercise.

At rest, expiration is a *passive* process whereby the elasticity of lung tissue and the chest wall restore the thoracic dimensions to resting values. During exercise, however, expiration is facilitated by accessory muscles that include the abdominal wall muscles (rectus abdominus, internal and external obliques). Abdominal wall muscles act to compress the contents of the abdomen and thereby push the diaphragm up. The internal intercostal muscles are oriented in the opposite direction from the external intercostals, and therefore when contracted they pull the ribcage downward toward its resting position. The advantage to using accessory muscles of expiration is to shorten expiratory time and thus increase ventilatory rate.

Case Conclusion   TS is able to do a total of 10 repetitions up the stairs within 50 minutes. His ventilatory rate and heart rate have changed little since the second repetition, and thus his oxygen consumption has remained fairly constant. However, the workload has exceeded the maximum possible energy produced from aerobic metabolism, and the excess work performed is compensated for by anaerobic metabolism at the level of the muscle. This has resulted in a high concentration of lactate in the muscle beds and a relative acidosis that later results in stiffness and fatigue. However, in the process his overall physical condition has improved due to optimizing the five components of oxygen delivery, especially his ability to increase cardiac output in the setting of high oxygen consumption.

Thumbnail: Oxygen Transport and Ventilation

Pathophysiology

The five steps of oxygen transport are ventilation, alveolar diffusion, hemoglobin binding, circulation, and peripheral diffusion

Circulation (i.e., cardiac output) is the rate-limiting step in oxygen transport

Inspiration is an active process mediated by respiratory centers in the medulla and pons

Diaphragm contraction pushes down on the abdomen and pulls up on the rib cage

Increases the vertical and horizontal dimensions of the thorax

Creates negative pressure

Accessory muscles of inspiration include external intercostal, scalene, and sternocleidomastoid muscles

Expiration is normally a passive process allowed by relaxation of the diaphragm

Accessory muscles of expiration include the abdominal wall muscles and the internal intercostal muscles

---

Key Points

- Exercise results in increased oxygen consumption, which requires increased oxygen delivery
- Increased minute ventilation (MV) = (respiratory rate) × (tidal volume)
  - Achieved primarily through increased respiratory rate
- Increased cardiac output (CO) = (heart rate) × (stroke volume)
  - Achieved primarily through increased heart rate
- Arterial oxygen content CaO_2 = [oxygen bound to hemoglobin] + [dissolved oxygen] = $[1.36 \times Hgb \times SaO_2] + [0.003 \times PaO_2]$
  - Hgb = hemoglobin concentration (13–15 mg/dL), SaO_2 = arterial oxygen concentration (98%), PaO_2 = arterial oxygen tension (80–100 mmHg)
  - CaO_2 = 20.0 + 0.3 = about 20 mlO$_2$/dL plasma
- Oxygen delivery = CO × CaO_2
  - Achieved primarily through increased CO
  - Oxygen delivery increases from about 0.5 L/min to 4 L/min

Questions

1. Which muscle is *not* used in forceful inspiration?
   A. Diaphragm
   B. Scalenes
   C. Sternocleidomastoids
   D. Internal intercostals
   E. External intercostals

2. Diffusion of gas across the alveolar capillary membrane is *inversely proportional* to which of the following?
   A. Area of the membrane
   B. Difference between partial pressures of the gas on both sides of the membrane
   C. A diffusion constant that is related to the solubility and molecular weight of the gas
   D. Thickness of the membrane
   E. Size of the alveolus

3. Which of the following has the *lowest* pressure in the cardiovascular system?
   A. Pulmonary arteries
   B. Pulmonary veins
   C. Systemic arteries
   D. Systemic veins
   E. Splanchnic vessels

4. Which of the following represents inspired air's partial pressure of oxygen at sea level?
   A. 760 mmHg
   B. 713 mmHg
   C. 160 mmHg
   D. 150 mmHg
   E. 100 mmHg

> **HPI:** When TS graduated from college he no longer had wrestling to stay in shape, so he took up mountain climbing. He and his wife, VS, went on a hike to Mt. Whitney (elevation 14,300 feet) in California with some friends. They left Santa Barbara at sea level on Friday morning and spent the night in the desert at about 1200 feet. The next day they drove to the trailhead at 6000 feet and began backpacking; VS carried a 40-pound pack. By 7:00 P.M. they had hiked eight miles and set up camp at 10,600 feet. VS had difficulty sleeping during the night. Even though they had stopped hiking 2 hours previously, she still felt short of breath and was breathing heavily. TS noticed that throughout the night her breathing pattern was very irregular with periods where she would stop breathing for a number of seconds. The next morning VS felt tired but, despite her fatigue, continued up the trail. After 4 hours they had hiked another three miles and reached 13,100 feet. By that time VS had a horrible headache, body aches, nausea, and she vomited.

Thought Questions

- What is the primary environmental change at high altitude responsible for VS's illness?

- What is the body's response to this change in the environment?

- Which two main chemoreceptors offer feedback to the respiratory centers?

- What acid-base alteration occurs during high-altitude adaptation?

- How does VS's body compensate for the primary acid-base disturbance?

Basic Science Review and Discussion

Partial Pressure of Oxygen in Inspired Air   Atmospheric pressure (or barometric pressure) is 760 mmHg at sea level. This pressure decreases at higher altitudes. At 11,000 feet—the height of many peaks in the Rockies, Sierras, and Cascades—the barometric pressure is about 500 mmHg. Atop Mount Everest (29,000 feet) the barometric pressure is about 250 mmHg. Water vapor pressure of inspired air is 47 mmHg and the fractional concentration of oxygen in dry air is 0.21 regardless of the altitudes. At 11,000 feet this results in a partial pressure of inhaled oxygen of $Pio_2 = (500 - 47 \text{ mmHg}) \times 0.21 = 95$ mmHg (compared to 150 mmHg at sea level), which translates directly to a decreased hemoglobin saturation and lower oxygen delivering capacity. The end result is hypoxemia, or a lower than normal blood oxygen content.

Regulation of Breathing   There are two primary locations for chemoreceptors that offer feedback to the respiratory centers in the medulla and pons. Central chemoreceptors are located in the ventral portion of the medulla and are surrounded by cerebrospinal fluid (CSF). These receptors are stimulated by CO_2 that crosses the blood-brain barrier and are responsible for the minute-to-minute regulation of respiratory rate and volume. Small increases in blood CO_2 tension translate into increases in CSF CO_2 tension and carbonic acid. Receptor stimulation activates the dorsal respiratory group in the medulla, increasing the respiratory rate. Hyperventilation lowers the partial pressure of CO_2 in the alveoli, which facilitates diffusion of CO_2 from the blood into the alveoli.

Peripheral chemoreceptors, which are primarily responsible for hyperventilation during hypoxemia, are located in the carotid bodies at the bifurcation of the common carotid arteries. These chemoreceptors are stimulated by both low oxygen tension (with maximal response at $Pao_2 < 70$ mmHg) and low pH. There are also receptors in the lungs that offer feedback to the respiratory centers, including pulmonary stretch receptors, irritant receptors, and juxta-capillary receptors (J receptors).

High-Altitude Hypoxia and Acid-Base Physiology   As VS gains altitude, she is exposed to a lower partial pressure of oxygen, causing her to become hypoxemic. Stimulation of peripheral baroreceptors causes her to hyperventilate. This facilitates equilibration of aveolar Pao_2 and $Paco_2$ with those of ambient air (i.e., Pao_2 increases and $Paco_2$ decreases). In serum, CO_2 exists in equilibrium with carbonic acid (H_2HCO_3) and bicarbonate (HCO_3^-). Their relationship is described by the Henderson-Hasselbach equation: $pH = pKA + \log\{[HCO_3^-]/[CO_2]\}$. This equation is depicted graphically by the Davenport diagram (Figure 2-1). As VS blows off CO_2, her blood becomes alkalotic. This is known as a primary respiratory alkalosis. All acid-base disturbances are the result of altering the ratio of $[HCO_3^-]/[CO_2]$, the driving factor in the Henderson-Hasselbach equation. $[CO_2]$ is regulated primarily by ventilation; therefore, acid-base disorders that stem from a change in $[CO_2]$ are referred to as respiratory acidosis or alkalosis. It is important to understand that

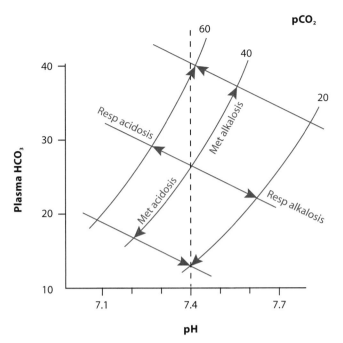

Figure 2-1. Davenport diagram shows how serum pH, [HCO$_3^+$], and PCO$_2$ change with the four primary acid-base disturbances (arrows originating from center) and how secondary compensation occurs (secondary arrows that push the pH back toward 7.4 [dotted line]).

O$_2$ and CO$_2$ are dissolved gases in serum and that their concentrations [O$_2$] and [CO$_2$] are measured by their partial pressures PaO$_2$ and PaCO$_2$. In contrast, HCO$_3^-$ is a dissolved ion in serum and its concentration [HCO$_3^-$] is measured directly.

[HCO$_3^-$] is regulated by the kidneys. Primary alterations in [HCO$_3^-$] occur via metabolic abnormalities and are therefore referred to as metabolic acidosis or alkalosis. Metabolic acidosis is typically caused by an excess of organic or exogenous acids that consume free HCO$_3^-$ (e.g., lactic acid in shock, ketoacids in diabetic ketoacidosis, toxic ingestions such as methanol, paraldehyde and others). Metabolic alkalosis is less common and usually results from excessive vomiting.

Once a primary acid-base disturbance exists, the buffering action of carbonic acid and its constituents carbon dioxide and bicarbonate will cause a secondary compensation to restore the pH back toward 7.4. It is simple to predict how compensation will occur by considering the ratio [HCO$_3^-$]/[CO$_2$] in the Henderson-Hasselbach equation. For example, in primary respiratory alkalosis [CO$_2$] decreases (PaCO$_2$ decreases) and the pH rises. In order to restore the pH toward its normal value, [HCO$_3^-$] must then decrease as well. This does in fact happen as bicarbonate is excreted from the kidneys; however, the process of bicarbonate excretion and complete compensation takes 2 to 3 days. Another example is metabolic acidosis where the primary disturbance is the consumption of bicarbonate by an organic or exogenous acid, resulting in a pH decrease. Again, looking at the ratio [HCO$_3^-$]/[CO$_2$] one predicts that in order to restore a normal pH that [CO$_2$] must decrease. This is accomplished by increasing minute ventilation, which excretes CO$_2$ via the lungs. It is important to note that compensation is never complete, meaning that the pH will trend back toward 7.4 but not fully reach it.

Case Conclusion Once VS became obviously ill, she and TS descended down to 9000 feet and spent the night. At that altitude, the increased partial pressure of inhaled oxygen enabled her to slow her breathing rate and allow her kidneys more time to excrete bicarbonate to compensate for the respiratory alkalosis that had developed. By the next afternoon VS felt well enough to resume the climb.

Thumbnail: High Altitude and Acid-Base

Pathophysiology

Partial pressure of oxygen in inspired air decreases as altitude increases

- Decreased PaO$_2$ results in hypoxemia (decreased PaO$_2$)
- Hyperventilation is triggered by peripheral chemoreceptors
- Increased minute ventilation decreases PaCO$_2$
- Decreased PaCO$_2$ allows for a relative increase in PaO$_2$

Respiratory alkalosis is a result of decreased PaCO$_2$, decreased serum [CO$_2$], and increased pH.

- Alkalosis and hypoxemia cause symptoms of acute mountain sickness
- Kidneys compensate by excreting HCO$_3^-$, which takes 2 to 3 days

Risk Factors

- Rapid ascent to altitudes greater than 8000 feet
- Unclear genetic predisposition to acute mountain sickness

Key Points

Central chemoreceptors in the medulla provide the primary regulatory feedback system for normal ventilation

- Respond to increases in CSF CO_2 levels

Peripheral chemoreceptors in the carotid bodies provide secondary feedback to respiratory centers in the medulla and pons

- Respond to decreased Pa_{O_2}, increased Pa_{CO_2}, and decreased pH

Acid-base disorders

- $[CO_2]$ regulated by lungs, and $[HCO_3^-]$ regulated by kidneys
- pH < 7.4 is acidosis
  - Pa_{CO_2} > 40 is primary respiratory acidosis
  - $[HCO_3^-]$ < 24 is primary metabolic acidosis
- pH > 7.4 is alkalosis
  - Pa_{CO_2} < 40 is primary respiratory alkalosis
  - $[HCO_3^-]$ > 24 is primary metabolic alkalosis

The ratio $[HCO_3^-]/[CO_2]$ predicts how the body will compensate for the primary disturbance

Questions

1. Peripheral chemoreceptors are activated by which of the following?
   A. Decrease in pH
   B. Increase in arterial Pa_{O_2}
   C. Decrease in arterial Pa_{CO_2}
   D. Increase in serum bicarbonate
   E. Hyperventilation

2. What is the physiologic advantage to hyperventilating at high altitude?
   A. Increases the partial pressure of oxygen in inspired air
   B. Creates respiratory alkalosis that facilitates oxygen-hemoglobin binding
   C. Decreases alveolar Pa_{CO_2} and thereby increases alveolar Pa_{O_2}
   D. Opens, or recruits, more alveoli for gas exchange
   E. Compensates for a primary metabolic acidosis

3. A patient presents to the emergency department with decreased mental status and the following arterial blood gas analysis is obtained: pH 7.26, Pa_{O_2} 100 mmHg, Pa_{CO_2} 26, $[HCO_3^-]$ 12. Which of the following is the primary acid-base disturbance and its accompanying compensatory mechanism?
   A. Respiratory acidosis with a compensatory metabolic alkalosis
   B. Metabolic acidosis with a compensatory respiratory alkalosis
   C. Respiratory alkalosis with a compensatory metabolic acidosis
   D. Metabolic alkalosis with a compensatory respiratory acidosis
   E. None of the above

4. A patient with long-standing chronic obstructive pulmonary disease presents to the emergency department with increased cough and difficulty breathing. The following arterial blood gas analysis is obtained: pH 7.34, Pa_{O_2} 76 mmHg, Pa_{CO_2} 60, $[HCO_3^-]$ 28. Which of the following is the primary acid-base disturbance and its compensatory mechanism?
   A. Respiratory acidosis with a compensatory metabolic alkalosis
   B. Metabolic acidosis with a compensatory respiratory alkalosis
   C. Respiratory alkalosis with a compensatory metabolic acidosis
   D. Metabolic alkalosis with a compensatory respiratory acidosis
   E. None of the above

HPI: BR lives in the city three blocks down the street from CA, her grandmother. The city was in the grips of the first cold weather spell of winter, and CA had turned on the gas furnace early in the morning. BR came to visit mid-morning and her grandmother complained of a headache and nausea. BR thought that because her grandmother looked pale, she would grocery shop for her while CA stayed home and rested. BR was gone for 2 hours and returned to find her grandmother asleep in bed. BR tried to arouse her but CA wouldn't open her eyes. BR quickly called 911 and the paramedics arrived shortly thereafter. After assessing that CA was breathing spontaneously, they placed her on 100% oxygen and a cardiac monitor. They also established an IV, drew several vials of blood, and administered glucose. As part of the initial blood analysis in the emergency department, one of the vials drawn by the paramedics was sent for a blood gas analysis and carbon monoxide level. The carbon monoxide level returned at 38% (may be as high as 10% in smokers but normal is 0%). BR's grandmother was kept on high-flow oxygen and arrangements were made for more definitive treatment.

Thought Questions

- When and where is carbon monoxide poisoning most often seen?

- How is oxygen transported in the blood to peripheral tissues?

- How is carbon dioxide transported from peripheral tissues back to the lungs?

- How does carbon monoxide interfere with the normal transport of oxygen?

- How does carbon monoxide affect the oxygen-hemoglobin dissociation curve?

- In which three forms is carbon dioxide transported from peripheral tissue back to the lungs?

Basic Science Review and Discussion

Carbon monoxide poisoning is most often encountered in building fires, leaking heating systems, and suicide attempts. The most common cause of unconsciousness and death in fires is carbon monoxide poisoning; therefore, all fire victims should be monitored and treated for carbon monoxide poisoning. Carbon monoxide poisoning is also common during winter months in large cities in cold climates such as Chicago, New York, or Boston. Poisoning typically affects the elderly who have little hypoxic reserve. Symptoms are initially vague and include headache, nausea, fatigue, visual disturbances, paresthesias, chest or abdominal pains, and/or diarrhea. Attaching a hose from a car's exhaust into the driver's compartment is a common method of committing suicide. Carbon monoxide is very insidious because it is colorless and odorless; therefore making its presence often difficult to detect.

Alveolar Gas Equation Inspired air has a partial pressure of oxygen of 150 mmHg, which is calculated based on sea level barometric pressure (760 mmHg), adjusted for the partial pressure of humidified air (47 mmHg), and the fractional component of oxygen in air (0.21). The alveolar gas equation is used to calculate the partial pressure of oxygen in the alveoli (P_{AO_2}) based on the oxygen partial pressure of inspired gas (P_{IO_2}) and the alveolar partial pressure of carbon dioxide (P_{ACO_2}): $P_{AO_2} = P_{IO_2} - (P_{ACO_2}/R)$, where P_{AO_2} is the actual partial pressure of oxygen in the alveoli, P_{IO_2} is the partial pressure of oxygen in inspired air (150 mmHg), P_{ACO_2} is the partial pressure of CO_2 in the alveoli (approximate to P_{ACO_2}, or 40 mmHg, which is the partial pressure of CO_2 measured in arterial blood), and R is the ratio of CO_2 produced to O_2 consumed and is approximately 0.8. Therefore $P_{AO_2} = 150 - (40/0.8) = 100$ mmHg.

Henry's Law Once oxygen transits the alveolar membrane it dissolves into the blood. Henry's law dictates that the concentration of dissolved gas (C_x) is proportional to its partial pressure (P_x): $C_x = K \times P_x$. For oxygen, 0.003 mL/dL will be dissolved for each mmHg of P_{O_2} (e.g., K = 0.003 mL/dL for oxygen), which translates into a blood oxygen concentration about 0.3 mL/dL given a partial pressure for oxygen of 100 mmHg in the pulmonary capillaries. The oxygen requirement during exertion is about 15 mL/dL; an alternative means of oxygen transport must therefore exist in order to supply this demand.

Hemoglobin: The Oxygen Carrier The alternative means of oxygen transport is facilitated by hemoglobin, which is a protein contained within red blood cells. The molecule consists of four globin chains each having an iron-porphyrin moiety that binds oxygen; therefore, four molecules of oxygen can bind to one hemoglobin molecule. The affinity of hemoglobin for oxygen rises as more oxygen-binding sites become filled, which explains the nonlinear shape of

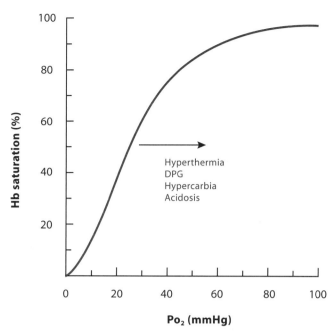

Figure 3-1. Oxygen-hemoglobin dissociation curve. Note the horizontal shape of the curve above oxygen saturation > 90% corresponding with Po_2 > 70 mmHg. Once the Po_2 drops below 70 mmHg, the oxygen saturation drops rapidly (steep portion of the curve). A shift to the right results in off-loading of oxygen from hemoglobin at higher Po_2.

the oxygen-hemoglobin dissociation curve (Figure 3-1). At Po_2 > 80 mmHg, the curve is essentially horizontal, which means oxygen is bound avidly to hemoglobin. Such a condition of high Po_2 exists in arterial blood where oxygen transport is desired. As the Po_2 declines, the curve undergoes a sharp descent, which means that oxygen is easily off-loaded. This condition exists in peripheral capillary beds where oxygen delivery to tissues is desired. In addition, there are certain factors that shift the curve to the right, which results in increased dissociation at a given Po_2. These factors include increased temperature, H+ concentration, Pco_2 concentration, and 2,3-DPG concentration. All of these conditions exist in peripheral muscle capillary beds during exertion, and thus facilitate in oxygen dissociation and delivery to tissues.

Carbon Dioxide Transport   Carbon dioxide (CO_2) is a normal by-product of cellular metabolism. It must be transported in the systemic venous system back to the heart, where it is pumped into the pulmonary capillary beds, diffuses across the alveolar-capillary membrane, and is exhaled by the lungs. CO_2 is transported in three forms: dissolved CO_2, carbamino compounds, and bicarbonate. The solubility of CO_2 is 20 times greater than that of oxygen; therefore, a larger proportion of CO_2 is dissolved in blood. Carbamino compounds are formed when CO_2 reversibly binds amine groups on circulating proteins. The most abundant of the CO_2-binding proteins is hemoglobin itself, which results in carbamino Hb. Deoxygenated Hb has a higher affinity for CO_2 than oxygenated Hb, which is referred to as the *Haldane effect*. Bicarbonate is generated from CO_2 in red blood cells by the following reaction: $CO_2 + H_2O \xleftarrow{CA} H_2CO_3 \longleftrightarrow H^+ + HCO_3^-$. The first reaction occurs in the presence of carbonic anhydrase (CA) in red cells, and the second reaction occurs spontaneously. Bicarbonate (HCO_3^-) diffuses out of the cells and is transported in blood plasma. Because H+ cannot freely cross the red cell membrane, chloride shifts into the cells to maintain electric neutrality. This is known as *chloride shift*. In total, 60% of CO_2 is transported as bicarbonate, 30% as carbamino compounds, and 10% as dissolved CO_2. This is in contrast to oxygen in which over 98% is transported by hemoglobin.

Pathophysiology of Carbon Monoxide Poisoning   As carbon monoxide enters the alveoli, it diffuses across the alveolar-capillary membrane similar to oxygen. Carbon monoxide reversibly binds hemoglobin at one of the oxygen-binding sites and converts the molecule into carboxy-hemoglobin (COHb). COHb binds the three remaining sites to oxygen; however, the conformation of the molecule is such that it does not release the bound oxygen. The oxygen saturation of hemoglobin therefore remains essentially the same (and measured oxygen saturation may in fact be normal), yet the oxygen cannot be off-loaded in peripheral tissues. For this reason, CO has the effect of shifting the oxygen-hemoglobin dissociation curve to the left. In addition, CO has 240 times the affinity for hemoglobin than oxygen. Thus, low concentrations of CO can have profound effects on oxygen-transport capabilities.

Case Conclusion   CA becomes minimally more responsive during the first 15 minutes in the emergency department with oxygen therapy alone. She is transported immediately to a hyperbaric oxygen chamber where she is placed at three atmospheres and continues to receive 100% oxygen. Because CO binds reversibly to oxygen receptors on the hemoglobin molecule, increasing the concentration of oxygen will reverse binding. Breathing 100% oxygen can achieve this; breathing 100% oxygen at three atmospheres greatly increases the delivered concentration of oxygen, in turn increasing alveolar Pao_2 The binding half-life of CO to hemoglobin is about 240 minutes while breathing room air, 80 minutes breathing 100% oxygen, and about 20 minutes breathing 100% oxygen at three atmospheres. After 2 hours in the chamber CA wakens and answers simple questions.

Thumbnail: CO Poisoning and Oxygen Transport

Pathophysiology

CO is an inhaled poison that binds hemoglobin

CO has 240 times the affinity of oxygen

Causes conformational change of hemoglobin

  Remaining sites bind oxygen tightly

Prevents oxygen off-loading in peripheral tissues

Results in tissue hypoxemia

Risk Factors

Smoke inhalation, leaking heating systems, car exhaust

Key Points

▸ Concentration of dissolved arterial oxygen is proportional to the oxygen tension in the alveoli according to Henry's law

  ▸ Dissolved oxygen accounts for only about 1.5% of arterial oxygen content

▸ Hemoglobin is a protein with four binding sites for oxygen

  ▸ Carries about 98.5% of oxygen in arterial blood

▸ Oxygen affinity is high at high oxygen tension (pulmonary capillaries) and low at low oxygen tension (peripheral capillaries)

▸ Oxygen-hemoglobin dissociation curve has a plateau at high oxygen tension

▸ Oxygen-hemoglobin dissociation curve is steep at lower oxygen tensions

▸ Shift to the right of the oxygen-hemoglobin dissociation curve results in off-loading of oxygen from hemoglobin

  ▸ Occurs in peripheral tissues as a result of increased temperature, increased P_{CO_2}, decreased pH, and increased 2,3-DPG

▸ Carbon dioxide is transported back to the lungs as bicarbonate, carbamino groups, and dissolved CO_2

  ▸ CO_2 is 20 times more soluble than O_2

  ▸ Higher percentage of CO_2 is in the dissolved form

  ▸ CO_2 diffuses across the alveolar membrane more readily

Questions

1. Approximately what percentage of oxygen is dissolved in arterial blood plasma?
   - A. 1.5%
   - B. 10%
   - C. 25%
   - D. 50%
   - E. 80%

2. Compared to carbon dioxide, what is the rate of diffusion of oxygen across the alveolar-capillary membrane?
   - A. Higher because of oxygen's smaller molecular weight
   - B. Higher because of oxygen's greater solubility
   - C. Higher because of oxygen's greater affinity for hemoglobin
   - D. Lower because oxygen is less soluble than carbon dioxide
   - E. Lower because of oxygen's greater affinity for hemoglobin

3. Which of the following conditions results in a *lower* arterial oxygen tension (mmHg)?
   - A. Anemia
   - B. Low cardiac output
   - C. CO poisoning
   - D. High altitude climbing
   - E. All of the above

4. Which of the following is *consistent* with a shift to the right of the oxygen-hemoglobin dissociation curve?
   - A. Increased affinity of hemoglobin for oxygen
   - B. Decreased P_{50}, or O_2 tension that produces 50% hemoglobin saturation
   - C. Facilitated off-loading of oxygen to peripheral tissues
   - D. Decreased temperature, increased pH, decreased P_{CO_2}, decreased 2,3-DPG
   - E. Carbon monoxide poisoning

HPI: EZ, a 67-year-old man, presents with dyspnea. He typically experiences shortness of breath on exertion such as walking up stairs, which has gradually worsened over the past 2 years. For 3 days, EZ has had an increased cough without sputum production and severe dyspnea when walking only a short distance. He has had no fevers or chills. EZ's chest feels tight when he takes a deep breath. He has also noted increased swelling in both feet. He has a history of hypertension, hyperlipidemia, and "asthma"; and he takes atenolol and lipitor. EZ has smoked two packs of cigarettes a day for 50 years.

PE: His vital signs are remarkable for a respiratory rate of 34 and a SaO_2 of 88%. On exam, he is thin, in moderate respiratory distress, and using accessory muscles to breathe. He has distended jugular veins. Despite EZ's overall thin appearance, his chest is large in diameter. His lung sounds are diminished and he has bilateral expiratory wheezes. He has mild peripheral cyanosis obvious around his fingernail beds. EZ also has 1+ peripheral edema.

Thought Questions

- How is the normal ventilatory cycle affected by obstructive lung disease? How are resting lung volume, vital capacity, and forced expiratory volume affected?

- What is the common characteristic feature for obstructive lung disease and what are the four major obstructive lung diseases?

- What are the pathophysiologic differences between emphysema and chronic bronchitis? How do these contribute to the obstructive pattern of COPD?

- What is the relationship between lung volume and compliance? How does this affect the work of breathing for someone with COPD?

- In which region of the lung is air trapping in COPD most predominant? How does ventilation, perfusion, and the ratio of ventilation to perfusion (V/Q ratio) differ between the lung base and apex? Why are these differences significant in COPD?

Basic Science Review and Discussion

Lung Volumes and Obstructive Lung Disease Normal ventilation consists of inspiratory and expiratory phases. Inspiration is an active process of expanding the chest cavity, creating increased negative intrathoracic pressure, and drawing air into the lungs. This is achieved mainly by contraction and downward deflection of the diaphragm, but also through expansion of the thoracic cage by the external intercostal, sternocleidomastoid, and scalene muscles. Exhalation occurs passively because of the inherent elasticity of lung tissue. Obstructive lung disease is characterized either by loss of lung elasticity (e.g., COPD) or increased airway resistance (e.g., asthma). The hallmark of obstructive lung disease is *reduction of expiratory flow rate.* As a result, air trapping occurs, causing an increase in the resting lung volume (i.e., increased functional residual capacity [FRC]) and end-expiratory volume (i.e., increased residual volume [RV]). Total lung capacity (TLC) is also mildly increased (Figure 4-1). As a result of the disproportionate increase in FRC, the vital capacity (VC = TLC − FRC) is drastically decreased. Forced expiratory volume in 1 second (FEV_1) is decreased as a result of both functional and mechanical obstruction, and is therefore a sensitive test for the presence of obstructive lung disease. Types of obstructive lung disease include chronic COPD, asthma, bronchiectasis, and cystic fibrosis.

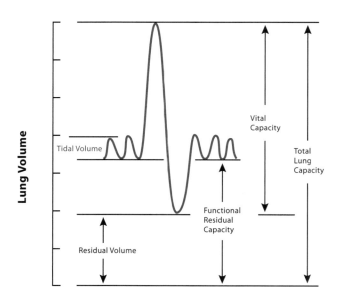

Figure 4-1. Graphical output of spirometer during normal breathing (TV), full inspiration (TLC), and full expiration (RV). FRC is the lung volume remaining after passive exhalation.

Pathophysiology of COPD Emphysema and chronic bronchitis are the two pathologic entities that comprise COPD. Often, these two entities coexist and patients will exhibit features of both; sometimes patients will exhibit a predominance of one or the other. Emphysema is caused by alveolar wall destruction as a result of excessive protease activity. Inhaled toxins, such as those in cigarette smoke, cause an increase in alveolar macrophages and neutrophils. The present hypothesis is that activated neutrophils release proteases that destroy interstitial elastin and cleave type IV collagen. Alveolar wall destruction leads to loss of pulmonary capillaries and a reduction of oxygen diffusing capacity. It also results in increased pulmonary artery pressure and right heart failure (cor pulmonale). Interstitial elasticity helps maintain patency of terminal and respiratory bronchioles in healthy adults. In emphysema, many of these bronchioles collapse without elasticity of the surrounding interstitium, thus creating obstruction to air outflow.

Chronic bronchitis is characterized by excessive mucus production in the bronchial tree. In response to inhaled toxins and irritants, epithelial goblet cells and subepithelial mucous glands proliferate and the number of ciliated epithelial cells decrease. This results in increased mucus production with chronic cough. Airway obstruction seen with chronic bronchitis is primarily due to bronchiolar inflammation and bronchospasm, both of which are triggered by inhaled irritants or acute respiratory infection. For this reason, systemic corticosteroids, inhaled β_2-agonists, and inhaled anticholinergics are helpful in COPD exacerbations.

Pressure-Volume Relationship Lung expansion is achieved through increasing the volume of the thoracic cage, which results in an increased negative intrapleural pressure. Compliance is a measure of the amount of volume change achieved by a certain amount of negative pressure (i.e., compliance = $\Delta V/\Delta P$). For example, stiff lungs (e.g., interstitial fibrosis) expand less for a given amount of pressure change; therefore, they have a low compliance. As lung volume increases, interstitial elastin becomes taut, and compliance decreases. For this reason, in COPD as FRC increases, lung expansion becomes more difficult because of the lower compliance at higher resting volumes (Figure 4-2). This leads to increased work of breathing that is characteristic with COPD.

Regional Variation in Ventilation Intrapleural pressure increases (i.e., it becomes less negative) toward the base of the lung due to the effects of gravity and the weight of the lung. For this reason, the alveoli at the base are less distended, and thus more compliant. During inhalation, higher compliance at the base results in greater expansion and thus greater ventilation compared to the apex. However, in COPD alveolar wall destruction and decreased elasticity of respiratory bronchioles results in alveolar collapse when

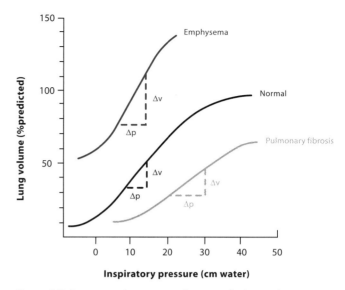

Figure 4-2. Pressure-volume curves for normal, obstructive (emphysema), and restrictive (pulmonary fibrosis) patterns. Note increased compliance ($\Delta v/\Delta p$) in emphysema versus pulmonary fibrosis. In general, compliance (slope of P-V curve) decreases at higher lung volumes as is seen by the flattening of the curves at high volumes.

increased thoracic pressure is created during exhalation. This collapse occurs preferentially at the bases because of their relatively higher compliance than at the apices. Therefore, patients with COPD ventilate the apices more than the bases, which is the opposite of normal physiology.

Regional Variation in Perfusion and Lung Zones Similar to the regional variation in ventilation, pulmonary capillary perfusion is greater at the lung base compared to the apex. In fact, the difference is even greater than that for ventilation because the pulmonary vascular pressure, which in effect acts like a column of fluid, varies largely from the bottom to the top of the lungs. Alveolar pressure, however, remains constant at atmospheric pressure throughout the lung regions. At the level of the alveolus, capillary flow is exposed to alveolar pressure and thus flow is dependent on relative pressure differences. At the apex where alveolar pressure exceeds pulmonary arterial and venous pressure (zone 1) there is practically no flow (Figure 4-3). Farther down, in zone 2, pulmonary arterial pressure exceeds alveolar pressure and the capillary flow is proportional to the difference of these two pressures. At the base, in zone 3, pulmonary venous pressure exceeds alveolar pressure and flow is proportional to the difference of pulmonary arterial and venous pressures. Because of the larger decrease in perfusion compared to ventilation from the base to the apex, the V/Q ratio is larger at the apex. However, this region contributes little to the total pulmonary capillary gas exchange because of its low perfusion.

In COPD, the shift of ventilation from the well-perfused bases to the hypo-perfused apices creates a pathologic V/Q mismatch. This impairs overall pulmonary gas exchange and results in hypoxemia. The inability to effectively expire alveolar CO_2 results in CO_2 retention, increased arterial $PaCO_2$, and respiratory acidosis. Noninvasive positive-pressure ventilation (NPPV) is a useful technique for treating acute exacerbations of COPD. NPPV consists of a tight-fitting, airtight face mask linked in series to a ventilator. The ventilator provides breaths to the patient at increased inspiratory pressures. This acts to open alveoli that have collapsed due to the increased compliance of the terminal and respiratory bronchioles.

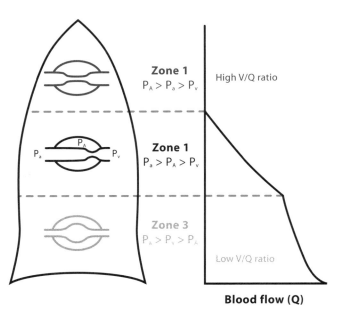

Figure 4-3. Depiction of the three lung zones where Pa is pulmonary arterial pressure, Pv is pulmonary venous pressure, and PA is alveolar pressure. PA is constant throughout all zones, whereas Pa and Pv decrease from zone 3 to zone 1 as a result of hydrostatic pressure.

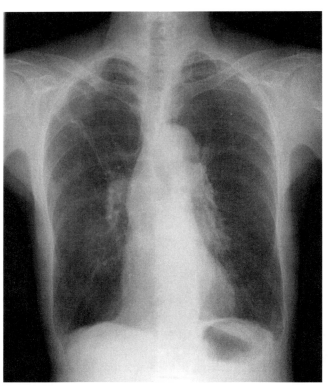

Figure 4-4. Chest x-ray showing characteristics of COPD: hyperinflated lungs, diaphragm flattening, and narrow cardiac silhouette.

Case Conclusion EZ is placed on 4 liters of oxygen by nasal cannula to keep his oxygen saturation above 92%; he is also placed on a cardiac monitor. An IV is obtained and he is given methylprednisolone 125 mg IV and continuous albuterol and ipratropium nebulizers. A chest x-ray shows hyperinflated lungs, flattening of the diaphragm, and narrowing of the cardiac silhouette (Figure 4-4). He continues to have difficulty breathing and is placed on NPPV via a tight-fitting facemask and a ventilator. An arterial blood gas is obtained prior to NPPV, which shows a pH 7.32, PO_2 56 mmHg, PCO_2 62 mmHg. He is admitted to the ICU where he continues to receive oxygen, nebulizers, and NPPV to which he gradually improves.

Thumbnail: COPD

Pathophysiology

Emphysema

Destruction of alveolar walls and elastin by chronic airway inflammation

Dilated airspaces and increased lung compliance

Cigarette smoke attracts neutrophils and macrophages

Increased protease activity

Respiratory bronchioles affected the most (centrilobular emphysema)

α_1-antitrypsin deficiency results in uncommon hereditary emphysema

Natural defense against proteolytic enzymes

Diffuse involvement of lung tissue (panacinar emphysema)

Chronic bronchitis

Proliferation of mucous glands and goblet cells in bronchi and bronchioles

Destruction of cilia and ability to clear secretions

Increased bronchospasm and airway resistance

Risk Factors

Smoking, air and environmental pollutants, respiratory infection

α_1-antitrypsin deficiency

Key Points

▶ Reduced expiratory flow rate (FEV_1)

▶ Patients exhibit features of both emphysema and chronic bronchitis

▶ Pulmonary function abnormalities

  ▶ Increased TLC, FRC, RV

▶ Decreased VC, FEV_1

▶ Ventilation-perfusion mismatch

  ▶ Alveolar collapse during exhalation

  ▶ Inadequate ventilation resulting in hypoxia and hypercapnia

Questions

1. COPD is characterized by which of the following?

   A. Increased lung compliance
   B. Increased vital capacity
   C. Decreased residual volume
   D. Decreased physiologic dead space
   E. Decrease in total lung capacity

2. In COPD, air trapping occurs

   A. more in the upper lobes.
   B. more in the lower lobes.
   C. centrally greater than peripherally.
   D. equally throughout.
   E. Cannot be determined

3. Which blood gas result represents compensated respiratory acidosis?

   A. pH 7.30; Pao_2 85; $Paco_2$ 30; HCO_3^- 12
   B. pH 7.24; Pao_2 60; $Paco_2$ 60; HCO_3^- 26
   C. pH 7.34; Pao_2 62; $Paco_2$ 60; HCO_3^- 28
   D. pH 7.48; Pao_2 70; $Paco_2$ 30; HCO_3^- 22
   E. pH 7.52; Pao_2 90; $Paco_2$ 48; HCO_3^- 48

4. As lung volume increases, lung compliance

   A. increases.
   B. decreases.
   C. stays the same.
   D. first increases, then decreases.
   E. cannot be determined.

HPI: JF, a 32-year-old woman, presents with shortness of breath. Two days ago she developed a runny nose, itchy eyes, and sore throat—all consistent with her typical allergic symptoms. JF has allergies every April and takes Claritin when the symptoms arise. Today, she began to wheeze and felt short of breath with exertion. She used her albuterol inhaler without improvement. JF's breathing got worse throughout the day. She has been hospitalized for asthma twice but never required intubation. She uses both beclomethasone and albuterol inhalers on a regular basis. She does not smoke, but has a dog at home.

PE: JF's vital signs are remarkable for a respiratory rate of 34 and a SaO_2 of 90% on room air. She is a healthy-appearing woman in moderate distress, using accessory muscles to exhale. On lung exam, JF has decreased air movement and both inspiratory and expiratory wheezes. She also has intercostal and supraclavicular retractions.

Thought Questions

- What are the structures in descending order of the conducting portion of the respiratory tract? How does the histology change at the different levels?

- What is the definition of *asthma*?

- What are the two distinct pathologic features of asthma?

- How is airflow in a tube related to the pressure gradient and resistance?

- Which law governs resistance of laminar flow in a tube?

- At which anatomic level does respiratory flow meet the greatest resistance?

- How are lung volumes affected during an asthma attack? Do altered lung volumes aid in ventilation?

- What effect does asthma have on the ventilation-perfusion ratio (V/Q ratio)? How are arterial PaO_2 and $PaCO_2$ affected during an asthma attack? What is the resulting acid-base disturbance?

- How do the medications used to treat asthma act to reverse the disease process?

Basic Science Review and Discussion

Pulmonary Anatomy and Histology Structures comprising the conducting portion of the respiratory tract include the trachea, large and small bronchi, and segmental and terminal bronchioles. The function of the conducting respiratory tract includes movement and conditioning of inspired air. The walls of these airways consist of cartilage, elastin, collagen, and smooth muscle to provide structural support and distensibility. The epithelium consists primarily of ciliated pseudostratified columnar cells from the trachea, bronchi, and into the bronchioles. This cell type transitions to ciliated simple cuboidal at the level of the respiratory bronchiole.

Mucous goblet cells are abundant in the trachea and decrease in number until they are absent in the terminal bronchioles. Mucous glands are present in the trachea and decrease in number until they are absent in the segmental bronchioles. The trachea contains C-shaped cartilage rings that persist as cartilage plates and islands to the level of the small bronchi. Smooth muscle and elastin fibers are present in the trachea and become more predominant as airway caliber becomes smaller. See Figure 5-1 for a summary of the histologic changes.

Pathophysiology of Asthma Asthma is characterized by airway obstruction primarily at the level of the bronchioles that is reversible with bronchodilator medication. The first component of this disease is *airway inflammation,* with cellular infiltration of the lamina propria, mucosal edema, and thick mucosal secretions. The second component is *airway hyperreactivity,* which is thought to be a consequence of the inflammatory response. In many cases an allergic stimulus exists, resulting in IgE-mediated mast cell degranulation with release of bronchoactive mediators (e.g., histamine, prostaglandins, leukotrienes) and migration of inflammatory cells. Common triggers include pollen, animal dander, dust, and mites. Other nonimmunogenic etiologies include exercise, cold temperature, cigarette smoke, other environmental pollutants, and viral upper respiratory illnesses.

Airflow Resistance For air to flow through a tube there must be a pressure gradient. If the flow through the tube is laminar, the flow is directly proportional to the pressure gradient and inversely proportional to the resistance in the tube ($V = \Delta P/R$). Laminar flow is characterized by the orderly arrangement of velocity vectors parallel to the walls of the tube, whereas turbulent flow is characterized by a chaotic, swirling movement through the tube. For laminar flow the resistance is determined by Poiseuille's law ($R = 8nl/\pi r^4$), where n = viscosity, l = length, and r = radius. Note that a decrease in tube radius will increase the resistance by a factor of 16. For turbulent flow, the above relationship is $V^2 = \Delta P/R$, therefore the

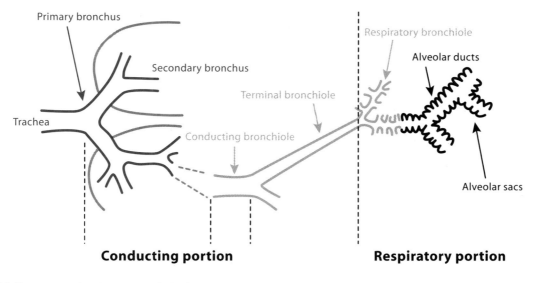

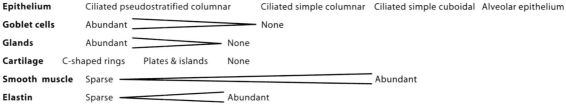

Conducting portion | | | **Respiratory portion**

Epithelium	Ciliated pseudostratified columnar		Ciliated simple columnar	Ciliated simple cuboidal	Alveolar epithelium
Goblet cells	Abundant ————————— None			
Glands	Abundant ————— None			
Cartilage	C-shaped rings	Plates & islands	None	
Smooth muscle	Sparse ————————————— Abundant			
Elastin	Sparse ————— Abundant			

Figure 5-1. Anatomy and histology of the respiratory tract. The conducting portion serves air conduction, humidification, and mucociliary clearance. The respiratory portion begins with the respiratory bronchioles and heralds the presence of alveoli and thus gas exchange.

flow velocity is far less for a given pressure gradient, or the effective resistance far greater. Whether the flow through a tube is laminar or turbulent depends on several flow characteristics, which are summarized by the Reynold's number (Re = 2rvd/n), where r = radius, v = velocity, d = density, and n = viscosity. The higher the Reynold's number, the more likely the flow will be turbulent; therefore, turbulence is more likely when the tube radius, flow velocity, and gas density are higher.

For this reason, flow in the trachea and bronchi tend to be more turbulent, whereas flow in the bronchioles tend to be more laminar. To understand the anatomic level of maximal resistance it is necessary to look at the total cross-sectional area of the conducting system at each level. At the level of the trachea, the cross-sectional area is several square centimeters. As the trachea branches into the main bronchi and further into smaller bronchi, the radius of the individual airways decrease but the total cross-sectional area actually increases. At the level of the tenth branch point (smaller bronchi), the total cross-sectional area begins to increase exponentially (Figure 5-2), so that the total area at the level of the bronchioles is several hundred times greater than that of the larger airways. Contrary to the increased resistance in the bronchioles expected by Poiseuille's law, the resistance is actually far less because of the parallel arrange-

ment of many bronchioles . Laminar flow and short length contribute largely to lower resistance in the bronchioles. The level of highest resistance in the normal lung is at the level of the medium-sized bronchi. In asthma, inflammation and bronchoconstriction at the level of the bronchioles is thought to have the greatest adverse effect on airway resistance, functionally decreasing the total cross-sectional area and eliminating the natural advantage of many bronchioles in parallel.

Obstructive Pattern of Disease Asthma, like COPD, is an obstructive process, meaning that the expiratory flow rate, or forced expiratory volume in one second (FEV_1) is reduced. The result is an increase in the total lung capacity (TLC), functional residual capacity (FRC), and residual volume (RV), and a decrease in the vital capacity (VC). These effects are secondary to early airway closure and air trapping that occurs during expiration as a result of bronchiolar constriction and edema. As discussed with COPD, the work of breathing is increased because lung compliance is lower at higher lung volumes according to the pressure-volume curve (see Figure 4-2). However, one advantage of higher lung volumes for asthmatics is that the tethering effect of expanded lung tissue helps expand the bronchioles, thus reducing airway resistance. Therefore, ventilation is more effective for asthmatics at higher lung volumes.

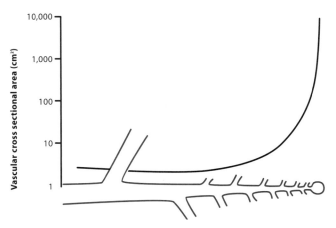

Figure 5-2. Total cross-sectional area of conducting airways as branching occurs.

Due to air trapping during an asthma attack, alveoli are underventilated. The result is a mismatch of ventilation and perfusion (V/Q mismatch) that leads to a decrease in arterial PaO_2. The physiologic response to hypoxemia is to increase minute ventilation (MV = tidal volume × respiratory rate). Since exchange of CO_2 across the alveolar membrane is more efficient than the exchange of oxygen, the effect of hyperventilation favors the elimination of CO_2. The result is a primary respiratory alkalosis that is typical for mild to moderate asthma. In severe asthma, ventilation is obstructed to the point where even the effective exchange of CO_2 is compromised. This results in increased arterial $PaCO_2$ and is a harbinger of respiratory failure and the need for mechanical ventilation. Increased $PaCO_2$ leads to a primary respiratory acidosis, which is characteristic of severe asthma.

Treatment of Asthma β-agonists (e.g., albuterol, metaproterenol, salmeterol) are the mainstay for asthma treatment. $β_2$ receptors are located on the surface of smooth muscle cells and their stimulation results in activation of adenylyl cyclase, increase of intracellular cAMP, and relaxation of smooth muscles. Albuterol and metaproterenol are short-acting agents used in nebulized form for acute asthma. Salmeterol is long-acting and used for maintenance therapy in inhaled form for prevention of acute exacerbations. For more severe asthma attacks, systemic β-agonists are used. Terbutaline is a $β_2$-selective agonist that is administered subcutaneously. Epinephrine is a nonselective α- and β-agonist that can be administered subcutaneously or intravenously. In addition to its therapeutic $β_2$ effects, epinephrine also results in $β_1$ (increased cardiac contractility and chronotropy) and α (increased peripheral vasoconstriction) agonist effects. Inhaled muscarinic anticholinergic agents (e.g., ipratropium bromide) are also useful in asthma because bronchoconstriction is modulated in part by local parasympathetic vagal tone. Methacholine is an inhaled procholinergic agent used to test airway reactivity in those with suspected reactive airways.

Corticosteroids are the second cornerstone of asthma therapy. Systemic steroids (e.g., prednisone, methylprednisolone, dexamethasone) are used during an acute attack to decrease airway inflammation. The effect of corticosteroids is seen in hours to days, in contrast to the immediate bronchodilatory effect of nebulized $β_2$-agonists and anticholinergics. Inhaled steroids (e.g., beclomethasone, fluticasone, triamcinolone) are a mainstay for maintenance therapy to prevent asthma exacerbations.

Other agents used in acute asthma include intravenous magnesium that is hypothesized to inhibit calcium-mediated smooth muscle contraction. Methylxanthines (e.g., theophylline, aminophylline) have anti-inflammatory and bronchodilatory effects but have fallen out of favor because of their toxicity. Cromolyn is a mast cell stabilizer that is used as maintenance therapy primarily in children. Leukotriene inhibitors (e.g., montelukast, zafirlukast) are newer agents being used for asthma prevention.

Case Conclusion JF is placed on 15 liters of oxygen by facemask. An IV is established and methylprednisolone 125 mg IV is administered. Her peak flow is measured at 180 liters (normal is about 10 ml/kg, or about 500–700 ml in an adult). JF is started on continuous albuterol and ipratropium bromide nebulizers. Her oxygen saturation increases to 95%, but her work of breathing does not improve. A chest x-ray is normal. She is given magnesium 2g IV and terbutaline 0.25 mg SQ. She begins to feel and look better, and her repeat peak flow is 280. JF is admitted for continued steroid and nebulizer therapy. The following day her peak flow is 480 and she is discharged home.

Thumbnail: Asthma

Pathophysiology

Characterized by inflammation of small bronchi and bronchioles

Response to environmental trigger

Mast cell degranulation, inflammatory cell migration

Release of histamine, prostaglandins, leukotrienes, chemotactic factors

Mucosal edema and lumenal secretions

Bronchospasm

Contraction of smooth muscle cells in bronchiolar cell walls

Response to increased vagal tone and inflammatory mediators

Chronically leads to smooth muscle hyperplasia

Risk Factors

Environmental allergens (pollen, animal dander, dust, mites)

Air pollutants, cold exposure, exercise, viral illness

Family history, history of atopy

Key Points

Features of Asthma

▸ Reversible airway obstruction caused by narrowed bronchi and bronchioles

▸ Pulmonary function abnormalities

  ▸ Increased TLC, FRC, RV

  ▸ Decreased VC, FEV_1

▸ Ventilation-perfusion mismatch (decreased V/Q ratio)

▸ Bronchiolar occlusion during exhalation causes air trapping

▸ Hypoxemia leads to increased minute volume and hypocapnea

▸ Respiratory alkalosis initially, then respiratory acidosis as condition worsens

▸ Reversible with medical treatment

▸ β_2-agonists, corticosteroids, anticholinergics, magnesium

Questions

1. Which factor has the *greatest* effect on laminar flow resistance in a tube?
   A. Length of the tube
   B. Diameter of the tube
   C. Viscosity of the gas
   D. Density of the gas
   E. Pressure differential

2. Air trapping in asthma occurs primarily as result of
   A. obstruction during inhalation and subsequent alveolar collapse.
   B. increased lung compliance caused by inflammation.
   C. the collapse of congested bronchioles during exhalation.
   D. shunting of ventilation to the upper lung fields.
   E. increased minute ventilation.

3. Which blood gas results would you expect in mild to moderate asthma?
   A. pH 7.30; PaO_2 85; $PaCO_2$ 30; HCO_3^- 12
   B. pH 7.24; PaO_2 60; $PaCO_2$ 60; HCO_3^- 26
   C. pH 7.34; PaO_2 62; $PaCO_2$ 60; HCO_3^- 28
   D. pH 7.48; PaO_2 70; $PaCO_2$ 30; HCO_3^- 22
   E. pH 7.52; PaO_2 90; $PaCO_2$ 48; HCO_3^- 48

4. Which of the following *favors* laminar flow as dictated by the Reynold's equation?
   A. Increased tube diameter
   B. Increased flow velocity
   C. Decreased gas density
   D. Decreased gas viscosity
   E. None of the above

HPI: JN, a 64-year-old man, has been an auto mechanic for 35 years. In his earlier years—before the risks of asbestos exposure were understood and before masks were worn—he had done a lot of brake jobs. While he replaced brakes, JN was always exposed to dust and fine particulate matter, but it never seemed to bother him. He had also been a one-pack per day smoker for 20 years, but he quit at age 40. JN now presents to his primary care doctor complaining of progressive dyspnea with exertion. He had always been very fit, but now has difficulty climbing a flight of stairs without becoming winded. He also tires quickly and fatigued when he goes on walks with his wife.

PE: JN is a healthy-appearing man with no respiratory distress. His vital signs are normal with the exception of a resting room-air oxygen saturation of 92%. His lung exam reveals fine crackles bilaterally that are louder at the bases. JN's extremities do not appear cyanotic but he has clubbing of his fingernails.

Thought Questions

- What is the fate of inhaled particles and how does particle size affect the location of deposition?

- How are deposited particles cleared from the conducting airways?

- How are deposited particles cleared from the alveoli?

- What is the definition of *pneumoconiosis* and what are the most common pneumoconioses?

- What is *pulmonary fibrosis* and how does it effect lung volumes and alveolar diffusion capacity?

Basic Science Review and Discussion

Inhaled Particulate Matter and Clearance Mechanisms

Deposition of aerosolized particles in the airways and alveoli depends largely on the diameter of the inhaled particles. The nasal passages and oropharynx are extremely effective at capturing particles as they are inhaled, and essentially all particles greater than 5 micrometers in diameter are captured. Extremely small particles (less than 1 micrometer) tend to remain suspended in air and are exhaled to a large extent, or diffuse through the terminal and respiratory bronchioles and into alveoli where they are deposited. Medium-sized particles (1–5 micrometers) are small enough to bypass the oronasopharynx, but are heavy enough so that they tend to deposit in small airways such as the terminal and respiratory bronchioles. These particles are too heavy to diffuse into the alveoli.

Particles that are deposited in the conducting airways are cleared by the mucociliary system. Mucus is produced both by seromucous glands and goblet cells. A muocus layer up to 10 micrometers thick is formed in the trachea, bronchi, and bronchioles. The outer gel layer is viscous, allowing it to trap deposited particles. The inner sol layer is very thin, which allows the cilia atop the epithelial cells to beat within it. The upward stroke of the cilia propels the gel layer superiorly toward the oropharynx. Once the mucus reaches the oropharynx it is either expectorated or swallowed. There are a number of disorders that alter the composition of the mucus layer and hinder the clearance of mucus and deposited particles. Toxic inhalants, such as those in cigarette smoke, can poison the epithelial cilia. Patients with chronic bronchitis produce an overabundance of thick, tenacious mucus that is too thick to be cleared by the cilia. Patients with asthma also have increased mucous production in small airways, which leads to mucous plugging and air trapping.

Particles that are able to reach the alveoli by diffusion are engulfed by alveolar macrophages that are amorphous cells that migrate along the surface of alveolar epithelia. Once phagocytized, particles are neutralized by lysozymal enzymes. These macrophages either migrate into larger airways where they can be cleared by the mucociliary system, or cross the alveolar wall into the lymphatic system where they can be drained. This is an important means of clearing bacterial and viral organisms and maintaining a sterile environment in the alveoli.

Pneumoconioses The term *pneumoconiosis* refers to parenchymal lung disease as a result of inhalation of inorganic dust. The most common pneumoconioses are asbestosis, coal workers' pneumoconiosis, and silicosis. The common pathophysiology of these disorders is the deposition of particles in the small airways and alveoli to the extent where they cannot be cleared. Some particles are phagocytized and cross the alveolar membrane into the interstitium. An inflammatory response results, with the migration of macrophages and fibroblasts and subsequent fibrotic reaction.

Pneumoconioses have varying pathologic attributes; however, these all result in pulmonary fibrosis. Pulmonary fibrosis is the accumulation of connective tissue in the pulmonary interstitium and subsequent destruction of the normal elastic quality of the lung parenchyma. The result is decreased alveolar expansion during inhalation leading to decreased total lung capacity (TLC), lower resting lung volumes or a lower functional residual capacity (FRC), decreased exhalation volume or functional vital capacity (FVC), and decreased forced expiratory volume (FEV_1). As compliance is decreased, increased intrathoracic negative pressure is required to expand the lungs during inspiration. Fibrotic tissue also increases the distance between the alveolar membrane and capillary endothelium; therefore, the diffusion of gases across the alveolar membrane is slowed. This has the greatest effect on the diffusion of oxygen across the membrane. In normal lungs, diffusion is rapid enough so that equilibrium occurs and hemoglobin in pulmonary venous blood is saturated. In pulmonary fibrosis, however, equilibrium does not occur and the PaO_2 of pulmonary venous blood is decreased. This is referred to as *diffusion limitation* and the result is arterial hypoxemia. Decreased oxygen content in arterial blood leads to drastically decreased exercise tolerance and peripheral ischemic changes such as cyanosis and fingernail clubbing. Alternatively carbon dioxide, as discussed previously, has 20 times the diffusing capacity as oxygen and CO_2

equilibrium is achieved despite the thickened alveolar membranes.

Restrictive Lung Disease Pulmonary fibrosis fits into a larger category of restrictive lung disease. Restrictive lung disease is a diagnosis made by pulmonary function testing, and it consists of the constellation of decreased lung volumes (TLC, FRC, FVC, and FEV_1). Restrictive lung disease can be either parenchymal or extraparenchymal. In parenchymal disease, decreased volumes result from interstitial fibrosis that causes the lungs to stiffen. Examples are idiopathic pulmonary fibrosis, pneumoconioses, sarcoidosis, and interstitial disease caused by certain drugs (e.g., amiodarone) or radiation. In extraparenchymal disease, there are external factors that limit lung expansion. Neuromuscular diseases in this category include myasthenia gravis, Guillain-Barré syndrome, muscular dystrophy, and cervical spine injuries that cause respiratory muscle paralysis. Other limitations to normal lung expansion include kyphoscoliosis, pes excavatum, and extreme obesity. Parenchymal restrictive disease is typically associated with a decreased alveolar diffusion capacity, whereas diffusion is unaffected in extraparenchymal disease.

Table 6-1. Pulmonary function tests in obstructive versus restrictive lung disease

	Normal	Obstructive	Restrictive
VC	4.8 L	3.5	3.5
FRC	3.8 L	6.0	2.2
TLC	6.0 L	8.0	4.5
FEV_1	3.5 L	1.5	3.0
Compliance	0.20 L/cm water	0.35	0.12

Case Conclusion JN's chest x-ray shows a diffuse interstitial pattern and the presence of pleural thickening. Pulmonary function tests show a restrictive pattern (Table 6-1) consistent with pulmonary fibrosis. Unfortunately, the pathologic changes that occur in asbestosis are irreversible and there is no specific treatment for JN's condition. Over the next 2 years he continued to have progressive dyspnea on exertion that eventually required supplemental oxygen at home.

Thumbnail: Asbestosis

Pathophysiology

Asbestosis and Other Pneumoconioses

Inhaled inorganic particles are phagocytized by macrophages and cross the alveolar membrane into the interstitium

Migration of inflammatory cells and release of mediators results in deposition of fibrotic connective tissue

The syndrome of asbestosis results in diffuse interstitial fibrosis, pleural thickening, and pleural plaque

Increased risk for bronchial carcinoma and malignant mesothelioma

Pulmonary Fibrosis

Deposition of fibrotic tissue in pulmonary parenchyma

Etiologies are many including idiopathic pulmonary fibrosis (IPF), pneumoconioses, sarcoidosis

Fibrotic tissue acts to inhibit normal expansion of alveoli

Lung volumes decreased including TLC, FRC, FVC, and FEV_1

Fibrotic tissue increases distance between alveolar membrane and capillary endothelium

Oxygen diffusion capacity is decreased, whereas CO_2 diffusion is only slightly affected

Diffusion limitation results in partially deoxygenated arterial blood and hypoxemia

Risk Factors

Asbestosis

Working in shipyards, exposure to insulating material, roofing material, and dust from brake lining

Silicosis

Exposure to rock quarry dust, mining, or sandblasting

Key Points

Restrictive Lung Disease
- Constellation of findings include decreased TLC, FRC, FVC, and FEV_1
- Disease processes with a restrictive pattern include idiopathic pulmonary fibrosis, sarcoidosis, pneumoconioses, and interstitial lung disease as a result of drugs or radiation

- Extraparenchymal processes can also lead to a restrictive pattern
  - Neuromuscular causes include myasthenia gravis, Guillain-Barré syndrome, muscular dystrophy, cervical spine injuries and respiratory muscle paralysis
  - Chest wall abnormalities include kyphoscoliosis and extreme obesity

Questions

1. Which of the following pulmonary function parameters may be *increased* in restrictive lung disease?
   A. FVC
   B. FRC
   C. TLC
   D. FEV_1
   E. FEV_1/FVC

2. Which of the following disease processes *does not typically result* in diffuse infiltrative disease and pulmonary fibrosis of the lungs?
   A. Pneumoconioses
   B. Chronic bronchitis
   C. Hypersensitivity pneumonitis
   D. Pulmonary vasculitides
   E. Sarcoidosis
   F. Collagen vascular diseases
   G. Pulmonary hemorrhagic disorders
   H. Drug- and radiation-induced fibroses

3. Which of the following statements is *false*?
   A. Asbestosis is associated with mesotheliomas.
   B. Pleural plaques imply asbestos exposure but not necessarily pulmonary disease.
   C. Silicosis is associated with a high incidence of tuberculosis.
   D. Silicosis is associated with quarrying, mining, and sandblasting.
   E. Coal workers' pneumoconiosis is often referred to as "Monday's disease."

4. Which of the following is *false* regarding sarcoidosis?
   A. It is characterized by noncaseating granulomas involving multiple organ systems.
   B. Chest x-ray often shows hilar adenopathy and diffuse interstitial disease.
   C. This occurs more frequently in black population.
   D. It is associated with bronchogenic carcinoma.
   E. It is associated with anterior uveitis, erythema nodosum, and polyarthritis.

HPI: SW, a 56-year-old woman, fractured her left ankle 2 weeks ago. A below-the-knee cast was placed and SW has been getting around using crutches. She was told to keep her left leg elevated as much as possible so SW has spent a lot of time at home watching TV with her leg propped up. She had been doing well until this morning when she developed a sharp pain in her right side that worsened each time she took a deep breath. SW got up several times to try and work out the pain but nothing relieved it. She felt short of breath every time she tried to walk.

PE: Other than her broken ankle, SW is a nonsmoking, healthy woman and only takes estrogen replacement. When she arrived in the emergency department she was mildly dyspneic. Her vital signs included a pulse of 110, blood pressure 118/68, respiratory rate 28, and Sao_2 of 92% on room air. On physical exam SW looked mildly uncomfortable but her color was good. Her heart and lung sounds were normal and no tenderness was elicited on palpation to her chest wall. She carried the cast on her left leg, and her left thigh did not appear any more swollen than her right. There was no thigh tenderness or palpable superficial veins.

Thought Questions

- How does pulmonary vascular resistance compare to systemic vascular resistance?

- What is the response of pulmonary vascular resistance to increased pulmonary artery pressure?

- How does pulmonary blood flow differ in different regions of the lung?

- What is the response of regional pulmonary vascular resistance to local alveolar hypoxia?

- What is the vascular response to a pulmonary embolus and how does it effect arterial Pao_2 and $Paco_2$?

Basic Science Review and Discussion

Pulmonary Vascular Resistance In general, flow resistance is defined as dP/flow rate; or in terms of blood flow, vascular resistance = (arterial pressure − venous pressure)/blood flow. Remembering the arterial and venous pressures of the pulmonary vasculature (15 mmHg and 5 mmHg, respectively) compared to the systemic vasculature (100 mmHg and 2 mmHg, respectively), and the same blood flow rate for both systems, the pulmonary vascular resistance is about one-tenth that of the systemic vascular resistance.

A pulmonary embolus, or blood clot, lodges in a portion of the pulmonary arterial system and creates a blockage to flow. This blockage increases local pulmonary vascular resistance and thus pulmonary arterial pressure. In response to increased pulmonary arterial pressure, however, the pulmonary vascular resistance tends to fall in unaffected portions of the lung by recruitment and distension. *Recruitment* is a process whereby capillaries—closed at normal pressures—become available for flow at higher arterial pressures. This results in a higher density of open capillaries,

decreased vascular resistance, and increased flow through these regions of the lung. In effect, the flow is shunted from the region of embolus to unaffected lung tissue, and the increased resistance caused by the embolus is blunted by the effect of recruitment. At higher pulmonary vascular pressures *distension* is a second mechanism by which the pulmonary vascular resistance falls in response to increased pulmonary vascular pressures. Pulmonary vessels are thin-walled, and at normal pressures are partially collapsed. At higher pressures these vessels have room to expand and thus facilitate higher flow rates at a lower resistance.

Pulmonary vascular resistance is also a function of lung volume. For example, during inhalation as alveoli expand the alveolar walls stretch and their contents are compressed. This has the effect of narrowing the diameter of the alveolar capillaries and increasing their resistance. In patients with chronic obstructive pulmonary disease (COPD) and chronic air-trapping, increased pulmonary vascular resistance leads to chronically increased pulmonary arterial pressures. The latter leads to cor pulmonale that is characterized by a thickened right ventricle and an enlarged right atrium. This condition eventually causes right-sided heart failure that is manifested by engorged neck veins, enlarged liver, and the accumulation of peripheral edema.

Physiologic shunting and ventilation-perfusion (V/Q) mismatch A previous case discussed the regional differences in ventilation (V) and perfusion (Q), and it introduced the concept of ventilation-perfusion ratio (V/Q ratio). Both ventilation and perfusion decrease from zone 3 (bottom) to zone 1 (top); however, the decrease in perfusion is far greater in the apices due to the gravitational effect on pulmonary artery pressures. For this reason, the V/Q ratio increases dramatically in the apices when compared to the bases (see Figure 4-3). Therefore, in the normal lung the apices are relatively overventilated, resulting in a higher Pao_2 and lower $Paco_2$.

A pulmonary embolism causes shunting of blood to both alveolar and extra-alveolar capillaries. Extra-alveolar capillaries are those that do not interface with alveolar gases; they therefore act as a physiologic shunt. In the normal lung, there is a small degree of physiologic shunt that accounts for the small decrease in tension between alveolar and pulmonary arterial oxygen ($PAO_2 - PaO_2$ = alveolar-arterial gradient, or A-a gradient that is about 5–10 mmHg in normal adults). Increased physiologic shunting in pulmonary embolism causes mixing of unventilated blood (PvO_2 of 40 mmHg) with ventilated blood (PaO_2 of 100 mmHg). The result is a lower PaO_2 (hypoxemia) and a greater A-a gradient. Similar to the body's response to high altitude, the relative hypoxemia of pulmonary embolism triggers a hyperventilatory response. This has the effect of increasing ventilation to those portions of the lungs with a higher V/Q ratio (e.g., the apices).

Intuition might lead one to believe that increased blood flow to regions of higher V/Q ratio (i.e., higher PAO_2) would counteract the hypoxemia caused by the increased physiologic shunt. The reason this is not true returns again to the nature of the oxygen-hemoglobin dissociation curve. Remember, at high oxygen tension (e.g., $PAO_2 > 90$ mmHg), the curve is nearly horizontal, meaning that any increase in PAO_2 above 100 mmHg results in only a slight increase in oxygen content (i.e., hemoglobin saturation) because the blood is, in effect, already saturated with oxygen. Alternatively, because of the more linear nature of the CO_2 dissociation curve, the lower $PACO_2$ of the hyperventilated regions of the lung results in a significant off-loading of CO_2, and thus a significant decrease in blood CO_2 content. The end result in pulmonary embolism is a decrease in both PaO_2 and $PaCO_2$. $PaCO_2$ results in a primary respiratory alkalosis that is typical of pulmonary embolism.

Case Conclusion Because of SW's mild dyspnea and hypoxia, an arterial blood gas was obtained that revealed pH 7.48, PaO_2 82 mmHg, $PaCO_2$ 30 mmHg, and $[HCO_3^-]$ 21. A chest x-ray was normal but a serum d-dimer was 876. She was sent for a ventilation-perfusion (V/Q) scan that showed a large right lower lobe ventilation-perfusion mismatch, consistent with pulmonary embolism. The source of the embolism was presumed to be her casted lower extremity. SW was started on heparin, admitted to the hospital, and later sent home on a 6-month course of warfarin.

Thumbnail: Pulmonary Embolism

Pathophysiology

Blood clot that forms in the pulmonary arterial system

Greater than 90% of cases are seeded from deep venous thrombosis (DVT) in lower extremities

Flow obstruction results in increased local resistance and pulmonary arterial pressure

Increased pressure results in both recruitment and dilatation of alveolar and extra-alveolar pulmonary capillaries

Despite this, the overall effect is an increase in pulmonary vascular resistance

Increased extra-alveolar flow results in increased physiologic dead space (high V/Q)

Mixing of deoxygenated and oxygenated blood leads to decreased PaO_2

Hypoxemia triggers hyperventilatory response that increases ventilation to unaffected lung

Ineffective in increasing PaO_2 because blood is already saturated with oxygen due to the nature of oxygen-hemoglobin curve

Lower $PACO_2$ has effect of rapidly unloading CO_2 from blood due to the linear nature of CO_2 dissociation curve

End result is an elevated A-a gradient with respiratory alkalosis

Risk factors

Recent surgical procedures or orthopedic injuries, postpartum, heart failure with low cardiac output, cancer, oral estrogen replacement or oral contraceptive pills (OCPs), smoking

Familial risk factors include deficiencies of antithrombin III, protein C, protein S, and the presence of lupus anticoagulant

Key Points

▸ Clinical features include dyspnea, tachypnea, tachycardia, and hypoxia

▸ Large pulmonary emboli lead to pulmonary hypertension and right heart strain

  ▸ EKG findings of rightward axis, RBBB, or $S_1Q_3T_3$ syndrome (i.e., deep S wave in lead I, Q wave in lead III, and an inverted T wave in lead III)

  ▸ Echo finding of right ventricular dilatation and wall motion abnormalities

▸ Clinical finding of elevated neck veins, hepatic congestion, peripheral edema

▸ Treatment includes anticoagulation with unfractionated heparin or low-molecular-weight heparin

▸ Systemic thrombolysis is indicated for signs of cardiopulmonary failure such as respiratory distress, hypotension, or cardiac arrest

Questions

1. Which of the following is the *strongest risk factor* for pulmonary embolism?
   A. Smoking
   B. Recent surgical procedure
   C. Postpartum
   D. Use of OCPs
   E. History of deep venous thrombosis

2. Which of the following causes a *reduction* in pulmonary resistance?
   A. Positive pressure ventilation
   B. Breathing gas with an FiO_2 of 0.10
   C. Acute aortic valve stenosis
   D. Pneumonectomy
   E. Forced exhalation

3. Acute pulmonary embolism causes which of the following?
   A. Acute left heart strain
   B. Vasodilation of effected capillary beds
   C. Vasodilation of unaffected capillary beds
   D. Decreased pulmonary capillary resistance
   E. Decreased A-a gradient

4. In the normal lung, which of the following is *true* regarding zone 1 compared to zone 3 ?
   A. Higher ventilation
   B. Higher perfusion
   C. Higher V/Q ratio
   D. Higher compliance
   E. Higher capillary pressure

HPI: GK, a 72-year-old woman, had a myocardial infarction 5 years ago and presently suffers from congestive heart failure. She was doing well until today when she entertained relatives for Thanksgiving dinner. They cooked a feast including turkey, stuffing, mashed potatoes, cranberry sauce, and apple pie. Several hours after dinner GK began to feel short of breath and fatigued. She laid down to rest and developed sudden worsening in her breathing, and called 911.

PE: Upon arrival to the emergency department GK was pale, cool, diaphoretic, and dyspneic. Her vital signs included a pulse of 98, blood pressure of 220/110, respiratory rate of 28, and an oxygen saturation of 88% on oxygen. Her physical exam revealed moist, cool skin. Her neck veins were engorged, her lungs with crackles bilaterally halfway up, her heart with an S3 gallop. GK had 2+ peripheral edema and good peripheral pulses.

Thought Questions

- Which equation governs the filtration of fluid across a semipermeable membrane and how does this translate to the pathophysiology of pulmonary edema?

- What are the most common precipitating etiologies of pulmonary edema?

- What is the effect of increased interstitial pressure on the alveolar membrane?

- Does alveolar edema result in an increase in anatomic dead space or physiologic shunt?

- What is the treatment for acute pulmonary edema?

Basic Science Review and Discussion:

Flow Across a Semipermeable Membrane Filtration of fluid across a semipermeable membrane is governed by the Starling equation: $Q_f = K_f [(P_p - P_i) - \sigma (\pi_p - \pi_i)]$, where Q_f = fluid filtration rate, K_f = filtration coefficient, P_p = pulmonary vessel hydrostatic pressure, P_i = interstitial hydrostatic pressure, σ = osmotic reflection coefficient, π_p = pulmonary vessel oncotic pressure, π_i = interstitial oncotic pressure. This equation basically states that the fluid balance across a membrane is determined by the difference in hydrostatic pressures and the difference in oncotic pressures across the membrane. Every membrane has a different permeability to fluid (K_f), and this coefficient increases as membrane damage occurs. Similarly, the contribution of oncotic pressure differences varies among membranes and is quantified by the coefficient σ. When $\sigma = 0$, a membrane allows free passage of proteins across it, and the contribution of oncotic pressure differences to fluid flow is zero. The alveolar membrane is relatively impermeable to protein, and the normal osmotic reflection coefficient is 0.8. Considering this equation, increased fluid flow (i.e., pulmonary edema) can be caused by an increase in pulmonary vessel hydrostatic pressure P_p (e.g., left heart failure, mitral or aortic valve stenosis) or a decrease in pulmonary vessel oncotic pressure π_p (e.g., hypoproteinemia from cirrhosis or renal failure).

Left-Sided Heart Failure and Pulmonary Edema Pulmonary edema is most often caused by a sudden increase in pulmonary capillary hydrostatic pressure that causes water and solutes to cross the capillary endothelial membrane into the alveolar interstitium. This is usually a result of left-sided heart failure, where decreased cardiac output causes left atrial and pulmonary venous pressures to rise. Left-sided heart failure is most typically a result of a myocardial infarction, although it can also be a result of mitral or aortic valve stenosis or insufficiency. Patients who have a history of left-sided heart failure may suddenly develop acute pulmonary edema in response to small increases in pulmonary venous pressure. Some of the more common etiologies include increase in salt intake, noncompliance with medications, overaggressive intravenous fluid resuscitation, administration of blood products, new atrial fibrillation, and new myocardial ischemia.

When alveolar interstitial pressure reaches a certain point, structural damage to the alveolar epithelium occurs. The epithelium consists of predominantly alveolar type I cells that normally provide a tight barrier to fluid and protein influx. These cells also contain Na-K ATPase channels that pump water out of the alveoli into the interstitium. Increased hydrostatic pressure damages the integrity of this barrier; this allows fluid, protein, and red cells to seep into the alveoli. These substances neutralize the effect of surfactant, thus increasing alveolar surface tension and causing their collapse.

Acid-Base Disturbance in Pulmonary Edema The presence of alveolar fluid prevents alveolar gas exchange and therefore creates a physiologic shunt. In other words, mixed venous blood flowing into the pulmonary capillaries is not properly ventilated and returns deoxygenated blood to the left heart. As discussed in the previous chapter, this results in decreased PaO_2 and arterial hypoxemia. In response to hypoxemia, or in part to the lactic acidosis created by end-organ hypoxia, hyperventilation occurs. As already discussed, this does not contribute significantly to the arterial oxygen content, but acts to excrete CO_2. Therefore, patients with acute pulmonary edema often present initially with a mixed acid-base disorder of metabolic acidosis (decreased $[HCO_3^-]$) and respiratory alkalosis (decreased

$Paco_2$). In severe cases, a respiratory acidosis is present (elevated $Paco_2$).

Treatment for Acute Pulmonary Edema   The treatment for acute pulmonary edema is to decrease pulmonary capillary hydrostatic pressure and thus reduce the pressure gradient that results in fluid flow across the endothelial membrane. Foremost is the correction of arterial hypoxemia that results from V/Q mismatching and physiologic shunting. This is accomplished by the administration of high-flow supplemental oxygen. Nitrates are a mainstay in pulmonary edema because these cause a pulmonary vasodilation that directly leads to decreased pulmonary vascular hydrostatic pressure. For mild pulmonary edema sublingual nitroglycerin or topical nitroglycerin paste can be used. For more severe pulmonary edema an intravenous nitroglycerin drip is typically used. Diuretics are also important in the treatment of acute pulmonary edema. Loop diuretics (e.g., furosemide) cause a rapid decrease in intravascular volume, which in turn decreases vascular hydrostatic pressure and results in fluid shift back from the interstitium into the vasculature. Mor-

phine also has the effect of vasodilatation of pulmonary capillary beds and is useful in acute pulmonary edema.

As in chronic obstructive pulmonary disease (COPD), noninvasive positive-pressure ventilation (NPPV) is very effective for oxygenating and ventilating a patient with acute pulmonary edema. A tight-fitting face mask is used in line with a ventilator to provide high Fio_2 mixture and pressure support to the patient's normal respirations. The positive pressure has the effect of opening a greater number of alveoli that tend to collapse in the presence of alveolar edema fluid, and the high Fio_2 is important in raising the arterial oxygen content and to help overcome physiologic shunting. Endotracheal intubation and mechanical ventilation may be required if NPPV fails to correct the arterial hypoxemia due to the overwhelming degree of edema fluid, or if the patient tires and cannot sustain the increased ventilatory rate at increased workload. Fortunately, acute pulmonary edema is reversible within hours if treated early with aggressive use of nitrates, diuretics, morphine, and NPPV; and endotracheal intubation can usually be avoided even in severe cases.

Case Conclusion   GK was placed on high-flow oxygen by facemask, intravenous nitroglycerin was started and she was given a dose of furosemide 60 mg IV. A 12-lead EKG was obtained that showed no evidence of acute myocardial ischemia; however, an aspirin was administered orally just in case an acute coronary syndrome was the precipitating cause. A Foley catheter was placed in order to monitor GK's urine output. A chest x-ray revealed diffuse interstitial edema characterized by indistinct vessel borders, peribronchial cuffing, and cephalization of vessels (Figure 8-1). NPPV was also started to increase her oxygenation and ventilation. Within 1 hour GK had put out 800 cc of urine, her oxygen saturation had increased to 96% on supplemental oxygen, and her respiratory rate had decreased to 18 per minute. She was admitted to a monitored bed for further diuresis and serial cardiac enzymes.

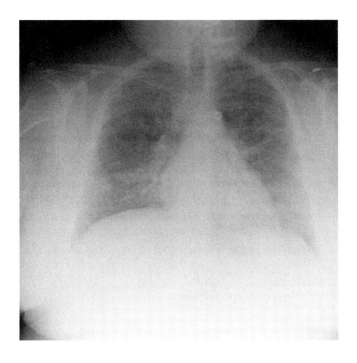

Figure 8-1. Chest x-ray showing pulmonary edema characterized by indistinct vessel borders, peribronchial cuffing, and cephalization of vessels.

Thumbnail: Pulmonary Edema

Pathophysiology

Starling equation governs fluid flow across a membrane

Pulmonary edema can result from increased pulmonary vessel hydrostatic pressure, decreased pulmonary vessel oncotic pressure, or increased membrane permeability coefficient

As pulmonary hydrostatic pressure increases, damage to alveolar wall membrane occurs

Increased permeability coefficient allows fluid, solutes, protein, and cells to enter alveoli

Surfactant neutralized and washed away

Alveolar surface tension increases, resulting in loss of structural integrity and tendency for alveolar collapse

Fluid-filled alveoli are underventilated and create areas of decreased V/Q ratio

Effective physiologic shunting results in arterial hypoxemia

Arterial hypoxemia causes increased minute ventilation

Fluid-filled interstitium and alveoli results in decreased pulmonary compliance and increased work of breathing

Increased work of breathing combined with increased minute ventilation lead to respiratory failure

Inability to compensate for arterial hypoxemia

Heralded by steadily rising $Paco_2$ and declining Pao_2 (respiratory acidosis)

Risk Factors

Increased pulmonary hydrostatic pressure

Left-sided heart failure due to myocardial infarction

Mitral or aortic valve stenosis or insufficiency

Medical noncompliance with diuretics, high-sodium diet

Decreased pulmonary oncotic pressure

Cirrhosis, chronic renal failure

Key Points

Pulmonary Edema

▸ Clinical features include dyspnea, tachypnea, diaphoresis, tachycardia, hypertension, hypoxia, diffuse pulmonary rales

  ▸ Often associated with signs of right-heart failure including jugular venous distension, hepatic engorgement, peripheral edema

▸ Treatment includes high-flow oxygen, nitrates, diuretics, and morphine

▸ Severe cases require NPPV

  ▸ Provide high Fio_2, pressure-supported respiration to maximize alveolar opening

Questions

1. Which of the following *counteracts* the flow of edema fluid across the pulmonary capillary endothelial membrane in pulmonary edema?

   A. Increased pulmonary vessel hydrostatic pressure
   B. Decreased interstitial oncotic pressure
   C. Decreased interstitial hydrostatic pressure
   D. Decreased membrane permeability coefficient
   E. Decreased cardiac output

2. Pulmonary edema has which of the following effects on pulmonary physiology?

   A. Increases alveolar wall surface tension
   B. Increases pulmonary compliance
   C. Overall increase in V/Q ratio
   D. Decreases ventilation to lung apices
   E. Decreases pulmonary artery pressures

3. Which of the following arterial blood gas results would be expected in early pulmonary edema?

   A. pH 7.28; Pao_2 64; $Paco_2$ 60; $[HCO_3{}^-]$ 18
   B. pH 7.34; Pao_2 92; $Paco_2$ 36; $[HCO_3{}^-]$ 20
   C. pH 7.48; Pao_2 72; $Paco_2$ 32; $[HCO_3{}^-]$ 22
   D. pH 7.52; Pao_2 86; $Paco_2$ 42; $[HCO_3{}^-]$ 30
   E. pH 7.30; Pao_2 86; $Paco_2$ 38; $[HCO_3{}^-]$ 16

4. Which of the following is *not* standard in treatment of acute pulmonary edema as a result of left-sided heart failure?

   A. High flow oxygen
   B. Positive-pressure ventilation
   C. Nitrates
   D. Diuretics
   E. β-agonist nebulizers

[handwritten: Acute → Bacterial]

[handwritten, top right: R mid lobe most common]

HPI: SS, a 26-year-old woman, smokes a pack of cigarettes daily but is otherwise healthy. She became ill one morning when she developed a sudden shaking chill and spiked a temperature up to 102.4°F. SS noted pain in her right chest when she took a deep breath but had no difficulty breathing. Later that morning she developed a dry cough and the pain increased. SS took acetaminophen for her fever but continued to feel worse. By afternoon, she had not eaten, her fever rose to 103.2°F, and she began to have shaking chills again.

[handwritten: Blood culture]

PE: Upon arrival in the emergency department, she looked ill and was mildly dyspneic. Her vital signs included a temperature of 102.8°F, pulse 118, blood pressure 112/74, respiratory rate 32, and oxygen saturation of 92% on room air. On physical exam, she had ronchi in the right lower lung field with egophony and transmitted upper airway sounds.

[handwritten: egophony]

[handwritten: Bronchophony egophony pectoriloquy]

Thought Questions

- How do classical and atypical presentations differ for pneumonia? What are the most common organisms causing each of these syndromes?

- What are some of the most common risk factors for pneumonia?

- Which features of pneumonia result in a worse outcome and subsequently require hospitalization and intravenous antibiotics?

- How are antibiotics selected to treat pneumonia?

Basic Science Review and Discussion

Classic versus Atypical Pneumonia The classic presentation for pneumonia is the sudden-onset of fever, chills, cough with or without purulent sputum, pleuritic chest pain, and dyspnea. This syndrome is most frequently caused by *Streptococcus pneumoniae*; however, *Haemophilus influenzae*, *Moraxella catarrhalis*, *Staphylococcus aureus*, or Gram-negative enteric bacteria may also be the culprit. When sputum is available, a diagnosis can be made by Gram stain

with an adequate specimen that contains greater than 25 neutrophils and less than 10 squamous cells. Gram stain findings and optimal antibiotic treatment are detailed for each organism in Table 9-1. The chest x-ray in classical pneumonia shows a focal consolidation confined to a particular lobe of the lung that correlates with location of pleuritic chest pain. A consolidation refers to alveolar infiltrates that consist of the bacterial pathogen and exudative inflammatory response, including inflammatory cells, cytokines, and proteinaceous fluid.

Atypical pneumonia usually occurs as a more indolent process that may progress over several days, and include more prominent constitutional symptoms such as a low-grade fever, myalgias, fatigue, arthralgias, headache, sore throat, or skin rash. Pulmonary complaints are often less marked, the cough is usually nonproductive, and pleuritic chest pain is often absent. Atypical pneumonia is most commonly caused by *Mycoplasma pneumoniae*; however, many organisms can possibly cause it, including other bacterial pathogens (e.g., *Chlamydia pneumoniae*, *Legionella*, *Mycobacterium tuberculosis*), viral pathogens (e.g., adenovirus, parainfluenza virus, respiratory syncytial virus), or fungal pathogens (e.g., aspergillosis, coccidioidomycosis, histoplasmosis, *Pneumocystis carinii*). The Gram stain in

[handwritten: "Walking" pneumonia]

Table 9-1. Gram stain findings and antibiotic treatment for common bacterial pathogens

Organism	Gram stain findings	First-line antibiotics
Streptococcus pneumoniae	Gram-positive cocci in pairs	Penicillin
Mycoplasma pneumoniae	Does not stain. Diagnosis with positive cold-agglutinin serology.	Erythromycin
Haemophilus influenzae	Gram-negative coccobacillus	Trimethoprim-sulfamethoxazole, ampicillin
Staphylococcus aureus	Gram-positive cocci in clusters	Nafcillin
Legionella pneumophila	Rare Gram-negative rods, numerous neutrophils. Diagnosis with positive urine *Legionella* antigen.	Erythromycin
Escherichia coli, Klebsiella pneumoniae, Pseudomonas pneumoniae	Gram-negative rods	Aminoglycosides, third-generation cephalosporin
Chlamydia pneumoniae	Giemsa stain shows cytoplasmic organisms within epithelial cells.	Erythromycin

atypical pneumonia contains fewer neutrophils and is less diagnostic. The chest x-ray findings vary but will often show bilateral patchy or interstitial infiltrates.

Risk Factors   As with many infectious diseases, risk factors for pneumonia include the elderly, debilitated, and immunocompromised. More specifically, patients with chronic lung disease, chronic renal failure, diabetes mellitus, and sickle-cell disease are more susceptible to pneumonia. Patients who suffer from alcoholism, seizure disorders, or chronic debilitating neurologic disorders are prone to aspiration pneumonia. Immunocompromised patients include those with AIDS or those taking immunosuppressive medications such as steroids or chemotherapeutic agents. These patients are susceptible to the common bacterial and viral agents, but consideration must also be given to opportunistic organisms such as tuberculosis, fungal agents (e.g., *Candida, Pneumocystis carinii*), or parasites.

Admission Criteria   The decision to admit a patient with pneumonia for intravenous antibiotics is multifactorial and based largely on clinical experience; however, there are several clinical features that portend a poor outcome and usually warrant admission. These include patients older than age 70 or those with significant comorbidity such as renal, heart, or lung disease. Patients who have failed outpatient antibiotic therapy or who cannot tolerate oral medication must also be admitted. Patients with evidence of respiratory failure or sepsis should definitely be admitted. This is evident by persistent tachypnea greater than 30 breaths/min, tachycardia greater than 120/min, hypotension less than 90 mmHg, hypoxia less than 90%, or changes in mental status. Patients with an empyema or large parapneumonic effusion should also be admitted.

Treatment   The selection of antibiotics is based on the suspected agent and whether the pneumonia was acquired in the community, in the hospital, or other chronic care facil-

ity. Community-acquired pneumonia in young healthy adults is usually one of the atypical organisms such as *Mycoplasma, Chlamydia,* or a virus. Smokers are more likely to harbor one of the typical bacterial pathogens such as *S. pneumoniae, H. influenzae,* and *M. catarrhalis.* Macrolide antibiotics (e.g., azithromycin, clarithromycin) provide good coverage against the typical and atypical organisms and are therefore the first-line against community-acquired pneumonia. Of course, if a sputum sample can be obtained and Gram stain performed in a timely fashion, then a specific organism may be identified and the antibiotic tailored (see Table 9-1). Commonly used second-line agents include a fluoroquinolone (e.g., levofloxacin), second-generation cephalosporin (e.g., cefuroxime), amoxicillin/clavulanate (Augmentin), or doxycycline.

Patients with community-acquired pneumonia who have significant comorbidities and require hospitalization should be covered more broadly for gram-negative pathogens. Therefore, in addition to a macrolide or fluoroquinolone, a third-generation cephalosporin (e.g., ceftriaxone, cefotaxime) should be administered intravenously. For hospital-acquired pneumonia, antibiotic coverage needs to be expanded to cover resistant strains of *Streptococcus* and *Staphylococcus, Pseudomonas,* gram-negative organisms, and anaerobes. Imipenem and meropenem as single agents provide good coverage for these organisms in addition to the typical bacterial pathogens. Despite their broad coverage, these drugs should not be used as first-line agents to avoid drug-resistance. A good choice is a third-generation cephalosporin with antipseudomonal activity (e.g., cefepime, ceftazidime) plus an aminoglycoside (e.g., tobramycin, gentamicin), which also possesses antipseudomonal activity. Antipseudomonal penicillins (e.g., ticarcillin, piperacillin) are also good options. Again, sputum and blood cultures are important in hospital-acquired pneumonia in order to specify the organism, identify drug sensitivities, and tailor antibiotic therapy.

Case Conclusion   SS has the typical symptoms for classic bacterial pneumonia. A chest x-ray showed a consolidation in the right middle lobe (see Figure 9-1). Given that she is a young, healthy smoker, the most likely pathogens are *S. pneumoniae, H. influenzae,* and *M. catarrhalis.* If she were treated as an outpatient, azithromycin would be a reasonable choice of antibiotics. However, because SS does not look well, is not tolerating fluids, and her oxygen saturation is in the low 90s, she is admitted for antibiotic treatment and intravenous rehydration. In the emergency department, she is able to provide a deep sputum sample, which is sent to the laboratory for Gram stain and culture. The Gram stain shows abundant neutrophils with gram-positive cocci in pairs. A diagnosis of pneumococcal pneumonia is made and SS is given intravenous penicillin G. Her fever breaks that evening and she feels better the next day. She is discharged home on the third day in good condition.

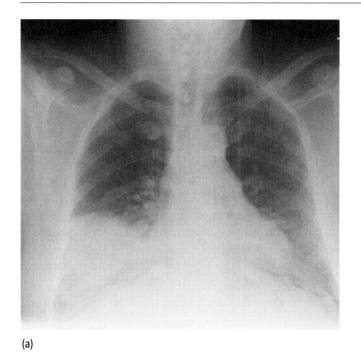

(a)

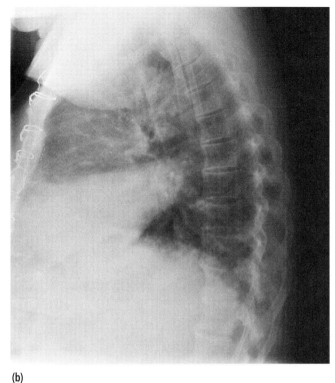

(b)

Figure 9-1. Chest x-ray showing a right middle lobe pneumonia. Note that the right heart border and right diaphragm are obscured on the PA view (a) and the wedge-shaped infiltrate on the lateral view (b) that corresponds to the right middle lobe.

Thumbnail: Pneumonia

Pathophysiology

Classic Pneumonia

Rapid onset of symptoms

   High fever, rigors, cough, pleuritic chest pain

Physical exam reveals tachycardia, tachypnea, hypoxia, focal ronchi, egophony, transmitted breath sounds

Chest x-ray shows focal consolidation

Most common pathogens are *S. pneumoniae, H. influenzae, M. catarrhalis*

Atypical Pneumonia

Symptom onset more gradual or indolent

   Low-grade fevers, myalgias and arthralgias, fatigue, headache, rash

Physical exam may reveal low-grade fever, tachycardia, mild hypoxia, diffuse rales

Chest x-ray shows diffuse interstitial infiltrates

Most common pathogens are *M. pneumoniae, C. pneumoniae,* or a virus

Risk Factors

Mucociliary dysfunction

   Smoking, chronic asthma or bronchitis, cystic fibrosis, bronchiectasis

Comorbid disease

   Heart disease, renal failure, chronic lung disease, diabetes mellitus

Immunocompromised

   Cancer, AIDS, chemotherapeutic agents, chronic steroid use

Key Points

- ▸ Identification of specific organism is important in tailoring therapy
- ▸ Empiric treatment is based on several factors
  - ▸ Community acquired, healthy adult
    - ▸ Macrolide, fluoroquinolone, second-generation cephalosporin, amoxicillin/clavulanate, doxycycline
  - ▸ Community acquired, but ill and requiring hospitalization

- ▸ Third-generation cephalosporin PLUS macrolide, fluoroquinolone, second-generation cephalosporin, amoxicillin/clavulanate, doxycycline
- ▸ Hospital acquired   *Gram negs*
- ▸ Requires double coverage for *Pseudomonas*
- ▸ Antipseudomonal penicillin (e.g., ticarcillin, piperacillin) or antipseudomonal cephalosporin (e.g., cefepime, ceftazidime) PLUS an aminoglycoside (e.g., gentamicin, tobramycin)

Questions

1. A 26-year-old healthy male smoker presents with sudden-onset shaking chills, fever to 103.0°F, cough, and left-sided pleuritic chest pain. A chest x-ray shows focal consolidation in the left lower lobe. Which organism is *least likely* to be causative?
   A. *Streptococcus pneumoniae*
   B. *Hemophilus influenzae*
   C. *Moraxella catarrhalis*
   D. *Mycoplasma pneumoniae*
   E. *Staphylococcus aureus*

2. An outbreak of illness occurs in a large apartment complex characterized by low-grade fevers, cough, malaise, and diarrhea. In one patient, a Gram stain of induced sputum reveals several Gram-negative rods and many neutrophils. What is the antibiotic of choice for this illness?
   A. Penicillin G
   B. Ciprofloxacin
   C. Erythromycin
   D. Gentamicin
   E. Cefaclor

3. A 22-year-old college student presents with 2 weeks of low-grade fevers, dry cough, malaise, myalgias, headache, and decreased appetite. A chest x-ray shows diffuse, interstitial, patchy infiltrates. What is the first-line antibiotic for this illness?
   A. Azithromycin
   B. Doxycycline
   C. Ceftriaxone
   D. Amoxicillin/*clavulanate*
   E. Levofloxacin

4. A 36-year-old man with AIDS presents to the emergency department with 10 days of a dry, nonproductive cough, intermittent fevers, malaise, and decreased appetite. Over the past 2 days he has developed difficulty breathing and severe dyspnea on exertion. His vital signs are significant for mild tachypnea and an oxygen saturation of 88% on room air. He has oral thrush, and his pulmonary exam reveals bilateral fine rales. A chest x-ray shows bilateral perihilar interstitial opacities. What is the first-line antibiotic agent for this condition?
   A. Penicillin G
   B. Trimethoprim/sulfamethoxazole
   C. Azithromycin
   D. Doxycycline
   E. Rifampin

> **HPI:** RJ, a 58-year-old man, immigrated to the United States from India 20 years ago. He never experienced health problems until 2 months ago when he began feeling ill. He has had chronic intermittent fevers, mostly at night and associated with drenching sweats. He has had a nagging cough with small amounts of blood-streaked sputum, a decreased appetite, and a 20-pound weight loss over the past 2 months. RJ has not recently traveled out of the country and has had no contacts with persons who were ill. He does not recall if he has ever had a skin test for tuberculosis or if he was ever immunized against tuberculosis in India.

Thought Questions

- Which organism is responsible for tuberculosis and what distinguishes it from other bacteria?

- What is the mode of transmission and the host's immunologic reaction to the bacterium?

- What is the difference between primary and secondary tuberculosis?

- What is the role of purified protein derivative (PPD) in the diagnosis of tuberculosis?

- How is tuberculosis treated?

Basic Science Review and Discussion

Pathophysiology and Transmission   Tuberculosis is caused by the bacterium *Mycobacterium tuberculosis,* which is one of many types of mycobacteria including *M. leprae* and *M. avium. Mycobacteria* are distinguished from other bacteria by their cell wall, which is acid-fast. Its cell wall has a high lipid content such that once it is stained it cannot be decolorized by acid alcohol. *M. tuberculosis* contains highly immunogenic proteins in its cell wall that activate cell-mediated immunity and account for the pathogenesis of the disease.

M. tuberculosis is contracted via respiratory droplets from a person with active tuberculosis. Desiccated bacilli can remain airborne for long periods of time. Once the bacilli are inhaled into the lungs, they are phagocytized by macrophages and carried to regional lymph nodes. This initial infection—or primary tuberculosis—usually occurs in the lower lobes of the lung where ventilation is highest. Macrophages release chemotactic factors that initiate a cell-mediated immunologic response. Lymphocytes and monocytes migrate to the focus of infection and create a granuloma; that is, an island of inflammatory tissue that contains macrophages with phagocytized bacteria and histiocytes. These lesions typically remain self-contained and heal, forming a ring of calcification that can be seen on chest x-ray. The bacteria, however, remain viable and latent within this granuloma.

Primary Tuberculosis   In most infected hosts, primary tuberculosis is asymptomatic. In patients who are immunocompromised, or in those who suffer from malnutrition and famine, the primary infection has a greater chance of spreading outside the initial site of infection. This is referred to as *disseminated tuberculosis,* and can manifest in many ways including miliary tuberculosis, which is characterized by numerous, small lesions distributed throughout the lungs, and simultaneous hematogenous spread with seeding of other organs. Extrapulmonary sites of infection include infected pleural effusions, pericarditis, lymph nodes (e.g., scrofula), bones and large joints (e.g., Pott's disease is cavitary lesion and destruction of vertebral body), kidneys, liver, adrenal glands, chorioretinitis and uveitis, and meningitis.

Secondary Tuberculosis   Tuberculosis usually manifests clinically as reactivation pulmonary disease many years after the initial infection. Typically, there is no inciting event, although reactivation occurs with a higher prevalence in the elderly, debilitated, undernourished, and immunocompromised. Reactivation tuberculosis tends to occur in the apical regions of the lung because of the higher V/Q ratio and the fact that *M. tuberculosis* flourishes in areas of higher oxygen tension. Reactivation tuberculosis can manifest as a focal lobar consolidation resembling other bacterial pneumonias. Classically, areas of focal inflammation result in caseating granulomas that appear nodular on a chest x-ray. These lesions may become necrotic and form cavitary lesions that can erode into bronchi. Erosion of lesions into blood vessels result in hemoptysis, which is a common feature of tuberculosis.

The diagnosis of pulmonary tuberculosis is made by sputum microscopic examination and culture. Under the microscope, *M. tuberculosis* appears as a slender, curved rod that is resistant to acid alcohol staining (i.e., acid-fast). *M. tuberculosis* is a slow-growing, aerobic microbe that can take 4 to 8 weeks for growth to occur on a classical culture medium. There are more selective media that facilitate growth in 1 to 2 weeks. Common clinical practice is to keep a patient in isolation if active tuberculosis is suspected until three sputum samples are negative on three separate days. The likelihood of identifying organisms by microscopy is related to the degree of disease. One-third of patients who ultimately have positive culture results will have negative microscopic smears even after multiple specimens. Therefore, patients with active tuberculosis will be missed; however, these are patients with a lower burden of bacteria in the respiratory airways and who are less contagious.

PPD Tuberculin PPD is a substance formed from a number of proteins associated with *M. tuberculosis,* and is used to identify persons with active tuberculosis or prior exposure. The PPD is placed subdermally on the forearm and a positive reaction will occur in 48 to 72 hours as a raised, discoid, erythematous patch. In patients with prior exposure to tuberculosis, memory T cells will be activated by the introduction of the PPD proteins, resulting in proliferation and infiltration into the tissues surrounding the injection. This is the result of a cell-mediated hypersensitivity reaction. A positive result depends on the diameter of the lesion; however, there are different thresholds for a positive result based on the patient being tested and their pretest likelihood of disease (Table 10-1). For immunocompromised patients (e.g., AIDS) any reaction is considered positive. For patients with a high likelihood of being infected (e.g.,

family member of someone with TB, healthcare worker), 5 mm or greater is considered positive. For persons who are at higher risk for TB (e.g., homeless, from an endemic region, institutionalized), 10 mm or greater is considered positive. For those with a low risk for TB, 15 mm or greater is considered positive.

Treatment for tuberculosis is difficult because of drug resistance, the required duration of treatment and compliance, and the cost of the drugs. There are a number of drugs available for the treatment of tuberculosis with varying toxicities (Table 10-2). When treatment is initiated, typically three agents are used simultaneously until culture sensitivities are obtained. This is done because of the prevalence of resistance. Resistant strains are typically found in populations from endemic regions of the world (e.g., Haiti, Africa, Southeast Asia) where the only available drug for treatment has been isoniazid. As a result, organisms resistant to isoniazid are very common in these regions. Multidrug resistance is becoming more common in the United States as well, where in New York City up to 25% of *M. tuberculosis* is resistant to both isoniazid and rifampin. Therefore, in addition to these two agents, usually pyrazinamide or ethambutol is added to the initial treatment regimen.

Table 10-1. Interpretation of PPD results

Result	Negative/Positive Interpretation
< 5 mm	Negative, except in HIV patients
5–10 mm	Positive in those likely infected (e.g., household contacts, known exposure, healthcare worker)
10–15 mm	Positive in those at elevated risk (e.g., homeless, endemic area)
> 15 mm	Positive for general population

Table 10-2. Drugs used to treat tuberculosis and common toxicities

Drug	Condition
Isoniazid	Hepatitis, peripheral neuropathy
Rifampin	Hepatitis, flu-like illness
Streptomycin	Hearing loss, renal impairment
Pyrazinamide	Hepatitis, hyperuricemia
Ethambutol	Optic neuritis

Case Conclusion RJ is admitted to the hospital to an isolation room. His chest x-ray shows a right upper lobe infiltrate that is concerning for secondary tuberculosis. He is started on isoniazid, rifampin, and pyrazinamide. A PPD was placed on admission, and by 48 hours a discoid lesion about 20 mm in diameter had formed at the injection site. On the second day RJ was able to produce sputum that showed several slender, curved organisms in clumps that were acid-fast. Several days after treatment he began to feel better and his cough decreased. After 14 days of isolation, antibiotic therapy, and several sputum samples that showed no organisms he was discharged from the hospital with a 6-month course of oral isoniazid and rifampin. The culture results came back subsequently showing *M. tuberculosis* sensitive to both isoniazid and rifampin.

Thumbnail: Tuberculosis

Pathophysiology

Primary Infection

Mycobacterium has a cell wall that is rich in lipids and is acid-fast

Proteins in cell wall are highly antigenic

Inhaled bacilli phagocytized by macrophages and carried to regional lymph nodes

Macrophages initiate inflammatory response by releasing chemotactic factors

Cell-mediated hypersensitivity results with influx of lymphocytes and monocytes

Primary granuloma is formed around initial site of infection that consists of macrophages, histiocytes, and lymphocytes

Latent Phase

Majority of primary infections are asymptomatic

Granuloma self-contained, heals, and forms calcified granuloma that is evident on chest x-ray

Calcified granuloma "dormant," but contains viable *Mycobacteria*

PPD test becomes positive several weeks after primary infection and remains so during the latent phase

Secondary (Reactivation) Tuberculosis

Disease manifests years later as a result of age, comorbid disease, or immunocompromised state

Reactivation occurs typically in apices and upper poles of lower lobes where the V/Q ratio is high

Spread of *Mycobacteria* outside the original granuloma results in formation of caseating granulomas that can necrotize and become cavitary granulomas

Cavitary granulomas erode into bronchioles and generate sputum with *M. tuberculosis*

Cavitary granulomas can also erode into blood vessels causing hemoptysis

Disseminated Tuberculosis

More common in immunocompromised and children

Result of hematogenous spread of *Mycobacteria* and seeding in various organs of the body

Risk Factors

Endemic regions of the world: Southeast Asia, Africa, India, Latin America

Overcrowded living conditions, homeless, inner-city urban dwellers, jailed or institutionalized

Key Points

- Presenting symptoms of reactivation tuberculosis include chronic cough, hemoptysis, intermittent fevers, night sweats, weight loss
- Chest x-ray may show any variety of infiltrate, although classically shows granulomatous or cavitary lesions in the upper lobes
- Patients with pulmonary infiltrates suspicious for tuberculosis must be kept in isolation until three sputum samples are negative for acid-fast organisms
- Positive PPD suggests prior infection with *M. tuberculosis,* but does not necessarily imply active tuberculosis
  - Any reaction in immunocompromised persons is positive

- For individuals at high risk, 5 mm is positive
- For individuals with several risk factors, 10 mm is positive
- For individuals at low risk, 15 mm is positive
- Initial treatment of active tuberculosis consists of a three-drug regimen
  - Duration of treatment at least 6 months due to large number of inactive organisms and poor drug penetration into caseating granulomas and cavitary lesions
- Treatment of asymptomatic patient with positive PPD and normal chest x-ray is typically rifampin for 6 months

Questions

1. Which of the following is *true* regarding primary tuberculosis?
   A. Usually progresses to fulminant disease
   B. Imparts transient immunity to host
   C. Invokes β-cell-mediated humoral immunity
   D. Characterized by granuloma formation
   E. Results in contagious host

2. Which of the following is *false* regarding secondary tuberculosis?
   A. Typically occurs in the lung apices
   B. Characterized by fevers, chills, night sweats, and weight loss
   C. PPD is usually negative during active disease
   D. Caseating granuloma can necrotize into adjacent bronchi
   E. Risk factors include elderly, debilitated, immunocompromise

3. An 18-year-old Hispanic woman lives with her father who was recently diagnosed with active tuberculosis based on symptoms of fevers, cough, weight loss, a chest x-ray showing a cavitary lesion, and a sputum sample with acid-fast bacilli. What size PPD skin reaction would be considered positive and mandate treatment for this woman?
   A. Any reaction
   B. 5 mm
   C. 10 mm
   D. 15 mm
   E. 20 mm

4. What is the *most common* side effect of drug therapy for tuberculosis?
   A. Hepatitis
   B. Peripheral neuropathy
   C. Thrombocytopenia
   D. Hyperuricemia
   E. Renal failure

HPI: LL, a 45-year-old diabetic woman, has had a nagging ulcer on her right big toe that has been slow to heal. One day she began to develop fevers and chills, and she vomited several times. That night LL missed her insulin dose because she did not feel well. The following morning she vomited three more times and called 911.

PE: Upon arrival to the emergency department LL was pale, mildly confused, her pulse was 126, blood pressure 86/42, respiratory rate 32, and oxygen saturation 98% on supplemental oxygen. Her physical exam was remarkable for only dry mucous membranes, and a nonhealing ulcer on her right toe. Two large-bore IVs were started, 2L of normal saline were administered rapidly, and a Foley catheter was placed.

Labs: LL's initial lab values showed a glucose of 520, an anion gap of 24 (Na 132, Cl 96, HCO_3 12), and 3+ urinary ketones and glucose. The initial chest x-ray was normal. She was started on an insulin drip and admitted to the ICU for close monitoring. Her blood pressure improved with fluid resuscitation but LL began to feel short of breath about 12 hours later. A repeat chest x-ray showed diffuse airspace disease bilaterally and her oxygen saturation decreased to 88% on supplemental oxygen. Her difficulty breathing increased to the point where LL needed intubation and mechanical ventilation to maintain oxygen saturations above 90%. Initial blood cultures grew gram-positive cocci in clusters, consistent with *S. aureus*, and broad-spectrum antibiotics were started.

Thought Questions

- What is the definition of *adult respiratory distress syndrome* (ARDS) and what are the most common causes?

- What is the effect of ARDS on lung mechanics and function?

- What is the effect of ARDS on the serum acid-base status?

- What is the advantage of mechanical ventilation in ARDS?

Basic Science Review and Discussion

Pathophysiology of ARDS ARDS is a generic term that refers to alveolar membrane damage resulting in increased membrane permeability to water, solutes, proteins, and cells. Alveoli become filled with cellular debris and proteinaceous fluid that leads to physiologic shunting of pulmonary blood, arterial hypoxemia, and respiratory distress. Chest x-ray shows diffuse bilateral pulmonary infiltrates (Figure 11-1) with an appearance similar to that of severe pulmonary edema. Etiologies abound, but the most common is pulmonary capillary endothelial damage as a result of sepsis. Even though the source of infection may not be pulmonary, endotoxins released in sepsis cause diffuse damage to capillary endothelium, including those in the pulmonary circulation. The result is extravasation of fluid and cells across the alveolar membrane. ARDS can be the result of direct damage to the alveolar membrane, such as that from diffuse pulmonary infections (e.g., bacterial, viral, or fungal pneumonias), aspiration (e.g., gastric contents or water),

inhaled toxins (e.g., chlorine gas or smoke), traumatic pulmonary contusion, narcotics overdose, high-altitude exposure, or diffuse immunologic response to disease (e.g., Goodpasture's syndrome or systemic lupus erythematosus [SLE]). Etiologies of ARDS are summarized in Table 11-1.

Similar to pulmonary edema, as the alveoli become filled with fluid, the function of alveolar surfactant is nullified. As discussed previously, the function of surfactant is to reduce the alveolar surface tension and prevent alveolar collapse. Therefore, in ARDS the alveoli collapse as they fill with fluid. In addition, the increased interstitial and alveolar fluid results in a large decrease in compliance. Decreased

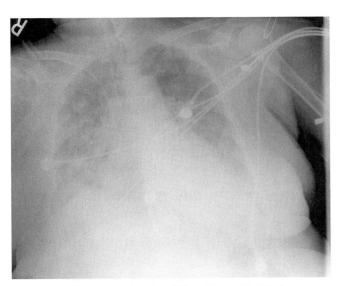

Figure 11-1. Chest x-ray showing diffuse bilateral infiltrates consistent with ARDS.

Table 11-1. Etiologies of ARDS

Systemic process	Sepsis, traumatic shock, hemorrhagic pancreatitis
Pulmonary infections	Bacterial, viral, fungal
Aspiration	Gastric contents, near drowning
Toxic inhalants	Smoke, high-concentration oxygen, chlorine gas
Narcotics overdose	Heroin, methadone, morphine
Immunogenic	Goodpasture's syndrome, systemic lupus erythematosis
Cardiopulmonary bypass	Postperfusion lung

compliance translates directly to an increase in the work of breathing. Arterial hypoxemia results from both the increased physiologic shunt due to underventilated alveoli and the decreased diffusion capacity due to interstitial edema. The physiologic response to hypoxemia is increased minute ventilation. Combined with the increased work of breathing, this results in rapid respiratory failure that requires intubation and mechanical ventilation.

In the early phase of ARDS, increased minute ventilation secondary to hypoxemia will result in overventilation of unaffected alveoli and the off-loading of CO_2. In a manner similar to that of acute pulmonary embolism or pneumonia, this will result in a respiratory alkalosis. However, as the disease progresses and more alveoli fill with fluid, effective ventilation decreases and CO_2 retention occurs. This eventually leads to respiratory acidosis.

Mechanical Ventilation Mechanical ventilation is essential once ARDS reaches the point where increased minute ventilation cannot compensate for the degree of physiologic

shunt, arterial hypoxemia, and CO_2 retention and acidemia. The major advantages to mechanical ventilation are that it eliminates the work of breathing for the patient, provides comfort under adequate sedation, allows delivery of a high FiO_2 if necessary, and enables the delivery of constant positive pressure that allows expansion of collapsed alveoli. Eliminating the work of breathing and improving patient comfort may be the most important of these advantages because it greatly decreases metabolic demand and oxygen consumption. Even though supplemental oxygen can be delivered to a patient by means of a nasal canula, facemask, or bag-valve mask, a nonrebreather facemask with oxygen flow of 15 liters/minute only provides an FiO_2 of about 0.40. In contrast, a cuffed endotracheal tube connected to a mechanical ventilator can provide an FiO_2 of 1.00. Minute ventilation can be adjusted by setting the ventilation rate and volume. Lung compliance can be discerned by measuring airway pressures at different lung volumes.

In addition to the pressure provided to initiate the inspiratory phase of ventilation, the ventilator can be set to provide a small amount of positive pressure during the expiratory phase. This is referred to as positive end-expiratory pressure (PEEP), and it is beneficial for patients with ARDS. During normal expiration, the intrathoracic pressure rises as the chest wall contracts. In ARDS, where alveolar surfactant has been washed out and the alveolar surface tension high, the increased intrathoracic pressure during expiration contributes to alveolar collapse. These alveoli also tend to be in the more dependent zone 3 areas where pulmonary circulation is greatest, and their closure contributes significantly to the physiologic shunt. PEEP counteracts this by providing additional intra-alveolar pressure. This allows oxygen delivery to a greater number of alveoli and decreases physiologic shunting.

Case Conclusion LL was mechanically ventilated with volume control at a rate of 12 per minute, a volume of 600 mL, PEEP of 10 mmHg, and a FiO_2 of 1.00. Before intubation, an arterial blood gas analysis showed a pH 7.22, PO_2 64, and PCO_2 68. After 2 hours of mechanical ventilation, a repeat blood gas showed pH 7.32, PO_2 92, PCO_2 48. The FiO_2 was decreased to 0.60, and further decreased to maintain a PO_2 of greater than 70 mmHg. LL remained ventilated for the next 6 days while her body slowly reabsorbed and cleared the pulmonary infiltrates. LL was extubated and was able to leave the hospital after 2 weeks and start pulmonary rehabilitation.

Thumbnail: ARDS

Pathophysiology

ARDS results from damage to the alveolar-capillary membrane and the exudate of fluid into the alveoli

Fluid contains water, solutes, proteins, cells

Alveolar filling washes away surfactant

Normal function of surfactant is to decrease surface tension of alveolar wall

Increased surface tension in ARDS results in alveolar collapse

Increased physiologic shunt and arterial hypoxemia

Decreased compliance as result of increased interstitial and alveolar fluid

Stiff lungs (decreased compliance) result in increased work of breathing

Response to hypoxemia is increased minute ventilation or hyperventilation

Increased minute ventilation combined with increased work of breathing results in respiratory failure

As more alveoli fill with fluid, and the patient tires and is no longer able to maintain high minute ventilation, respiratory acidosis occurs

Risk Factors

Most common etiology is sepsis, releasing endotoxin and damaging pulmonary capillary endothelium

Other causes that lead to direct damage to alveolar epithelium include diffuse pulmonary infections, aspiration of caustic substances, inhalation of toxins, traumatic pulmonary contusions, immunologic conditions

Key Points

▶ Clinical features include dyspnea, tachypnea, tachycardia, and hypoxia

　▶ Onset may be delayed behind primary process (i.e., sepsis or pancreatitis) but progression of symptoms very rapid once they start

▶ Early mechanical ventilation is a life-saving intervention for ARDS

▶ Eliminates work of breathing for the patient, provides comfort under adequate sedation, allows delivery of a high FiO_2, and enables the delivery of PEEP

▶ PEEP prevents alveolar collapse during expiration and increases the number of ventilated alveoli

Questions

1. Which of the following is *not* a known etiology of ARDS?

   A. Bacterial sepsis
   B. Aspiration pneumonitis
   C. Smoke inhalation injury
   D. Severe asthma attack
   E. Acute necrotizing pancreatitis

2. Considering the Starling equation for fluid flow across a semipermeable membrane, a change in which of the following variables is at the root of the pathophysiology of ARDS?

   A. Capillary hydrostatic pressure (P_p)
   B. Interstitial hydrostatic pressure (P_i)
   C. Filtration coefficient (K_f)
   D. Capillary oncotic pressure (π_p)
   E. Interstitial oncotic pressure (π_i)

3. Which of the following arterial blood gas results is consistent with ARDS?

   A. pH 7.28; Pao_2 64; $Paco_2$ 60; $[HCO_3^-]$ 18
   B. pH 7.34; Pao_2 92; $Paco_2$ 36; $[HCO_3^-]$ 20
   C. pH 7.48; Pao_2 72; $Paco_2$ 32; $[HCO_3^-]$ 22
   D. pH 7.52; Pao_2 86; $Paco_2$ 42; $[HCO_3^-]$ 30
   E. pH 7.30; Pao_2 86; $Paco_2$ 38; $[HCO_3^-]$ 16

4. Which of the following is *not* a beneficial effect of increased PEEP in ARDS?

   A. Increased inspiratory tidal volume
   B. Increased cardiac output
   C. Increased alveolar recruitment
   D. Decreased peak inspiratory pressures
   E. Increased minute ventilation

HPI: HF, a 52-year-old man, is a 30-year smoker and was doing well until about 2 months ago when he began feeling fatigued, general malaise, developed a chronic nonproductive cough, and lost his appetite. HF assumed he had a viral illness and wasn't worried until yesterday when he noticed some blood in his sputum. Today he coughed up about a teaspoon of blood and decided to go see his doctor. He reports that he has lost 25 pounds over the past 6 weeks.

PE: HF's vital signs are unremarkable but he looks pallid and thinner than normal. His chest exam reveals decreased breath sounds over the superior left lung field.

Thought Questions

- What are the four types of primary lung cancer?

- What is the incidence of metastatic lung cancer compared to primary lung cancer, and which primary cancers metastasize most often to the lung?

- Which paraneoplastic syndromes are often associated with lung cancer?

- Which lung cancers are amenable to surgical resection?

- What are the two most common types of benign pulmonary tumors?

Basic Science Review and Discussion

Types of Lung Cancer   There are four major types of primary lung cancer (Table 12-1) based on their cell type. Squamous cell carcinoma is the most common. It tends to be located centrally, and histologically is characterized by keratin formation and intracellular bridges. Adenocarcinoma consists of malignant glandular cells that produce mucin. Adenocarcinoma is located peripherally and, unlike the other types of cancer, appears to have no link to smoking. Large-cell carcinoma is also peripheral and consists of poorly differentiated cells; it is likely an undifferentiated form of adenocarcinoma. Small-cell carcinoma is a central tumor that behaves differently from other bronchogenic cancers. It consists of many cells about twice the size of lymphocytes that multiply rapidly making it highly invasive. Metastasis has usually occurred by the time of diagnosis. Alternatively, metastatic

spread to the lung from a primary site outside the lung is actually more common than bronchogenic carcinoma itself. Common sites of the primary tumor include breast, ovary, kidney, thyroid, pancreas, testicles, and bone.

Clinical Findings   Patients with lung cancer usually present with a history of weight loss, fatigue, cough, hemoptysis, chest pain, and dyspnea. Patients with adenocarcinoma present with increased sputum production. Pancoast's syndrome refers to an apical tumor that compresses the sympathetic cervical chain and leads to Horner's syndrome (ptosis, myosis, and anhydrosis). Superior lobe tumors can also lead to superior vena cava (SVC) syndrome as a result of compression of the SVC. These patients have swelling of the face and upper extremities because of venous engorgement. Many bronchogenic cancers are diagnosed because of a pneumonia that is refractory to antibiotic therapy. Tumors commonly cause bronchial obstruction and a postobstructive pneumonia. Patients with refractory pneumonia should undergo CT scan or bronchoscopy to search for an obstructive lesion.

There are several paraneoplastic syndromes associated with bronchogenic tumors. Squamous cell carcinoma typically results in hypercalcemia as a result of bone involvement. As tumor invades bone, osteoclastic activity releases parathyroid hormone (PTH)-like factors that results in the liberation of calcium. Small-cell carcinoma is most often associated with paraneoplastic syndromes including syndrome of inappropriate antidiuretic hormone (SIADH), resulting in water retention and low serum sodium. Small-cell carcinomas can also cause Cushing's syndrome by means of ectopic adrenocorticotropic hormone (ACTH) production and various neuromuscular disorders by unknown means.

Table 12-1. Four major types of lung cancer

	Histologic Findings	Other Characteristics
Squamous cell carcinoma	Keratin producing, intercellular bridges	Central, cavitates
Adenocarcinoma	Gland/mucin formation	Peripheral
Large-cell carcinoma	Poorly differentiated	Peripheral, cavitates
Small-cell carcinoma	Packed lymphocyte-like cells	Central, rapid metastasis

Diagnosis and Work-up The approach to diagnosis of a lung mass depends on the location. The easiest way of making a diagnosis is by sputum cytology. However, the sensitivity is relatively low, especially for peripheral lesions. If the lesion is central, the next approach to diagnosis is bronchoscopy. The sensitivity of bronchoscopy for making the diagnosis for central lesions is about 90%. Peripheral lesions can often be approached with percutaneous CT-guided needle biopsy, which has a diagnostic accuracy of about 80%. However, patients with significant risk factors for lung cancer may go directly to open thoracotomy and resection given a single peripheral lesion.

Once a diagnosis of cancer is made, the next step is to determine whether metastasis has occurred. This is best achieved by a CT scan of the chest. Lymph nodes greater than 1.5 cm suggest metastatic spread and, in that case, mediastinoscopy is indicated for lymph node biopsy to confirm the diagnosis. If mediastinal metastasis has occurred then the patient is likely no longer a candidate for surgery. There is no need to look for extrathoracic metastases unless there are specific symptoms (e.g., neurologic deficits, bone pain) or lab abnormalities (e.g., hypercalcemia, liver function abnormalities) that may suggest so. Pulmonary function tests are also part of the preoperative work-up because patients with lung cancer often have concomitant lung disease such as chronic obstructive pulmonary disease (COPD). A postoperative pre-dicted FEV_1 is calculated based on the current FEV_1 and the planned amount of lung resection. If the reserve function is adequate and there is no evidence of metastasis, then the patient is a surgical candidate. Surgical techniques continue to improve, and in recent years there has been success with resection of affected ipsilateral hilar and mediastinal lymph nodes.

Benign Pulmonary Tumors Common benign pulmonary tumors include bronchial adenomas and pulmonary hamartomas. Bronchial adenomas are intrabronchial tumors that can cause chronic cough, hemoptysis, and obstructive symptoms. Diagnosis is made by bronchoscopy, and treatment is surgical resection because these tumors have the potential for malignant transformation. About 80% of bronchial adenomas are carcinoids that can be locally invasive and often secrete hormones such as ACTH or antidiuretic hormone (ADH). Carcinoids may also metastasize to the liver and cause carcinoid syndrome consisting of cutaneous flushing, bronchoconstriction, and diarrhea. Pulmonary hamartomas are benign, peripheral tumors consisting of smooth muscle and collagen. Their classic appearance on chest x-ray includes small, rounded size with distinct, well-demarcated borders. These typically have central, speckled calcifications known as the "popcorn" pattern. If a nodule on chest x-ray is consistent with these findings, then a repeat x-ray is indicated every 6 months for 2 years to confirm its stability.

Case Conclusion HF's chest x-ray showed a large mass in the left superior lobe consistent with bronchogenic carcinoma. A chest CT showed diffuse mediastinal adenopathy. Labs showed a calcium of 10.0, which is consistent with early bone metastasis. On the basis of these findings HF is not a candidate for surgery. Over the next several months he received radiotherapy to the left superior lobe and systemic chemotherapy. His condition continued to worsen until he developed pneumonia and sepsis requiring endotracheal intubation. After discussion with the family and the patient's previous wishes, HF was withdrawn from the ventilator and expired soon after.

Thumbnail: Bronchogenic Carcinoma

Pathophysiology

Squamous Cell Carcinoma

Centrally located, consists of keratin and intracellular islands

Often cavitary, locally invasive, bone metastasis (hypercalcemia)

Adenocarcinoma

Peripherally located, glandular cells that produce mucin

No apparent link to smoking

Large-Cell Carcinoma

Peripherally located, likely undifferentiated form of adenocarcinoma

Small-Cell Carcinoma

Centrally located, islands of numerous lymphocytic-appearing cells

Highly invasive, usually metastatic at time of diagnosis

Often associated with paraneoplastic syndromes due to secretion of hormones such as ADH, ACTH

Risk Factors

Smoking increases risk 13-fold, long-term passive exposure increases risk 1.5-fold

Dose-response relationship such that 40 pack-year smoker has 60-fold risk increase

Asbestos exposure has synergistic effect with smoking increasing risk 200-fold

Other industrial exposures and air pollution

Key Points

- Benign-appearing peripheral nodules on chest x-ray can be followed with repeat chest x-rays at 6-month intervals for 2 years
- In high-risk patients or with suspicious-appearing masses, tissue biopsy required
  - Bronchoscopy for central lesions
  - CT-guided needle biopsy for peripheral lesions
  - Open thoracotomy and wedge resection if suspicion very high
- Anatomic staging determines extent of disease and metastasis

- CT scan of chest defines tumor size, location, and presence of mediastinal lymph node involvement
  - Suspicious-appearing lymph nodes require mediastinoscopy for biopsy
- CT scan of abdomen often done to assess for liver or adrenal metastases
- Physiologic staging involves pulmonary function tests (PFTs)
- In general, cancer that is contained within a single lung with minimal hilar and mediastinal lymph node extension is amenable to surgery

Questions

1. Which of the following will *most likely* present with massive hemoptysis?
   - A. Squamous cell carcinoma
   - B. Adenocarcinoma
   - C. Large-cell carcinoma
   - D. Small-cell carcinoma
   - E. Metastatic lung cancer

2. Which of the following manifests as a peripheral lesion and can present as diffuse, multifocal pneumonia-like infiltrates?
   - A. Squamous cell carcinoma
   - B. Adenocarcinoma
   - C. Large-cell carcinoma
   - D. Small-cell carcinoma
   - E. Metastatic lung cancer

3. A 72-year-old smoker develops a left lower lobe pneumonia that is treated with a 5-day course of azithromycin. His symptoms and lobar infiltrate do not improve and he is admitted to the hospital for intravenous antibiotics. Upon further inquiry, he has also had blood-streaked sputum and lost 25 pounds over the past 2 months. Which of the following is a reasonable next test that will most likely yield a specific diagnosis?
   - A. CT scan of thorax
   - B. MRI of thorax
   - C. Bronchoscopy
   - D. Mediastinoscopy
   - E. Open biopsy

4. Which finding is *not* known to be associated with bronchogenic carcinoma?
   - A. Eyelid drooping
   - B. Hoarseness
   - C. Facial swelling
   - D. Leg swelling
   - E. Hematuria

HPI: SO, a 19-year-old man, was first diagnosed with cystic fibrosis (CF) at age 2 when he developed multiple respiratory infections and suffered from malnourishment. Since then, he has had multiple hospital admissions for *Pseudomonas* pneumonias and has been started on insulin and pancreatic enzymes for pancreatic insufficiency. SO has been well over the past months until today when he started to develop low-grade fevers; increased cough; and thick, green, foul-smelling sputum.

PE: His vital signs include a temperature of 100.6°F, pulse 102, blood pressure 114/82, and oxygen saturation of 94% on room air. SO is thin, but nontoxic appearing. His sinuses are nontender and his oropharynx is clear. He has coarse breath sounds in both lung bases. He also has clubbing of his fingernails.

Thought Questions

- What is the genetic anomaly in CF and how is this abnormal gene expressed?

- How would you describe the pathophysiology of CF in the lungs?

- What is *bronchiectasis* and how does it occur in CF?

- Is CF classified as an obstructive or restrictive disease?

- How is a presumptive diagnosis of CF made?

Basic Science Review and Discussion

Pathophysiology of CF CF is an autosomal recessive disease that has been linked to the deletion of position 508 on the long arm of chromosome 7, which is thought to be associated with chloride channels. Patients with CF have abnormally functioning chloride channels on the apical membranes of certain exocrine epithelial cells that make them impermeable to chloride. As a result, sodium and water is reabsorbed from the lumen and the secretions are abnormally thick and viscid.

Although CF has multi-organ effects, its pulmonary manifestations are the primary reason for hospitalization and the ultimate cause of mortality for the majority of patients. CF highlights the importance of an intact mucociliary system in the respiratory airways. Thick secretions in the bronchi and bronchioles impair ciliary function and prevent the upward migration of mucus. As a result, the patient suffers from recurrent bacterial and viral respiratory infections, chronic inflammation, bronchial plugging, and subsequent bronchial wall destruction.

Bronchiectasis *Bronchiectasis* refers to a persistent dilatation of the bronchi due to destruction of the elastic and muscular layers of the bronchial wall. These changes occur as a result of the chronic inflammation and deposition of lysozymal enzymes. Bronchiectasis is classically seen in patients with CF, although other conditions may also lead to bronchiectasis. It can be a result of prolonged, untreated, necrotizing pneumonia; chronic fungal infections such as aspergillosis or histoplasmosis; or chronic obstruction due to bronchial tumors. Bronchiectasis results in chronic obstruction as a result of thick immobile secretions, dilated bronchi, and mucus plugging. Therefore bronchiectasis—as well as CF—is classified as an obstructive pulmonary disorder. Patients with these conditions have characteristic obstructive lung volumes including elevated total lung capacity (TLC) and functional residual capacity (FRC), and decreased vital capacity (VC) and forced expiratory volume (FEV_1)

Diagnosis of CF CF should be considered in an infant who suffers from meconium ileus, steatorrhea or malabsorption syndrome, or diabetes mellitus. After infancy, CF manifests as recurrent sinus and respiratory infections, typically with *S. aureus* in childhood and then the mucoid strain of *P. aeruginosa* in adolescence and adulthood. These patients become chronic carriers of these pathogens and total eradication becomes impossible. The presumptive diagnosis of CF can be made with the sweat test. Because of the abnormal chloride channels in exocrine glands of the skin, patients with CF excrete much higher concentrations of sodium and chloride in their sweat. Levels greater than 60 meq/L are considered diagnostic for CF.

Case Conclusion SO was started on continuous saline nebulizers with an occasional albuterol and atrovent nebulizer treatment in attempts to loosen his secretions. He was empirically given tobramycin and ceftazidime intravenously to cover *P. aeruginosa*. SO was able to produce thick, green sputum that was sent to microbiology for culture. He was admitted to the hospital where he received aggressive pulmonary toilette including saline nebulizers and chest physical therapy. The sputum culture eventually produced *P. aeruginosa* sensitive to tobramycin.

Thumbnail: CF

Pathophysiology

Deletion of position 508 on the long arm of chromosome 7

Results in abnormal chloride channels throughout the body

Pulmonary manifestations arise due to abnormal sodium chloride content of bronchial secretions making them thick and tenacious

Abnormal ciliary function prevents upward migration of mucus

Patients suffer from chronic pulmonary infections and bacterial colonization

Recurrent infections cause chronic inflammation, lysozymal enzymes, and bronchial wall destruction

Bronchiectasis results from destruction of elastin and muscular layers of bronchi

Increased TLC and FRC, and decreased FEV_1 and VC, consistent with COPD

Extrapulmonary manifestations include meconium ileus, pancreatic dysfunction (steatorrhea, malabsorption, vitamin deficiencies, diabetes mellitus), biliary cirrhosis and chronic fatty liver, infertility in men, and chronic sinusitis

Risk Factors

Autosomal recessive disease; 5% of the white population are carriers

Approximately 1:2500 white people have the disease; carriers are entirely asymptomatic

Family history is a risk factor but lack thereof does not exclude disease

Rare in other races; 1:17,000 black Americans, 1:90,000 Asians

Key Points

▸ Recurrent pulmonary infections with *S. aureus* in childhood and mucoid strain of *P. aeruginosa* in adolescence and adulthood

  ▸ Antibiotic treatment should first include double-coverage for *Pseudomonas* that usually includes an aminoglycoside and a third-generation cephalosporin

  ▸ Antibiotics should be adjusted based on culture sensitivities

▸ Other treatment modalities for acute pulmonary exacerbations

▸ Saline and albuterol/atrovent nebulizers to loosen secretions and maximally dilate plugged bronchi

▸ Chest physical therapy to loosen secretions

▸ Human recombinant DNAase nebulized has been shown to loosen secretions

▸ Pulmonary complications of CF include atelectasis, pneumothoraces, hemoptysis, and cor pulmonale, respiratory failure

▸ The only effective treatment for respiratory failure is lung transplantation

Questions

1. Which of the following is *false* regarding the respiratory epithelia of patients with CF?
   A. Abnormal CF transmembrane regulator (CFTR) protein
   B. Chloride channel dysfunction
   C. Decreased chloride secretion into mucus
   D. Decreased sodium reabsorption into cells
   E. Abnormally thick respiratory mucus

2. Which of the following is *false* regarding the gastrointestinal effects of CF?
   A. Hypersecretion and depletion of pancreatic enzymes
   B. Obstruction of intestinal crypts
   C. Decreased biliary secretions
   D. Steatorrhea due to malabsorption
   E. Meconium ileus and bowel obstruction

3. Which of the following is *true* regarding the respiratory pathology of CF?
   A. Usually manifests after age 5
   B. Airway colonization typically with *Streptococcus*
   C. Chronic airway inflammation results in a restrictive pattern of disease
   D. Pneumothorax is a common complication
   E. Chronic bronchiectasis is atypical

4. Which of the following antibiotics is *not* effective against *Pseudomonas*?
   A. Piperacillin
   B. Aztreonam
   C. Levofloxacin
   D. Cefepime
   E. Tobramycin
   F. Azithromycin

Case 1

1. D
2. D
3. D
4. D

Case 2

1. A
2. C
3. B
4. A

Case 3

1. A
2. D
3. D
4. C

Case 4

1. A
2. B
3. C
4. B

Case 5

1. B
2. C
3. D
4. C

Case 6

1. E
2. B
3. E
4. D

Case 7

1. E
2. C
3. C
4. C

Case 8

1. B
2. A
3. C
4. E

Case 9

1. D
2. C
3. A
4. B

Case 10

1. D
2. C
3. B
4. A

Case 11

1. D
2. C
3. A
4. B

Case 12

1. A
2. B
3. C
4. E

Case 13

1. D
2. A
3. D
4. F

Part II

Gastrointestinal

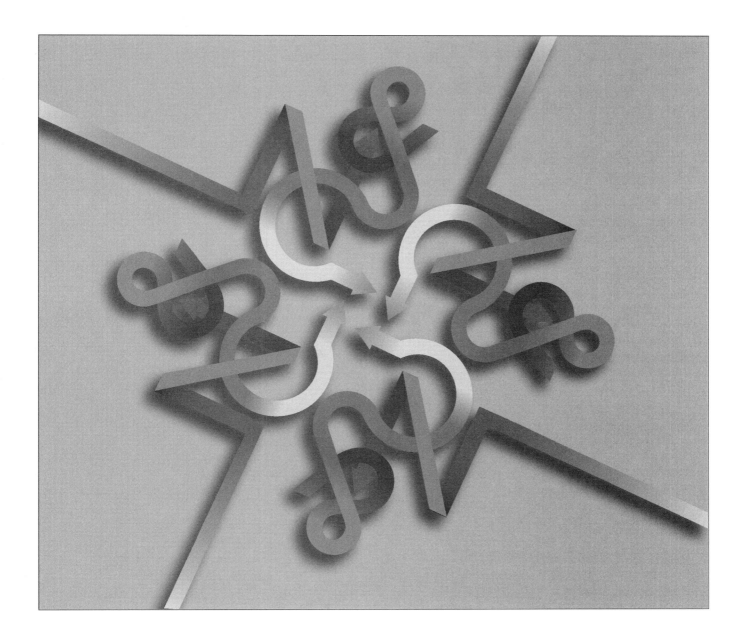

HPI: JS a 45-year-old man, complains about his inability to eat. He reports that, over the past 12 months, he has had difficulty swallowing. JS has lost approximately 40 pounds over the past 8 months. He reports that it "feels like food is getting stuck in my throat." During the first few months of this problem, JS was able to drink increasing amounts of liquids to "push it [the food bolus] through" into his stomach. He was able to eat soups to get nutritious benefit but now he is unable to swallow soup. Over the past few weeks JS has noted that when he leans forward he regurgitates small bits of partially digested and foul-smelling food. Coworkers have always joked about his "bad breath" (halitosis). JS denies any pain associated with swallowing (eating or drinking); he does not vomit. He notes no blood in his regurgitated foods. JS's past medical history is notable for scleroderma, pneumonia treated with antibiotics, and hypertension treated with atenolol.

PE: JS is 5'8" tall and weighs 189 pounds. His blood pressure measures 138/90. The rest of his vital signs are normal. The physical exam is notable for JS's skin—there is sclerosis and atrophy of the skin over his fingers, arms, and shoulder. The lung examination reveals crackles bilaterally at both bases. His abdominal exam is normal; his extremity exam is significant for the skin changes listed above; otherwise there is no cyanosis, clubbing, or edema. Peripheral pulses are intact; fingers move easily.

Labs: Albumin 2.0 (3.5–5.5 g/dL) In order to work up his symptoms further, you order an upper gastrointestinal (GI) endoscopy. The study reveals no cancerous lesions, large amount of food in dilated esophagus, and no peristalsis. The specialists follow this abnormal result with manometry, which shows increased basal pressure and inability of the lower esophageal sphincter (LES) to relax. Finally, JS undergoes a barium swallow (BS) with telling results: dilated esophagus with "bird's beak" and distal stenosis.

Thought Questions

- What is the *most likely* diagnosis for this patient?

- What is the relevant anatomy and microanatomy?

- How does normal swallowing proceed; what are the functions of the LES?

- What are the proposed etiologic agents and how is JS's past medical history linked to his new complaint?

- Which other diseases may present with the complaint of dysphagia? Is all painless dysphagia achalasia?

Basic Science Review and Discussion

The most likely diagnosis for JS is **achalasia.** The combination of progressive painless dysphagia associated with a history of scleroderma and abnormal lab data and imaging studies ensure the diagnosis. The muscular tube of the esophagus is bordered by two rings of muscle: the **upper** and **lower esophageal sphincters** (UES, LES). These act as opening and closing doors that allow food to travel through while protecting the lining of the esophagus. The UES and LES work in conjunction with the peristaltic smooth muscle of the body of the esophagus. If these are synchronous, food reaches the stomach; if not, major problems result.

Anatomy of the Esophagus   The physiology of swallowing is complicated and framed by examining the form and function of the esophagus. Like other components of the GI tract, the esophageal wall is composed of the mucosa, submucosa, muscularis propria and adventitia. The **mucosa** (or inner lining of the esophagus) is composed of stratified squamous epithelial cells. Beneath it lies the **lamina propria** (mostly connective tissue) and **muscularis mucosa** (thin layer of longitudinal muscle). The next layer is the **submucosa,** which consists of a layer of blood vessels, inflammatory cells, lymphoid follicles, and nerve fibers including **Meissner's plexus.** Following the submucosa is the **muscularis propria,** which includes the inner circular layer and outer longitudinal layer of smooth muscle. The **myenteric (Auerbach's) plexus**—believed to be dysfunctional in achalasia—is located in this layer. Of note, the upper third or approximately 6–8 cm of the esophagus includes a layer of striated muscle.

Physiology of Swallowing   The bolus of food or drink in the oropharynx sets off a chain reaction beginning with relaxation of the UES followed by waves of coordinated peristalsis that propels the bolus to the lower esophagus; with its relaxation, the bolus enters the stomach. Extrinsic and intrinsic innervation, smooth muscle properties (response to distension), and humoral properties are all involved in the coordination of this event. The LES must open at the correct moment to allow the bolus of food to enter the stomach and close to prevent reflux of the acidic gastric contents that are under positive pressure relative to the esophagus.

Pathophysiology of Achalasia Because the LES does not relax in achalasia, JS suffers from dysphagia. Many patients find that drinking large quantities of liquids immediately after food can overcome the abnormalities of achalasia. Abnormalities verified by manometry include: the lack of peristalsis, incomplete relaxation of the LES with swallowing, and increased resting tone of the LES. Some hormones and other chemical agents (gastrin, acetylcholine, histamine, prostaglandin $F_{2\alpha}$) can increase the resting tone of the LES. Leading to progressive dilation, the wall of the esophagus may thicken secondary to hypertrophy of the muscularis or later become thinner after marked dilatation and stretching of the fibers. The ganglia of the myenteric plexus are absent in the body of the esophagus; in the LES these may be absent or present and dysfunctional. The pathophysiology of these abnormalities is poorly understood; however, it appears that the ganglion cells that normally secrete vasointestinal peptide are destroyed or are absent from the myenteric plexus. One theory purports that a virus infects the dorsal vagus motor nucleus, another theory links LES dysfunction to increased sensitivity to gastrin. Less commonly, achalasia can result from an identifiable cause such as advanced scleroderma. Secondary achalasia can arise from infection with *Trypanosoma cruzi* resulting in Chagas' disease. Chagas' disease causes widespread destruction of myenteric plexus in many portions of the GI tract resulting in progressive dilation. Other causes of secondary achalasia may result from sarcoid, amyloidosis, paraneoplastic syndromes or even diabetic autonomic neuropathy.

Achalasia Patients with this rare (1:100,000) disorder may suffer from a collagen vascular disease such as **scleroderma** or **calcinosis,** *Raynaud's* **phenomenon, esophageal disease, sclerodactyly, telangiectasia (CREST) syndrome,** malnutrition, or aspiration secondary to nearby gastric contents and subsequent aspiration pneumonia. These patients also experience an increased incidence of abscess, bronchiectasis, pulmonary fibrosis, candidal esophagitis, lower esophageal diverticula, and esophageal ulceration. The most worrisome are those patients who develop esophageal squamous cell carcinoma (5%).

Case Conclusion JS questions the association between the scleroderma and achalasia. He wants to know more about the disease, as well as treatment options. You explain that in patients with scleroderma, the muscularis layer progressively atrophies and is slowly replaced by collagen. As the disease progresses the fibrosed esophageal wall leads to atony and dilatation, associated with the "bird's beak" finding on imaging. Late scleroderma achalasia may be complicated by gastroesophageal reflux disease (GERD) as the LES becomes atrophic.

Treatment options for primary achalasia include both medical and surgical. Medical options are calcium channel blockers, nitrates or botulinium toxin injection via endoscopy to relax the LES. The surgical options include balloon dilation, fundoplication, or cardiomyotomy, which is an incision in the LES muscle. JS chose conservative medical management.

Thumbnail: Achalasia

Epidemiology

Men > women, middle-aged, incidence 1:100,000

Pathogenesis

Decreased numbers of ganglion cells in body of esophagus with decreased/normal nonfunctioning ganglion in LES

Impaired inhibitory innervations of myenteric (Auerbach's) plexus

No peristalsis, poor relaxation of LES, increased resting tone of LES; progressive dilatation of esophagus "bird's beak" sign on BS, malnutrition

Uncertain etiology

Secondary causes

Chagas disease, collagen vascular disease (especially scleroderma and CREST syndrome), diabetes with autonomic neuropathy, paraneoplastic, sarcoidosis, amyloidosis, invasion of nerve ganglion by virus (polio)

Imaging

Upper GI/barium swallow—"bird's beak" (stenosis) with dilatation

Sequelae

Aspiration pneumonia, esophageal diverticula, esophageal ulceration candidal esophagitis, pulmonary fibrosis, bronchiectasis, abscess, 5% risk of squamous cell carcinoma

Key Points

- Presents with progressive painless dysphagia, regurgitation of foods, halitosis
- Often diagnosed in middle-aged males
- Differential diagnosis: Primary achalasia with no other comorbidity, etiology often unknown

- Secondary achalasia is often associated with scleroderma and CREST syndrome, dermatomyositis, Chagas disease, diabetes mellitus, paraneoplastic syndromes, amyloidosis, and sarcoid

Questions

1. Which of the following is *less likely* to occur with achalasia based on the abnormality of the LES?
   A. Scleroderma
   B. GERD
   C. *H. pylori* dyspepsia
   D. Hiatal hernia
   E. Mallory-Weiss tears

2. Hirschsprung's disease and achalasia both have which of the following in common?
   A. Increased risk of gastrointestinal cancers (e.g., squamous cell cancer of the esophagus)
   B. Congenital loss of bowel function
   C. Absence of ganglion cells
   D. Increased incidence of collagen vascular disease
   E. Inability to pass stool normally

3. Which of the following is *not* a sequela of achalasia?
   A. Collagen vascular disease
   B. Pulmonary fibrosis
   C. Esophageal diverticula
   D. Aspiration pneumonia
   E. Squamous cell esophageal cancer

4. Which of the following is *not* a component of CREST syndrome?
   A. Esophageal dysmotility
   B. Raynaud's disease
   C. Congenital megacolon
   D. Calcinosis
   E. Telangiectasia

HPI: DH, a 48-year-old, self-described, "high powered" executive has complained of terrible heartburn for many years. This pain interferes with his ability to "work 12 hours a day and 6 days a week." The heartburn worsens at night when DH lies down to go to sleep and occasionally results in the regurgitation of sour, blood-stained pieces of food. He notes that he has a cough at night. DH smokes about 10 cigarettes a day, drinks about six cups of coffee each day, and drinks four to six glasses of scotch on weekends. His past medical history is significant for hypertension for which he takes a nifedipine.

PE: DH is 5'11" tall and weighs 183 lbs. His blood pressure measures 145/92. His other vital signs are unremarkable. Overall, DH's physical examination is unremarkable. Because of DH's complaints, you decide to order an upper gastrointestinal (GI) endoscopy. The photographs and biopsy results reports show gross hyperemia (increased blood flow often seen in inflammatory conditions) with several ulcerations; the biopsy reveals severe acute inflammation with superficial necrosis, areas of ulceration with formation of granulation tissues, and no fibrosis is apparent. Hematoxylin and eosin staining reveals areas with increased numbers of eosinophils and neutrophils in the epithelial layer, elongation of lamina propria papillae, and basal zone hyperplasia.

Thought Questions

- What is the *most likely* diagnosis for this patient?

- Which factors are associated with the above diagnosis?

- What are the common etiologies for this disorder?

- What do all these etiologies lead to histologically?

- How can DH modify his risk factors/behaviors to lessen his symptoms?

- What is the major sequelae of this illness?

Basic Science Review and Discussion

The diagnosis for DH is inflammatory esophagitis, likely secondary to reflux esophagitis known as **gastroesophageal reflux disease (GERD).** There are many associated origins for inflammatory esophagitis but GERD is by far the most common. **Esophagitis** has a prevalence in the United States between 10% and 20%; the prevalence is far higher in Iran and China likely secondary to lifestyle factors (e.g., ingestion of scalding-hot tea). Esophagitis is caused by many etiologies but they all lead to a common histologic characterization of severe acute inflammation with superficial necrosis and ulceration with late formation of granulation tissue debris and finally fibrosis.

Pathophysiology of GERD Many of the etiologies of esophagitis have similar pathophysiologic alterations that lead to an environment in the distal portion of the esophagus, which irritates the mucosal squamous cells. Several etiologies can result in an inflamed esophagus including decreased efficacy of the antireflux mechanism, increased time to clear refluxed material, presence of anatomic abnormalities such as a sliding hiatal hernia, increased gastric volume, and decreased ability of esophageal mucosa to undergo repair.

Etiologies of Esophagitis Causes of esophagitis can be further categorized related to their primary method of damage. Viruses, fungal agents and bacteria are common causes of esophagitis in patients who are in an immunocompromised state following a period of viremia, fungemia or bacteremia. Viruses like **herpes simplex virus (HSV)** and **Cytomegalovirus (CMV),** as well as the fungal species **Candida, Mucor,** and **Aspergillus,** often infect immunocompromised individuals (e.g., AIDS, chronic steroids). The infectious agent can often be identified based on gross or microscopic appearances. HSV and CMV will cause small ulcerations with evidence of microscopic nuclear inclusions, whereas *Candida* species will present with a gray-white pseudomembrane observed visually on endoscopy. Bacterial insults will reveal invasion into the lamina propria on biopsy.

Similarly, the history may lead to the diagnosis in patients suffering from cancer or who have ingested corrosive substances. Patients who are treated with cytotoxic chemotherapeutics and radiation for cancer may develop esophagitis with characteristic fibrosis of the submucosa and atrophy of the mucosal layers. In those patients who have ingested corrosive agents by mistake or in an attempt to commit suicide, characteristic morphologic changes to the epithelial lining of the esophagus occur. This is also apparent in individuals who smoke chronically and ingest large amounts of alcohol or even scalding-hot tea. More specifically, ingestion of acidic or alkaline agents results in coagulative or liquefactive necrosis respectively, of the mucosa. Alcohol, smoking, and scalding-hot tea cause the most common changes to the mucosa as well as decreasing

LES tone, which will be illustrated in the specifics of DH's case.

Less commonly, inflammatory esophagitis can be linked to other illnesses or comorbid conditions. Patients with hypothyroidism, as well as those with systemic sclerosis, pemphigoid, epidermolysis bullosa, and pregnant women may have decreased lower esophageal sphincter tone leading to esophagitis.

Diagnosis, Risk Factors, and Treatment   DH has **GERD** in which there is transient relaxation of the **LES** resulting in the regurgitation of stomach contents (acid and bile) leading to inflammation. Grossly (seen by endoscopy), the first sign is hyperemia and later ulceration with microscopic infiltration of the epithelial layer of the mucosa with eosinophils and later neutrophils, basal zone hyperplasia, and elongation of the lamina propria papillae. Later, the debris accumulates secondary to the superficial necrosis and ulceration with culmination in granulation tissue formation and eventual fibrosis. DH indulges in several behaviors that can worsen his symptoms including smoking, caffeine, and alcohol intake. Education is of paramount importance in resolution of this patient's symptoms. DH takes a calcium channel blocker for hypertension which, in addition to being a third-line medication for hypertension, can cause relaxation of the LES and exacerbate DH's heartburn. Changing his medication to a beta-blocker or diuretic may improve his symptoms. Although DH is not taking any β_2-adrenergic or anticholinergic agents, in other patients discontinuation of these agents also limit symptoms. Other, more conservative measures such as raising the head of the bed for sleeping, limiting fatty food intake (secondary to decreased cholecystokinin levels and gastric transit time), and not eating within an hour of going to bed may alleviate DH's symptoms.

Case Conclusion   DH returns in 3 months and has acted on all of your recommendations; he quit smoking cigarettes, limited his alcohol and caffeine intake, raised the head of his bed, and stopped eating prior to going to bed. His symptoms have almost completely resolved and his blood pressure is well controlled on a beta-blocker. DH wonders what his ultimate fate would have been had he not heeded your recommendations; therefore, you inform him regarding **Barrett's esophagus,** which can occur in approximately 10% of patients with chronic GERD. With the presence of gastric contents in the distal esophagus, the squamous mucosal cells are injured and are replaced by metaplastic columnar epithelium. This change does not affect all patients with GERD but appears to target those with more severe forms. It is theorized that inflammation leads to ulceration, followed by healing that is accomplished by re-epithelialization and growth of stem cells which, in a low pH environment, regrow as columnar cells. Because these columnar cells are more resistant to the acidic injury and are common in the stomach, Barrett's leads to an increase in the incidence of adenocarcinoma of the esophagus by 30 to 40 times compared to the general population.

Thumbnail: Varieties of Inflammatory Esophagitis

Agent	Gross/Microscopic Findings	Risk Factors	Treatments
Candida, Mucor, Aspergillus	Gray-white pseudomembrane	Immunosuppression Treatment with broad-spectrum antibiotics Debilitation	Antifungal
HSV, CMV	Punched out ulcers with microscopic nuclear inclusion	Immunosuppression AIDS	Antiviral
Bacterial	Invasion into lamina propria		Antibacterial
Radiation	Submucosa—fibrosis Mucosa—atrophy	Treatment for cancer	
Chemical Ingestion (corrosive-acid, alkali)	Liquefactive necrosis (alkaline) Coagulative necrosis (acids)	Accidental ingestions Suicide attempts	Gastric lavage
Chronic Alcohol, Smoking (GERD)	Hyperemia, ulcer typical Microscopic invasion of epithelium with eosinophils and neutrophils, basal zone hyperplasia and elongation of lamina propria papillae		Smoking cessation, treatment of alcoholism

Key Points

- Presents with heartburn, sour taste in mouth, nocturnal cough
- Often diagnosed in those over age 40; persons on calcium channel blockers, β_2-agonists, or anticholinergics; individuals with anatomic risks (hiatal hernia); chronic caffeine, alcohol, or scalding-hot tea drinkers, smokers, and pregnant women
- Common pathology includes severe acute inflammation, superficial necrosis, ulceration with granulation tissue, debris, fibrosis

- Treatment includes education, removal of inciting agents, treatment of comorbid illness (e.g., *Candida* in AIDS patient), H_2 blocker, proton pump inhibitor
- Chronic conditions include squamous metaplasia with resulting columnar cells and increased risk of Barrett's adenocarcinoma

Questions

1. Which of the following would a 16-year-old woman display after ingestion of a large amount of lye?
   A. Liquefactive necrosis
   B. Coagulative necrosis
   C. Gangrenous necrosis
   D. Fat necrosis
   E. Radiation necrosis

2. Which of the following pathologic cell types occur in patients with long-standing and severe GERD?
   A. Transitional
   B. Squamous
   C. Metaplastic squamous
   D. Metaplastic columnar
   E. Microvilli

3. A 38-year-old man with temporal wasting, a history of pneumonia, Kaposi's sarcoma, and new heartburn and cough presents. When considering long-term patient care, which of the following is the single *most important* test?
   A. CBC with differential
   B. TSH
   C. Chest x-ray
   D. Sputum culture
   E. Enzyme-linked immunosorbent assay (ELISA) test for HIV

HPI: BL, a 57-year-old male, presents complaining that his stomach has been hurting for years. On further questioning, you sort out that he has a 5-year history of chronic nausea and vomiting, dyspepsia, and occasional epigastric pain. BL denies constipation, diarrhea, fever or chills, hematemesis or melena, or cough. He recently watched a television show that focused on ulcers. BL is sure he has one and wants some treatment. A review of his medical history reveals he has hypertension treated with hydrochlorothiazide, smokes about 10 cigarettes a day, and drinks three to six cans of beer each day.

PE: BL is 5'11" tall and weighs 167 pounds. His blood pressure measures 134/78. The rest of his vital signs are normal. On abdominal examination, he has normoactive bowel sounds and epigastric tenderness to deep palpation without guarding or rebound. The rest of his exam is unremarkable.

Labs: WBC 5.5 (4.5–11 $\times$ 10^3 per μL); diff-neutrophil 59% (57% to 67%); Seg 56% (54% to 62%); bands 1% (3% to 5%); hemoglobin 14.9 (12–16 g/dL); hematocrit 45 (35% to 45%); platelet 234 (159–450 $\times$ 10^3 per μL); bilirubin (tot), 0.2 (0.2–1.0 mg/dL); bilirubin (dir) 0.0 (0–0.2 mg/dL); AST/SGOT 34 (7–40 U/L); ALT/SGPT 27 (7–40 U/L); GGT 8 (8–40 U/L); Alk phos 123 (70–230 U/L); amylase 64 (25–125 U/L); lipase 78 (10–140 U/L).

An upper gastrointestinal (GI) endoscopy reveals a stomach, which is erythematous with thinning of mucosa and flattening of rugae. No obvious erosions or areas of hemorrhage are evident. A biopsy of a characteristic area is obtained, which shows silver-stained Gram-negative S-shaped rods, many lymphocytes and plasma cells. There is also evidence of urease on the biopsy specimen. For completeness, a urease breath test was performed that is positive.

Thought Questions

- What is the *most likely* diagnosis for this patient?

- What is the relevant anatomy, microanatomy, and physiology of this disease?

- How would you describe the presentation of the acute and chronic form of this illness?

- What are the modifiable risk factors?

- Does this illness predispose the patient to other sequelae?

Basic Science Review and Discussion

BL most likely has **chronic gastritis.** His symptoms (chronic dyspepsia, nausea and vomiting) as well as the physical exam (normal except for epigastric tenderness) lead us to perform the appropriate diagnostic tests to reveal chronic gastritis secondary to infection with *Helicobacter pylori.* As expected, his laboratory values are normal and the diagnosis results from delineation of his history—including risk factors—and is confirmed by biopsy. Gastritis is classified as acute or chronic. Within those groups there are various etiologies and associations that can lead to appropriate diagnosis, treatment, and resolution of the illness.

First, we must review the anatomy, microanatomy, physiology, including the prominent cell types in the stomach. Normally, on gross inspection, the stomach has coarse rugae that are most prominent in the proximal stomach; these flatten when the stomach is distended and full of food. On closer inspection, there is a fine "mosaic pattern" that is characterized by the gastric glands or "pits." As expected, the mucosal surface is lined by tall columnar cells with fine microvilli and a film of glycocalyx on the luminal side.

Stomach Physiology There are four regions in the stomach based on anatomic location and predominant cell types (Figure 16-1). Distal to the **gastroesophageal junction** lies the **cardiac** portion of the stomach that is dominated by many glands containing mucous cells. **Mucous cells** are responsible for secreting mucus to protect the stomach surface from the acidic environment. Bordering the cardiac portion is the **fundus** with high concentrations of **parietal** and **chief cells.** Parietal cells have large numbers of mitochondria, resulting in bright eosinophilia on hemotoxylin and eosin (H&E) stains. Parietal cells make **intrinsic factor** and hydrochloric acid; intrinsic factor binds to **vitamin B$_{12}$** to allow ileal absorption. A deficiency in B$_{12}$ leads to macrocytic and megaloblastic **anemia** as well as neurologic signs and symptoms. HCl is produced via the hydrogen-potassium-ATPase that exchanges H$^+$ ions for K$^+$ ions. The acid is produced to aid in food digestion by lowering the pH so that **pepsin,** a protein cleaving enzyme, is activated.

Chief cells, which also reside in the fundus, lie at the base of the glands and produce **pepsinogen** that is cleaved to pepsin in acidic environments (pH 1–3) to allow for digestion of proteins. Chief cells are large basophilic cells with apically-oriented zymogen granules. The distal portion of the fundus is bordered by the **body** (or **corpus**). The most distal portion of the stomach—the **antral**—is rich in **mucous**

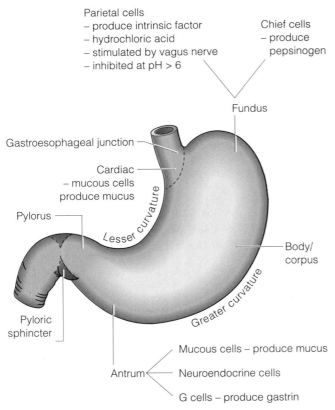

Parietal cells
– produce intrinsic factor
– hydrochloric acid
– stimulated by vagus nerve
– inhibited at pH > 6

Chief cells
– produce
  pepsinogen

Fundus

Gastroesophageal junction

Cardiac
– mucous cells
produce mucus

Lesser curvature

Pylorus

Body/
corpus

Greater curvature

Pyloric
sphincter

Mucous cells – produce mucus

Antrum — Neuroendocrine cells

G cells – produce gastrin

Figure 16-1. Physiology of the stomach. Major anatomic divisions of the stomach with important cell types and their products.

and **G cells,** as well as neuroendocrine cells. The mucous cells produce mucus to increase the pH of the food bolus about to enter the duodenum; the G cells produce **gastrin**—a 17 or 34 amino acid peptide—that stimulates gastric motility and secretions of acid, intrinsic factor, and pepsinogen I and II. Of note, the entire gastric mucosal surface is replaced approximately every 2 to 6 days.

Also important in our understanding of basic stomach physiology is elucidation of the response to various stimuli by the parietal and chief cells. Parietal cells increase HCl production in response to neural stimulation via the vagus nerve, endocrine stimulation with gastrin or local concentrations of histamine on mast cells. Similarly, chief cells are stimulated by the vagus and low local pH (inactivated at a pH > 6).

Pathophysiology of Gastritis **Acute gastritis** is defined as the transient inflammation of the gastric mucosa, typically with neutrophils. This inflammation may be accompanied by hemorrhage into the mucosa as well as sloughing of the mucosa that can be a life-threatening source of an **upper GI bleed.** These patients may present with **hematemesis** (vomiting bright-red blood) or **melena** (black, tarry stools). Acute gastritis is most often caused by heavy use of nonsteroidal anti-inflammatory drugs (NSAIDs) especially aspirin (e.g.,

patients with rheumatoid arthritis). These patients may complain of nausea, vomiting, dyspepsia, and epigastric pain. In NSAID use the agents decrease synthesis of prostaglandins; there is an inability to maintain the bicarbonate rich (buffer) mucus barrier. Other risk factors include heavy alcohol use, smoking, uremia, those persons on chemotherapy or after radiation, infection with *Salmonella* (low pH allows for dissemination of the bacteria), ischemia, infection (Cytomegalovirus [CMV] in AIDS), high stress (trauma, burns, postoperative), ingestion of corrosive substances (acid/alkaline), mechanical trauma. Although there are many inciting agents for acute gastritis, several must be classified as "idiopathic" because no known etiologic event is elucidated.

Many of the above risk factors lead to a common pathophysiology that may include one or more of the following: increased acid secretion, decreased bicarbonate buffer, decreased blood flow, disruption of mucosal layer, direct damage to the epithelium. On microscopic evaluation of the mild acute gastritis there is neutrophilic invasion of the lamina propia above the basement membrane. In more severe forms of the illness, there can be specific areas of erosion or loss of the superficial epithelium, without crossing the muscularis mucosa. The inflammatory reaction becomes more intense with purulent exudate into the lumen. There may be concurrent hemorrhage leading to acute erosive hemorrhagic gastritis. The condition is self-limiting; resolution obviously relies on removal of the inciting agent(s) or pathologic condition(s).

Similar to acute gastritis, patients with **chronic gastritis** may present with nausea, vomiting, and upper abdominal discomfort. Specifically, chronic gastritis is characterized by gland and mucosal atrophy and epithelial metaplasia secondary to chronic inflammation, typically with lymphocytes and plasma cells. The mucosa in chronic gastritis is usually devoid of erosions; however, it may progress to dysplasia and carcinoma. The risk of **gastric carcinoma** in long-standing gastritis may be as high as 4%, illustrating the importance of detecting and treating this common malady.

There are many etiologies for chronic gastritis; however, two warrant special consideration for they account for many of the cases: infectious, with *Helicobacter pylori,* and immunologic with accompanying **pernicious anemia.** Other causes of chronic gastritis include alcohol abuse and smoking, mechanical or motor disorders (bezoar, obstruction, gastric atony), cancer (treatment with radiation), Crohn's disease (granuloma formation), and postoperative with reflux of bile (after antrectomy and gastroenterostomy). The bulk of our discussion, however, revolves around infectious and immunologic etiologies.

Heliocobacter Pylori The incidence of *Helicobacter pylori* is estimated at approximately 50% in Americans over age 50.

Helicobacter pylori is a Gram-negative rod that commonly colonizes the antrum or both the antrum and the body-fundus areas of the stomach. It is theorized that *H. pylori* colonizes injured mucosa leading to increased healing time and inflammation, which produces symptoms. As in BL, detecting *H. pylori* by biopsy or the urease breath test accommodates diagnosis, treatment, and resolution of symptoms. Typical treatments include: (1) proton pump inhibitor, amoxicillin, and clarithromycin; or (2) bismuth, tetracycline, metronidazole, and proton pump inhibitor for varying times. These treatments are approximately 80% to 99% effective in patients with an ulcer (see peptic ulcer disease case).

Patients with *H. pylori* have an increased risk of **peptic ulcer disease (PUD)** and consequently gastric carcinoma. In addition to *H. pylori* gastritis, another common etiology for chronic gastritis is an immunologic variety associated with autoantibodies to the gastric gland parietal cells and **intrinsic factor** resulting in gastritis with pernicious anemia. These antibodies attack mainly in the fundus and corpus, but their effects may be observed globally. The antibodies destroy the glands leading to decreased HCl production and mucosal atrophy. Additionally, intrinsic factor is lost, paralyzing the GI tract form absorbing vitamin B_{12} in the distal ileum. This type of gastritis is associated with other immunologic diseases such as Hashimoto's thyroiditis and Addison's disease. This form of gastritis seems to be associated with an increase in adenocarcinoma of the stomach.

Pathology   The morphology of chronic gastritis, like acute gastritis, is similar on gross examination and microscopically in many of the etiologies. On gross inspection, the stomach may appear erythematous and coarse with accompanying flattening of the mucosa or boggy mucosa with thick rugae. Late in the disease, the mucosa thins and becomes flat as the rugae disappear. On microscopy, plasma cells and lymphocytes predominate in the lamina propria. The proportion of the mucosa involved indicates the severity of the inflammation. The histology goes through four other distinct phases depending on the natural course of the disease:

1. Regenerative changes in response to chronic injury the gastric glands increase mitotic activity
2. Metaplasia whereby portions of the mucosa are replaced by columnar and goblet cells
3. Atrophy when parietal cells decrease in number with a compensatory increase in number of gastrin producing cells
4. Dysplasia that may progress to carcinoma

Case Conclusion   BL is treated with antibiotics and an acid reducer (proton pump inhibitor) for 2 weeks and his symptoms begin to resolve. Additionally, he is educated on the environmental agents that may result in recurrence of his symptoms such as alcohol abuse and smoking.

Thumbnail: Two Types of Gastritis—Immunologic (Pernicious Anemia) versus Infectious (*Helicobacter pylori*)

	Immunologic	Infectious
Major Etiologic Agent	Auto-antibodies to parietal cells (H^+ K^+-ATPase) and intrinsic factor.	Infection with *Helicobacter pylori*
Also Known As	Autoimmune gastritis Diffuse corporal atrophic gastritis	*H. pylori* gastritis
Locale	Diffuse, body	Antrum and body
Leads to	Gland destruction $\Rightarrow$ decreased acid production	Slowed healing/chronic inflammation
Frequency	Less common	> 50% asymptomatic adults > age 50
Associated	Hashimoto's thyroiditis, Addison's, pernicious anemia	
Increased Risk of	Adenocarcinoma, carcinoid	PUD, chronic atrophic gastritis, gastric CA

Key Points

▶ Presents with acute or chronic complaints of nausea, vomiting, dyspepsia, epigastric tenderness ± hematemesis, melena.

▶ Risk factors are NSAID (especially aspirin) use, alcohol abuse/dependence, immunologic disorders (Hashimoto's, Addison's), stress (burns, ICU admission), ingestion of caustic substances (acid/alkali), chemotherapeutics and radiation in oncologic patients, uremia, AIDS, central nervous system (CNS) injury, and mechanical disorders (bezoar, etc.).

▶ Increased risk for gastric adenocarcinoma in those with chronic atrophic gastritis, pernicious anemia, antrectomy, gastroenterostomy (with gastric remnants); PUD; pernicious anemia (immune etiology); megaloblastic/macrocytic anemia, neurologic changes

Questions

1. A patient presents with what you suspect is acute gastritis without acute bleeding and negative rectal heme test. Which of the following is the *most likely* supporting pathology result from a biopsy specimen?
   A. Loss of superficial epithelium, with hemorrhage, purulent exudate
   B. Thinned and flattened rugae and mucosa
   C. Thinned and flattened mucosa in the presence of many S-shaped gram-negative rods
   D. Many neutrophils above the basement membrane, none below the muscularis mucosa
   E. Dysplasia

2. The Schilling test is helpful in determining the etiology of a megaloblastic and macrocytic anemia. If you are ordering this test for a patient with chronic gastritis, which other immunologic illnesses would also be *important* to screen?
   A. HIV and Addison's
   B. Hyperthyroidism and hypothyroidism
   C. HIV and hyperthyroidism
   D. Sarcoid
   E. Hyperthyroidism, hypothyroidism, and Addison's

3. Which gastric hormone is *increased* in chronic gastritis?
   A. Cholecystokinin
   B. Gastrin
   C. Pepsin
   D. Pepsinogen I and II
   E. Somatostatin

4. What is the associated risk of gastric carcinoma in a patient with chronic gastritis?
   A. 2% to 4%
   B. None
   C. 5% to 8%
   D. 10% to 20%
   E. 8% to 10%

HPI: GS, a 40-year-old male, complains of an intermittent gnawing, aching, and burning pain in his abdomen. He characterizes his pain eloquently while pointing to his epigastrium. Although GS is uncertain, he reports that the pain worsens at night and occasionally after meals—usually 2 or 3 hours afterward. His wife takes Tums (calcium carbonate) on a regular basis (to prevent osteoporosis). GS has symptomatic relief using two to three of these tablets. He denies deep or "penetrating" pain to his back or left side, and does not report weight loss, nausea, or vomiting. GS also denies hematemesis or melena. His past medical history is significant for chronic headaches, stress type for which he takes ibuprofen, approximately 3 to 4 days a week.

PE: GS is 5'6" tall. His blood pressure measures 112/59 and his pulse is 76. In general, he is in no acute distress, his cardiovascular and pulmonary exams are unremarkable. Abdominally, GS has normal bowel sounds, mild epigastric pain, no guarding or rebound; his rectal exam is significant for normal tone, but positive for microscopic blood (heme +).

Labs: WBC 8.5 (4.5–11 $\times$ 10^3 per μL); hemoglobin 12 (12–16 g/dL); hematocrit 35 (35% to 45%); platelet 215 (159–450 $\times$ 10^3 per μL); MCV 77 (80–100).

To complete his workup, GS undergoes an upper gastrointestinal (GI) series that reveals a gastric ulcer with gastric folds radiating to the base of the ulcer, as well as, a thick radiolucent edematous collar around a smooth appearing crater. Following the upper GI series, an endoscopy is ordered, which is also abnormal. On gross inspection, the endoscopic exam reveals an oval sharply punched out defect in the antrum near the lesser curvature, with no active bleeding or clotted blood. The pathology report describes penetration into mucosa, muscularis mucosa and partially into the muscularis propria. Additionally, there are no features of malignancy. Biopsy of characteristic areas are stained with silver and reveal many gram-negative S-shaped rods along the gastric epithelial cells. An urease breath test is positive.

Thought Questions

- What is the *most likely* diagnosis for this patient?

- What are the risk factors for GS's illness?

- Which bacterial agent is commonly associated with this illness?

- How can this agent be identified and eradicated?

- How would you describe the pathogenesis of this illness?

- What are the major sequelae of this illness?

- What is *acute gastric ulceration*?

Basic Science Review and Discussion

GS has **peptic ulcer disease (PUD)**—a gap in the mucosa of the stomach or duodenum that extends through the muscularis at varying depths. PUD is a chronic disease, characterized by periods of relapse and occurs only in the presence of acid and **pepsin**. Almost exclusively, ulcers are solitary and present in the duodenum or the stomach and are exceedingly rare in other parts of the GI tract. Patients who suffer from PUD have characteristic symptoms: The ulcer pain is often characterized as gnawing, burning or aching with worsening symptoms at night and vary in relation to meals dependent upon the location of the ulcer

(duodenum vs. gastric). If a patient describes a penetrating pain or referral to the back, chest, or right upper quadrant, as well as nausea and vomiting, this suggests a perforation of the stomach or duodenal wall. Weight loss—always a "red flag" for its association with cancer—should alert the clinician to a possible malignancy.

Epidemiology and Risk Factors PUD is a common illness seen more often in men than in women (duodenal 3:1 and gastric 3:2 in favor of men) often diagnosed in middle age. PUD is not associated with genetics or race and can be frustrating to a patient because it often has no obvious precipitating factor, heals spontaneously, and later recurs. However, PUD is associated with *Helicobacter pylori*, alcoholic cirrhosis, chronic obstructive pulmonary disease (COPD), chronic renal failure (CRF), and hyperparathyroidism. Additional risk factors include cigarette smoking, chronic nonsteroidal anti-inflammatory drug (NSAID) use, chronic corticosteroid use, and psychologic stress.

Duodenal and gastric ulcerations can often be differentiated based on the history of the illness. More common in incidence, duodenal ulcers often have decreased pain coincident with a meal; the pain recurs 1 to 3 hours following the meal. The theory is that the increased pH of the food bolus soothes the ulcer as it exits the stomach at the pylorus. These patients often complain that they are awakened at night from the gnawing pain. Duodenal ulcers are frequently associated with increased acid, increased parietal cell mass, and impaired mucosal barrier. Gastric ulcers, on the other hand, are less common and associated with burning upon eating and relieved with antacids. These are more common in the setting of a defective mucosal barrier secondary to *H. pylori,* bile reflux, alcoholic cirrhosis, and COPD. Gastric ulceration is associated with an increased risk of gastric cancer; duodenal ulcer is not.

Anatomy and Histology   Most patients with PUD have a single ulcer, but up to 20% have two or more ulcers; most ulcers are in the first part and anterior location of the duodenum. Stomach ulcers are often in the antrum region along the lesser curvature but can occur anywhere in the stomach. Other less-common locations include within Barrett's mucosa, at the margin of a gastroenterostomy site, near Meckel's diverticulum with ectopic gastric mucosa or in patients who suffer from Zollinger-Ellison syndromes. On visual inspection—often during endoscopic examination—the ulcers are small (6 mm in diameter) but can be up to 4–6 cm in diameter and appear to be "punched out" of the epithelial lining. The depth of the ulcer varies from shallow—through only the mucosa, to penetration—through the gastric or duodenal wall.

On microscopic examination, the margins are often level with the mucosa or slightly elevated, but a clear drop off from the nearby epithelial lining is apparent. The nearby gastric mucosa is almost always hyperemic likely secondary to concurrent gastritis. Histologically, there are three common considerations: active necrosis, inflammation, and healing. The active ulcer has several characteristics that are seen on biopsy specimens: fibrinoid debris at the margins and base of the ulcer, neutrophilic infiltration, granulation tissue with a proliferation of monocytes, and a fibrinous or collagenous layer resting on scar. In addition to the characteristics of the ulcer itself, there are typically signs of chronic gastritis, as well as *Helicobacter pylori* infection. After reading Case 16, one may wonder how to distinguish between gastritis and peptic ulcer disease. It should be noted that chronic gastritis is usually absent in cases of **acute erosive gastritis** or in acute ulceration secondary to stress but is consistently present in patients with peptic ulcer disease.

Pathophysiology of PUD   Despite much interest in PUD, little is known about the pathogenesis; in the simple terms, the mucosal defense is outmatched by the damaging forces. However, the presence of gastric acid and pepsin are neces-sary for ulcer formation. The specifics are not entirely clear but the association with acid is obvious by examining the situation in patients suffering from **Zollinger-Ellison syndrome.** This is most commonly caused by a pancreatic tumor that secretes **gastrin**, leading to markedly increased acid levels and peptic ulcerations. Several broader theories exist regarding the specific cause of ulcers: increased basal acid secretion or increased parietal cell mass. Other theories point to increased sensitivity or limited inhibition of regulatory mechanisms controlling acid secretion or rapid stomach emptying leading to increased exposure to acid.

In addition, the bacterium *Helicobacter pylori* is known to produce urease that produces ammonia, as well as a protease that breaks down proteins important to the function of the mucus barrier. *H. pylori* and its association with PUD are well described accompanying nearly 100% of duodenal and many gastric ulcers. Another theory purports an impaired mucosal defense (i.e., those patients with normal acid and pepsin and void of *H. pylori*). Unfortunately, no clear defects in the mucosal barrier, bicarbonate, or in blood flow can be elucidated clearly.

Some of the risk factors associated with PUD have clearer links to a weakened mucosal defense or possibly a stronger offense. NSAID use inhibits prostaglandin synthesis—an important factor of the mucus barrier. Smoking slows healing of existing ulcers, is thought to suppress prostaglandin synthesis, and favors more frequent recurrence. In GS, elimination of the smoking could have a beneficial affect on his illness. Corticosteroids and increased psychologic stress have been clearly shown to increase ulcer formation.

Acute Gastric Ulceration   Acute gastric ulceration occurs following severe stress and often encompasses multiple ulcers in all portions of the stomach. Typically, this is thought of as an extension of severe acute gastritis. Acute gastric ulceration is common in the intensive care unit and often occurs in patients with the following risk factors: shock, sepsis, burns (result in Curling's ulcers), trauma, conditions with increased intracranial pressure (Cushing's ulcers). Several common processes can occur in one or several of these conditions: impaired oxygenation of the tissue, vagal stimulation resulting in increased acid productions, or systemic acidosis. Commonly, patients who are acutely ill requiring intensive care are prescribed a proton pump inhibitor or H_2 blocker as prophylaxis, However, the only treatment is to correct the underlying condition.

Case Conclusion GS is diagnosed with PUD and begins treatment with bismuth, tetracycline, metronidazole, and proton pump inhibitor for varying times. The treatment is effective and GS asks about the potential sequelae of peptic ulcer disease with a gastric ulcer. Complications can be serious but, fortunately, are uncommon. The most common complication is bleeding and can occur in up to one-third of all patients with PUD. With this patient, it is likely the source of his microcytic anemia. Another serious complication is perforation, which can occur in approximately 5% of patients with PUD; this complication is the cause of death in two-thirds of patients with PUD. Additionally, obstruction from scarring can occur, typically in duodenal ulcers with vomiting and crampy abdominal pain.

Thumbnail: Gastrointestinal Pathophysiology—Duodenal versus Gastric Ulcer

	Duodenal	Gastric
Location	Duodenum, first portion Often the anterior wall	Between the body and antrum, along the lesser curvature
Assoc. with *H. pylori*	Yes, 90% to 100% of cases	Yes, 70%
Associations	COPD, alcoholic cirrhosis, chronic renal failure, hyperparathyroidism	Bile reflux, smoking, COPD, alcoholic cirrhosis
Frequency	Up to 80% of PUD	Up to 20% of PUD
Pathogenesis	Excess acid production, increased parietal cell mass, decreased bicarbonate in the mucus barrier (*H. pylori*)	Defective mucosal barrier secondary to *H. pylori,* reduced prostaglandin secondary to ischemia
Male:Female Ratio	3:1	1.5–2:1
Complications	Recurrence, hematemesis, melena, perforation into pancreas	Recurrence, hematemesis melena, perforation (air under diaphragm)
Associated with Cancer	No	Yes, −1% to 4%
Symptoms that may Differentiate	Pain 1 to 3 hours after eating Pain relieved by food, antacids	Pain aggravated with meals Pain relieved by antacids

Key Points

▶ Presents with chronic intermittent epigastric pain

▶ Often diagnosed in young adults or middle-aged men with alcoholic cirrhosis, COPD, chronic renal failure, hyperparathyroidism, NSAID use, smokers, those infected with *H. pylori,* corticosteroids, psychologic stress

▶ Etiology determined by history and physical exam, endoscopy, biopsy results, urease breath test

▶ Differentiate from acute gastric ulceration by nearby gastric tissue (unremarkable margins); comorbid conditions such as shock, sepsis, burns, trauma; increased intracranial pressure, location (throughout the stomach), number (often > 2)

Questions

1. A common treatment for PUD is the H_2 blocker cimetidine, which has several side effects including tremor, confusion, inhibition of the cytochrome P_{450} system, and which of the following?
   A. Stevens-Johnson syndrome
   B. Agranulocytosis
   C. Gynecomastia
   D. Microcytic anemia
   E. Depression

2. Aspirin and other NSAIDs *most likely* promote ulcer formation by which of the following pathogenic mechanisms?
   A. Ischemia
   B. Suppression of mucosal prostaglandin
   C. Increased acid production via stimulation of parietal cell mass
   D. Increasing parietal cell mass
   E. Increasing gastric emptying

3. Gastric ulcers *increase the risk* of which of the following cancers?
   A. Liver
   B. Pancreatic
   C. Duodenal
   D. Esophageal
   E. Gastric

4. A patient with a known history of PUD presents with acute abdominal pain. The kidney ureter and bladder (KUB) x-ray reveals free air under the diaphragm. What is the next best step in management?
   A. Barium swallow
   B. Outpatient management with proton pump inhibitor
   C. Outpatient management with H_2 blockade
   D. Emergency surgery
   E. Admission with serial abdominal examinations

> **HPI:** DO, a 3-week-old male neonate, has infrequent bowel movements. His mother, PO, had a normal antenatal course and delivery. DO did not pass stool in the first 24 hours of life and has had few bowel movements since; rectal stimulation is needed to induce bowel movements. His mother is breast-feeding but the DO is feeding less and less and is fussy. PO has noted DO's increasing abdominal girth as well as green-stained vomit over the past week.
>
> **PE:** Birth weight 3291 g, currently 3400 g; temperature 37.1°C; generally colicky, inconsolable; abdomen has decreased bowel sounds, nontender, distension, palpable stool through abdomen, no stool in rectum.
>
> After history and physical, an ordered abdominal radiograph reveals no stool or gas in the rectum and marked distension of the proximal bowel. Following the abnormal x-ray, an anal manometry is taken that shows no relaxation of the internal sphincter with balloon distension of the rectum. At the time of manometry, a rectal biopsy was performed that reveals no ganglion cells. In addition, there are hypertrophied nerve trunks.

Thought Questions

- What is the *most likely* diagnosis for this patient?

- What is the relevant anatomy and neuroanatomy?

- What are the major sequelae?

- What other etiologies are associated with this illness?

Basic Science Review and Discussion

DO is suffering from **congenital aganglionic megacolon** or **Hirschsprung's disease,** which is suspected in any neonate who does not pass stool within 24 hours of life. Hirschsprung's disease afflicts up to 1:5000, has an unclear hereditary component, and is more common in males and in those with Down's syndrome. Of those afflicted, 5% also have other severe neurological abnormalities.

Colonic Anatomy and Histology The colon or large intestine is approximately 1.5 meters long and stretches from the small intestine to the anus as it traverses the peroneal muscles at the level of the rectum. Its primary function is to reclaim water and electrolytes and is clear from the histology; the mucosal layer is flat and lined with columnar absorptive cells without prominent villi. Prolonged contact of luminal contents with the mucosa is achieved anterograde and retrograde peristalsis of the colon. In addition to maximizing contact to increase absorption, neuromuscular function of the colon is important to the removal of solid wastes. Peristalsis is mediated by the intrinsic (**myenteric plexus**) and extrinsic (autonomic-parasympathetic) neuronal control. The intrinsic portion is made up of two neural networks: one located in the base of the submucosa, called **Meissner's** plexus; the other located between the inner circumferential and outer longitudinal muscle layers, known as **Auerbach's** plexus.

Colonic Innervation The neuronal plexus of the colon derives from **neural crest cells** that migrate in the cephalad to caudad direction in the bowel wall. In patients with Hirschsprung's disease, the neural crest cells do not migrate to the distal portion of the colon. Therefore, a variable length of colon exists without any myenteric plexus (Meissner's or Auerbach's) leading to the inability to coordinate peristalsis followed by obstruction and colonic dilation proximal to that segment. Histologically, as in DO, the affected portions in congenital aganglionic megacolon have absent ganglion cells and ganglia in the submucosa and muscle walls. Less severe cases include only the rectum and may have intermittent stools or diarrhea when the pressure mounts. Other cases can be more severe spanning nearly the entire colon; luckily these are a small percentage of the cases. In all cases, the areas proximal to the aganglionic segment hypertrophy and dilate; in the most severe the dilation can be up to a diameter of 15–20 cm, which is termed megacolon.

The sequelae of congenital aganglionic megacolon are severe and include perforation of the colon, peritonitis, sepsis, enterocolitis, and water and electrolyte disturbances such as hypokalemia and hypoalbuminemia. Acquired megacolon may be detected in any age and can be caused by several differing etiologies. Chagas' disease is the only etiology that has neural abnormalities; the others are negative on rectal biopsy. Chagas' disease occurs when parasites—*Trypanosoma cruzi*—invade and destroy the plexuses. This illness is endemic in Latin America where reduviid bugs live in the cracked walls of homes. These bugs pass the parasite via a bite (or other break in the skin) and excrement. Other causes of megacolon include obstruction via neoplasm or stricture, as well as a late complication of ulcerative colitis or Crohn's disease. A functional psychosomatic disorder may also cause megacolon.

Case Conclusion   DO underwent two surgeries to correct the problem beginning at age 12 months. First, a diverting colostomy was created with the bowel containing ganglion cells that allows for decompression of bowel with the neuronal innervation. The second operation involved removing the aganglionic segment by pulling the innervated segment through the rectum and closing the colostomy. DO suffered no complications and is doing well.

Thumbnail: Congenital Hirschsprung's Disease

Epidemiology

Male > female (4:1), 1:5000–8000 live births, increased incidence in siblings of affected (4%), Down syndrome (10%), other neurologic abnormalities present (5%).

Pathogenesis

Failure of migration of neural crest cells, resulting in aganglionic portion of the rectum and colon; followed by functional obstruction and dilation of colon proximally.

Imaging

Abdominal x-ray—no gas/feces in rectum, proximal bowel distension.

Barium enema—"transition zone" between narrowed abnormal distal segment and dilated portion of bowel.

Anal manometry—no relaxation of internal sphincter with balloon distension of rectum.

Definitive Diagnosis

Rectal biopsy with stain for ganglion cells negative and positive for hypertrophied nerve trunks.

Sequelae

Intestinal obstruction, enterocolitis with bloody diarrhea, bowel perforation, sepsis, electrolyte abnormalities.

Key Points

- Presents with inability to pass stool within first day of life, poor feeding, neonatal obstruction and bilious vomiting, failure to thrive in older children (late diagnosis)
- Often diagnosed in males, children with Down syndrome, siblings of those with diagnosis
- Can progress to megacolon

Differential diagnosis of megacolon:

- Congenital megacolon—abnormal as neonate, young child, aganglionic segment

- Acquired megacolon—destruction of myenteric plexus Chagas' by trypanosomes, endemic locale
- Obstruction (neoplasm, etc.)—age, hallmarks of neoplasm, no evidence of plexus involvement
- Toxic—history of ulcerative colitis or Crohn's, no mural evidence
- Functional/psychosomatic—history of discord (school, home), no evidence of plexus involvement

Questions

1. A 41-year-old male presents complaining of fatigue, constipation, and inability to swallow food. A recent emigrant to the United States from Brazil, he has multiple bug bites on his face. You suspect Chagas' disease and consequent dilation of the esophagus and the colon. Which other major organ system must you investigate for sequelae of chronic Chagas' disease?
   A. Skin for gummas
   B. Heart for endocarditis
   C. Lungs for interstitial fibrosis
   D. Heart for myocarditis and cardiomyopathy
   E. Skin for evidence of scabies infestation

2. A concerned mother brings a 6-month-old male neonate who has rectal biopsy proven Hirschsprung's disease who, while awaiting the maturity to undergo corrective surgery, has had increasing difficulty feeding and maintaining proper hydration. He is floppy in his mother's arms and on examination his muscles are weak and his reflexes are decreased. Which of the following is the *most likely* abnormality associated with Hirschsprung's disease?
   A. Hypokalemia
   B. Hypoalbuminemia
   C. Hyperkalemia
   D. Insufficient caloric intake
   E. Dehydration

3. Neural crest cells derive from the ectoderm of a developing embryo. The neural crest is a band of cells that extend longitudinally along the neural tube. Which of the following structures does *not* originate from the neural crest?
   A. Cranial ganglia
   B. Autonomic ganglia
   C. Spinal ganglia
   D. Odontoblasts (form the dentin of the tooth)
   E. Skin

HPI: BG, a 29-year-old male, presents with a 3-day history of watery, voluminous diarrhea, abdominal cramping, and weakness. He does report that his partner, JB, has experienced similar symptoms although they seem milder. BG and JB shared a meal five nights ago that consisted of seafood and vegetables. BG describes the diarrhea as watery without any mucus or blood; he is thirsty and feels dizzy and weak. He has not eaten any meals or had anything to drink in approximately 24 hours, but his symptoms have not improved. BG denies fever, chills, or previous history of diarrhea or abdominal disease.

PE: Weight 155 pounds; BP 108/65 sitting, and after 5 minutes of standing, 92/58; pulse 92 sitting and 116 standing; generally ill appearing; HEENT—mucous membranes are dry, eyes sunken; skin, tenting on dorsum of hands; heart is RRR (seated); abdomen, hyperactive bowel sounds, nontender, nondistended, no hepatosplenomegaly; rectal, normal tone, heme negative; extremities, nontender, no edema.

Labs: WBC 8.2 (4.5–11 $\times$ 10^3 per μL); hemoglobin 17 (12–16 g/dL); hematocrit 48 (35% to 45%); platelet 327 (159–450 $\times$ 10^3 per μL); bilirubin (tot) 0.2 (0.2–1.0 mg/dL); bilirubin (dir) 0.1 (0–0.2 mg/dL); AST/SGOT 32 (7–40 U/L); ALT/SGPT 23 (7–40 U/L); alk phos 81 (70–230 U/L); sodium 135 (135–145 mmol/L); potassium 3.8 (3.5–5.0 mmol/L); chloride 100 (98–108 mmol/L); bicarbonate 24 (24–32 mmol/L); analysis of stool reports no gross or microscopic blood, no white blood cells.

Thought Questions

■ What is the *most likely* diagnosis for this patient?

■ What is the specific etiology?

■ What are the keys to appropriately diagnosing this illness?

■ What are the sequelae?

■ What are the similarities and differences in varying etiologies of enterocolitis and diarrhea?

Basic Science Review and Discussion

BG suffers from acute diarrhea. **Diarrhea** is a very common illness and the differential diagnosis is exhaustive; the etiologies vary greatly and are the focus of several different cases. Often the history and physical lead to a likely agent but in approximately 50% of cases an agent is not identified. Important to defining an etiology is a solid foundation in the types of diarrhea and clues that lead to the pathophysiologic process—whether it is microbiologic, malabsorptive or inflammatory in nature.

A working definition of diarrhea must be established because individuals vary widely in "normal" habits. Of the 9 liters of fluid presented to the intestines 200 g/d of stool is considered normal. When this volume is estimated to be greater than 250 g/d, the diagnosis of diarrhea is made. There are several classifications of **diarrhea: secretory, osmotic, exudative, deranged motility,** and **malabsorption;** malabsorption (sprue) is covered in future cases. **Deranged**

motility (intestinal stasis, decreased transit time) often accompanies diabetic neuropathy or other neurologic abnormalities; however, this is a diagnosis of exclusion. **Secretory** (infectious) diarrhea is characterized by stool volumes of greater than 500 cc/d with net intestinal secretion of electrolytes and water; this stool is isotonic with plasma and does not typically improve with fasting. In contrast, **osmotic** (lactase deficiency) diarrhea results from extra osmotic forces in the lumen that often resolves with a fast; as expected, stool osmolality is greater than plasma concentration. Finally, **exudative** (e.g., *Shigella*) diarrhea is often purulent, bloody, and does not improve with fasting; stool volumes vary but are often small and frequent.

Secretory Enterocolitis   **Infectious enterocolitis** can be viral, bacterial, or parasitic. The diagnostic possibilities may be minimized by considering the patient's age, immune status, nutritional status, environmental conditions (contaminated food or water sources) or predisposing factors (hospitalization, camping, foreign travel). Infectious enterocolitis is most commonly caused by rotavirus, Norwalk virus, and enterotoxigenic *E. coli*. Viral enterocolitis is most often caused by **rotavirus** in young infants that produces vomiting and diarrhea about 2 days after innoculation—typically with 10 particles. Rotavirus destroys only mature enterocytes and not crypt cells. This results in an overall secretion of electrolytes and water. Additionally, foodstuffs are not absorbed (secondary to enterocyte destruction) resulting in an osmotic component as well. **Norwalk** virus is a common nonbacterial food-borne diarrhea in children and adults exposed to contaminated food. This diarrhea begins less than 2 days from exposure and results in several days of painful nausea, vomiting, and diarrhea. **Adenovirus,**

another cause of viral diarrhea and vomiting, has a longer incubation (1 week) and 10 days of symptoms. Pathologically, these illnesses are similar with shortened villi and lymphocytic infiltration of the lamina propria.

It is clear from the history that BG suffers from secretory diarrhea; the diarrhea could be described as the classic "rice water" stools and likely results from the stimulation of cyclic adenosine monophosphate (cAMP) and subsequently adenylate cyclase via the enterotoxin produced by *Vibrio cholerae*. From the physical examination, it is clear that BG is dehydrated and needs aggressive hydration. The stool examination reveals no evidence of an inflammatory, exudative, or osmotic diarrhea.

Physiology   Various organisms cause **bacterial diarrhea** and **enterocolitis** by a few pathogenic mechanisms: ingestion of preformed toxin, infection by a toxin-producing organism, or infection by an invading organism. Ingestion of a **preformed toxin** (gastroenteritis) is commonly known as food poisoning; that is, symptoms develop rapidly after ingestion with painful abdominal cramps and explosive diarrhea. Frequent culprits are *Staphylococcus aureus, Bacillus cereus,* (contaminated rice), *Vibrio* species and *Clostridium perfringens* and *botulinum* (canned food). The ability to stick to enterocytes by fimbriae or pili affords advantage (*E. coli,* shigella) and prevents bacteria from being washed away, allowing these to replicate, produce toxin, or invade. This is termed bacterial **adhesion**. Similarly, bacteria gain advantage and cause disease by adherence and production of polypeptides—called **enterotoxins**—that bind to enterocyte causing a secretory diarrhea with electrolytes and water producing a net intestinal secretion. Necessary for **invasion** into enterocytes, is the ability to fool the enterocyte into endocytosis or transcytosis, allowing bacterial proliferation, cell lysis and cell to cell invasion. *Salmonella* and *Yersinia* both employ this technique to result in inflammatory diarrhea.

Bacterial Diarrhea   Pathologically, bacterial diarrhea is relatively nonspecific and may not indicate the severity of the diarrhea. In fact, cholera, which can cause a profound dehydration and is responsible for many deaths globally each year, has no specific abnormalities. Typically, there is damage to enterocytes and neutrophilic infiltration of the lamina propria and epithelium. However, *Campylobacter, Shigella, Salmonella,* and *Yersinia*—all common sources of bloody diarrhea (**dysentery**)—may have characteristic lesions. *Campylobacter* often has multiple superficial ulcers from the small intestine to the colon with crypt abscesses. Shigella infects the distal colon with characteristic inflammation, purulent exudate, and erosions. In contrast, *Salmonella* infects primarily the ileum and colon with linear ulcers; when producing systemic dissemination, it is referred to as **typhoid fever**. During the first week, the bacteria invades Peyer's patches and then disseminates; blood cultures are frequently positive at this stage. The following week is characterized by diarrhea and hepatosplenomegaly, neutropenia, and bradycardia. Typhoid fever may produce a chronic carrier state—often in the gallbladder. *Yersinia* diarrhea causes mucosal hemorrhage and ulceration.

E. coli produces toxin-induced and invasive diarrhea. The **enteropathogenic** type produces a nontoxin variety of mild diarrhea often in children. The **enterotoxigenic** strains produce a heat labile toxin (LT) which results in a secretory diarrhea via stimulation of cAMP; the heat stable toxin (ST), commonly referred to as "traveler's diarrhea," also results in a secretory diarrhea by stimulating guanylate cyclase. The **enteroinvasive** model produces an invasive enterocolitis. **Enterohemorrhagic** *E. coli* O157:H7 is found in raw ground beef and is associated with hemorrhagic diarrhea and hemolytic uremic syndrome.

Necrotizing enterocolitis (NEC) is severe acute infection in premature or low birth weight infants when they begin oral intake—often in the first 2 or 3 days of life. The pathophysiology revolves around immaturity of the neonatal gut, ischemic injury, the feeding (protein substrate in the lumen), and colonization by pathogenic organisms. The illness may be mild but more commonly is severe with dysentery and may progress to gangrene, perforation, and sepsis.

Pseudomembranous colitis is caused by the toxins of *Clostridium difficile*, a normal gut enteric that proliferates secondary to broad-spectrum antibiotic treatment. Nearly all antibiotics have been implicated but the most commonly cited are ampicillin and clindamycin. When suspicious, check a toxin assay for the diagnosis and, when positive, begin treatment with oral metronidazole or vancomycin.

Case Conclusion   BG received several liters of intravenous fluids and within 12 hours his diarrhea and cramping began to improve. After the fluid, his blood pressure and heart rate did not change appreciably. Checking orthostatic blood pressure and pulse readings lying and standing can indicate a patient's fluid status, which, in this case, is severe dehydration. Patients with cholera are at risk of death from the severe dehydration. BG improved with more intravenous fluids and was discharged without further problems.

Thumbnail: Enterocolitis—Differentiating Viral versus Food Poisoning versus Bacterial

Organism	Spread	Age, Incubation/Duration, Comments
Rotavirus	Person to person, food, water infective inoculum = 10 particles Infects enterocytes, not crypt cells	6 months to 2 years; 2d/5d; watery nonbloody diarrhea, vomiting
Norwalk	Food-borne, exposure to common source	Older children, adults; 2d/12–60h diarrhea, nausea, vomit, abdominal pain
Adenovirus	Person to person, shellfish, water	Children; week/week; diarrhea, vomit
Vibrio cholerae	Person to person, seafood, water, secretagogue enterotoxin	Any; 1 to 3 days watery diarrhea pandemic spread, no fecal WBCs, life threatening, needs IV hydration
Bacillus cereus	Reheated fried rice; preformed toxin	Any; 2 to 8 hours/24h vomit, then diarrhea
S. aureus	Meats, dairy preformed toxin	Any; 2 to 6 hours; sudden onset, vomit, abdominal pain, diarrhea
Clostridium perfringens	Meats, poultry, fish; enterotoxin without invasion	Any; 8 to 12 h/24h; watery diarrhea, abdominal cramping
Salmonella spp.	Poultry, eggs	Any; 1 to 2 days/variable; invasion, diarrhea, fever translocation, lymphoid inflammation, dissemination (5% to 10%); diarrhea and fever
E. coli subtypes: -toxigenic	Food contaminated with feces, water, "Traveler's" cholera-like	Any; 1 to 3 days/variable; watery diarrhea, no invasion
-hemorrhagic	Rare beef; shigella-like toxin	Any; 1 to 3 days/variable; hemorrhagic colitis, hemolytic uremic syndrome, no invasion
-pathogenic	Food, water	Infants; 1 to 3 day/variable; no invasion but enterocyte effacement
-invasive	Person to person, water, dairy	Any; variable/variable; invasion with local spread; fever, abdominal pain, dysentery
Campylobacter spp.	Animal contact, milk, poultry	Invasive and toxin mediated fever, pain, dysentery
Shigella spp.	Fecal–oral, person to person, low inoculum needed	Any; 1 to 3 days/variable; invasion with local spread; fever, pain, dysentery
Clostridium difficile	Broad-spectrum antibiotic therapy	Any; up to 4 weeks following antibiotics; forms pseudomembrane

Key Points

▶ Diarrhea—Defined as passage of more than 250 g of stool in 24 hours; accompanied by pain, urgency, perianal discomfort

▶ Dysentery—low volume, painful, bloody

Types of Diarrhea:

▶ Osmotic—Large volume; water is drawn into lumen by solutes; osmotic gap; no inflammation; improves with fasting (e.g., lactase deficiency malabsorption, antacids (magnesium)

▶ Secretory—Large volume, increased cAMP mechanism; isotonic with plasma; no inflammation; persist with fasting (e.g., infectious [enterotoxin, viral], neoplasm)

▶ Invasive/Exudative—Low volume; invasion of intestinal mucosa; purulent, bloody, inflammation (fecal white blood cells); persist with fast (e.g., infection [*Salmonella, Shigella, Entamoeba, Campylobacter*], IBD)

▶ Malabsorption (focus of future case)—Large volume, chronic, weight loss, bulky; increased osmolarity secondary to unabsorbed nutrients; improves with fasting; excess fecal fat

Questions

1. A 6-month-old child, born at 31 weeks of gestation, is brought to the emergency room with diarrhea and a temperature of 37.1°C. His vital signs are normal as is the rest of the physical examination. The diarrhea has no blood or mucus associated with it. Which of the following is the *most likely* etiologic agent?
   A. Rotavirus
   B. Adenovirus
   C. Salmonella
   D. Norwalk
   E. Necrotizing enterocolitis

2. A 35-year-old patient presents with fever, abdominal pain, and bloody diarrhea. She reports consuming some milk and chicken that was left on a counter top on a hot summer day. You know that *Campylobacter* is one of the most common causes for bloody diarrhea. Which of the following would you expect to find on a tissue biopsy that would confirm your diagnosis of *Campylobacter*?
   A. Purulent exudate and erosions in the distal colon
   B. Widespread mucosal hemorrhage and ulceration
   C. Shortened villi and lymphocytic infiltration of the lamina propria
   D. Linear ulcers in the ileum and colon
   E. Multiple superficial ulcers from the small intestine to colon with crypt abscesses

3. A 34-year-old male presents with copious diarrhea and cramping of 2 days' duration. He reports 10 to 12 episodes over the past 24 hours. He denies bloody diarrhea and reports that the diarrhea looks like water at this point. Which of the following mechanisms is *most likely* at work?
   A. Adhesion of a heat labile toxin
   B. Stimulation of adenylate cyclase
   C. Stimulation of guanylate cyclase
   D. Adherence and endocytosis of bacteria
   E. Destruction of mature enterocytes

HPI: TV, a 43-year-old female, complains of years of diarrhea and belly pain. She has had diarrhea with abdominal pain and bloating for as long as she can remember. TV says that her stomach always sticks out, she has flatus and bulky greasy stools, which, upon query, are described as always floating in the toilet. TV also reports decreased appetite secondary to the abdominal pain, and notes chronic fatigue and itchy red skin.

PE: Height 5'4"; weight 95 pounds; normal VS; Gen, thin; HEENT, temporal wasting; skin, erythema, excoriation of abdomen and legs; abdomen, positive bowel sounds, soft, nontender, distended, no rebound, no guard; extremities, 2+ pitting edema to the knees.

Labs: WBC 6.5 (4.5–11 $\times$ 10^3 per μL); hemoglobin 9 (12–16 g/dL); hematocrit 26 (35% to 45%); platelet 243 (159–450 $\times$ 10^3 per μL); bilirubin (tot) 0.2 (0.2–1.0 mg/dL); bilirubin (dir) 0.1 (0–0.2 mg/dL); AST/SGOT 12 (7–40 U/L); ALT/SGPT 23 (7–40 U/L); Alk Phos 100 (70–230 U/L); amylase 34 (25–125 U/L); lipase 65 (10–140 U/L); albumin 2.0 (3.5–5.5g/dL).

TV undergoes several diagnostic examinations to better elucidate the source of her symptoms. A 72-hour stool sample analysis is performed that reveals elevated fecal fat content without other abnormalities. A D-xylose test reveals decreased uptake of sugar. A tissue sample of the small intestine is obtained that shows marked atrophy and blunting of villi, increased numbers of intraepithelial lymphocytes and other immune cells (plasma cells, macrophages), but normal mucosal thickness.

Thought Questions

- What is the *most likely* diagnosis for this patient?

- What are the necessary physiologic steps to digestion of nutrients?

- What key components of the history and lab results lead to this diagnosis?

- What are the common and rare sequelae of this disorder?

- What is the etiology?

Basic Science Review and Discussion

TV has **malabsorption** (decreased absorption of nutrients), secondary to **celiac sprue.** Malabsorption is a general term that refers to the decreased absorption of proteins, carbohydrates, fats, electrolytes, water, vitamins, and minerals. Simply, it results from a disturbance in one or more of the following components: (1) intraluminal digestion, (2) terminal digestion (i.e., brush border of intestine), or (3) transepithelial transport. In some cases of malabsorption, there is a single, identifiable cause that can be identified at biopsy (e.g., parasitic infection); however, the clinical picture is often similar and in some cases of malabsorption the etiologies may be multiple. In the United States, the most frequent causes of malabsorption are **Crohn's disease, pancreatic insufficiency** (e.g., chronic pancreatitis), **bile salt deficiency** (e.g., cirrhosis, cholestasis), and celiac sprue.

Celiac Sprue   TV suffers from chronic celiac sprue, an autoimmune disorder with a prevalence of 1:3000 whites (nonexistent in native Africans, Japanese, Chinese) that is theorized to begin in childhood with introduction of wheat **gluten.** Antibodies are developed against a component of gluten—**gliadin**—that leads to immunologic destruction of the villi in the small intestine (atrophy) as well as hyperplasia of the intestinal crypts. There is a hereditary component to celiac sprue with clusters in families with **DQw2 histocompatibility** antigen, which is linked to **B8. Dr3** also increases an individual's risk. In addition to a familial component, there may be an important environmental factor as a protein from **adenovirus** 12 cross-reacts with gliadin antibodies. The immune response in the small intestinal mucosa leads to the congregation of B-lymphocytes and other immune cells. In the long term, celiac sprue is associated with an increased incidence of T-cell lymphomas and gastrointestinal and breast carcinomas.

Physiology of Digestion   The physiology of digestion of nutrients is salient to a discussion of the causes of TV's malabsorption and ensuing symptoms. One of the digestive tract's objectives is to cleave foodstuffs into assimilable forms that can cross the gut epithelium to be used for energy metabolism (fat, carbohydrates, proteins) or other metabolic processes (electrolytes, minerals, water). This process begins in the mouth and ends in the colon. In the mouth, the salivary glands produce **amylase** that begins the process of digesting starch. Amylase hydrolyzes α **1,4 bonds** resulting in maltose, maltotriose, and α limit dextrins. This process continues with the aid of pancreatic amylase that encounters food in the duodenal lumen, which results in more maltose, maltotriose, and oligosaccharides. Digestion of starches by **disaccharidases** concludes at the brush border of the small intestine producing glucose, galactose, and fructose, which are all monosaccharides and capable of transepithelial transport. Protein digestion begins in the stomach with **pepsin**, after the chief cell secreted pepsinogen is cleaved by a pH of < 2.

The pancreas also secretes **zymogens** as a part of its exocrine function as trypsinogen. In this case, **trypsin**, which is hydrolyzed from its precursor trypsinogen by **enterokinase** (enteropeptidase) along the brush border of the small intestine, breaks down peptides into smaller polypeptides and amino acids. **Bile salts** and pancreatic enzymes couple to break down fats into absorbable fatty acids. Bile salts, an integral part of bile secreted by hepatocytes, emulsify larger fat globules into smaller, uniformly distributed particles by lowering the surface tension. The fat particles are then cleaved by pancreatic enzymes such as **phospholipase A, lipase,** and **colipase** into absorbable fatty acids. The fatty acids undergo transepithelial transport and are converted to triglycerides which, with the addition of cholesterol, are converted into chylomicrons for lymphatic transport.

Malabsorption   The broad consequences of malabsorption include obvious findings such as pain and diarrhea but also endocrine disorders, skin abnormalities, and nervous system changes that may lead to diagnosis and illustrate the importance of nutrients. **Diarrhea**, distension, and pain stem from the inability of the gut to absorb nutrients with increased intestinal secretions; this creates an **osmotic diarrhea.** The endocrine consequences result from decreased absorption of calcium and vitamin D leading to **osteopenia** and **tetany.** Additionally, individuals may suffer from **amenorrhea, impotence,** and **infertility** secondary to generalized malnutrition and **hyperparathyroidism** from calcium and vitamin D deficiencies. Patients with malabsorption may suffer from **anemia** from low levels of iron, folate, and B$_{12}$; also, increased bleeding with **purpura** and **petechiae** secondary to vitamin K deficiency. B$_{12}$ and vitamin A deficiency result in peripheral **neuropathy.** Vitamin A deficiency coupled with zinc, essential fatty acids, and niacin can lead to **dermatitis.** TV had pitting edema because of her low protein state and hypoalbuminemia.

Case Conclusion   TV started a diet without oats, barley, rye, and so on, and had resolution of symptoms and signs of her illness. Her follow-up biopsy was negative. TV's case illustrates the hallmarks of the illness that can be diagnosed correctly only after the following three criterion are met: The patient has sprue with clinical documentation of malabsorption (fecal fat/pentose tests), tissue diagnosis with characteristic findings, and improvement in symptoms and mucosal histology on gluten withdrawal of the diet.

Thumbnail: Gastrointestinal Pathophysiology—Malabsorption

Epidemiology

Infancy to adulthood, fifth decade; incidence approximately 1:2000–3000

Pathogenesis

Poor intraluminal digestion secondary to defective hydrolysis or solubilization (e.g., pancreatic insufficiency, bacterial overgrowth)

Mucosal cell abnormality (enzyme deficiency, vitamin B$_{12}$ malabsorption due to pernicious anemia, abetalipoproteinemia)

Reduction in intestinal surface area (celiac sprue, Whipple's, Crohn's, lymphoma associated enteritis)

Infection (parasite)

Lymphatic obstruction (lymphoma)

Drug induced (cholestyramine)

Unexplained (endocrine disorders: diabetes mellitus, hypo/hyperthyroid, hypoparathyroid, hypoadrenocorticism)

Sequelae by System and Deficiency in Parentheses

Gastrointestinal: Diarrhea, pain, increased flatus, stool bulk

Mucositis (vitamin A, E)

Blood: Anemia (iron, pyridoxine, folate, B$_{12}$); increased bleeding (K)

Musculoskeletal: Osteopenia (calcium, vitamin D); tetany (Ca^{++}, Mg^{+}, vitamin D)

Endocrine: Infertility, impotence, amenorrhea (malnutrition); hyperparathyroidism (vitamin D, Ca^{++})

Skin: Petechiae, purpura (vitamin K); edema (protein); dermatitis (niacin, vitamin A, zinc, fatty acids)

Nervous System: Neuropathy (B$_{12}$)

Key Points

▶ Malabsorption is increased fecal fat, with malnutrition and vitamin/mineral deficiencies

▶ Presents with diarrhea, weight loss, bloating, increased flatus, pain

▶ Failure to thrive in infants

▶ Contributing genetic factors are 90% to 95% of patients with DQw2 histocompatibility antigen; HLA B8, DR3

▶ Often diagnosed in infants, those exposed to adenovirus 12, adults up to age 50

▶ Increased incidence with T-cell lymphoma of small bowel, GI and breast carcinoma

▶ Determine etiology with tissue biopsy, fecal fat test, absorption of sugars (D-xylose test)

Questions

1. Fat-soluble vitamins can be poorly absorbed in a case of malabsorption. Of the following, which deficiency is *correctly matched* to the fat soluble vitamin?
   A. Vitamin A—arthralgia
   B. Vitamin D—hypercalcemia, anorexia
   C. Vitamin E—dermatitis
   D. Vitamin K—elevated PT, aPTT resulting in abnormal bleeding
   E. Folic acid—macrocytic, megaloblastic anemia

2. A patient tells you she has been suffering from chronic celiac sprue. She reports bulky stools, with distension, flatus, fatigue and bleeding from her gums. She has red spots on her abdomen, arms, and legs. She has not adhered to her diet for some time. What is the most important *immediate* step to take?
   A. A shot of vitamin K
   B. You should have a long discussion with her about the importance of her adherence to her diet and participation in her health care
   C. Small intestinal biopsy
   D. Screen other family members for sprue
   E. Test stool for fecal fat

HPI: TB, a 38-year-old male, presents with chronic diarrhea, fevers, and joint pain. Although he has seen many doctors for his complaints, has neither received effective treatments nor what seems to be a clear diagnosis. TB has a 3-year history of bulky, voluminous stool with increased flatulence and a progressive weight loss (20 pounds over the past 2 years). The chronicity of these symptoms combined with a lack of diagnosis or treatment has left him quite frustrated. When he describes his symptoms, he also reports intermittent fevers and pain in his wrist, knee, and shoulder joints. He has also noted a couple of lumps in his neck. TB is currently taking no medications because he says that they haven't worked.

PE: TB is 5'8" tall and weighs 120 pounds. His temperature is 37.6°C and his vital signs are normal. His skin has a gray-brown pigmentation and he has palpable supraclavicular, submandibular, and cervical adenopathy. On abdominal exam, TB has positive bowel sounds; his abdomen is soft, nontender, slightly distended, without rebound or guarding. He also has diffuse joint tenderness and inguinal adenopathy.

Labs: WBC 10 (4.5–11 $\times 10^3$ per μL); hemoglobin 10 (12–16 g/dL); hematocrit 30 (35% to 45%); platelet 290 (159–450 $\times 10^3$ per μL); bilirubin (tot) 0.4 (0.2–1.0 mg/dL); bilirubin (dir) 0.1 (0–0.2 mg/dL); AST/SGOT 35 (7–40 U/L); ALT/SGPT 30 (7–40 U/L); Alk Phos 213 (70–230 U/L); amylase 78 (25–125 U/L); albumin 2.9 (3.5–5.5 g/dL); lipase 110 (10–140 U/L); small intestinal biopsy, blunting of mucosa; mucosa with distended macrophages in the lamina propria; by electron microscopy (EM), macrophages are periodic acid Schiff (PAS) positive and have gram stain positive rod-shaped bacilli inside; no evidence of inflammation; TB's blood and tissue bacterial cultures are negative for bacterial growth.

Thought Questions

- What is the *most likely* diagnosis for this patient?
- Which key laboratory and pathologic results lead to this diagnosis?
- What are other causes of malabsorption?
- What is the treatment?

Basic Science Review and Discussion

Malabsorption Syndromes Whipple's disease is a rare chronic condition that may affect many organ systems in the body but is most commonly characterized by malabsorption accompanied by chronic diarrhea, weight loss, joint pain, and obscure central nervous system (CNS) complaints; other patients have lymphadenopathy and hyperpigmentation. TB's history is consistent with Whipple's disease as well as a microcytic anemia (likely due to poor iron absorption) and a tissue biopsy that is pathognomonic for Whipple's disease. The illness is predominantly seen in white males 10:1 (male:female ratio) in their 30s and 40s (4th or 5th decade of life). Whipple's disease is caused by a bacterium, *Tropheryma whippelii*, and is diagnosed by biopsy of any affected tissue with macrophages that stain PAS positive and evidence rod-shaped bacilli by EM. The bacteria and heavy macrophage infiltrate fill the lamina propria and block lymphatic uptake of fat resulting in malabsorption. There are other causes of malabsorption; a short description of a few of the most important follows.

Bacterial Overgrowth Syndrome An uncommon cause of malabsorption is **bacterial overgrowth syndrome**, which occurs when the small bowel contains an abnormally large number of both aerobic and anaerobic bacteria. Typically, the small intestine keeps the bacteria numbers low by peristalsis, immunoglobulins, and other immunologic defenses, as well as, the nearby acidic environment of the stomach. Patients with intestinal strictures, diverticula, fistulas, or surgically denervated bowel are at risk for stasis and bacterial overgrowth syndrome. Anything that lowers the hydrochloric acid level (antacid therapy, gastric mucosal atrophy) predisposes to increased bacterial growth, often as numerous as in the colon. These risk factors are thought to contribute to malabsorption on the basis of several theories including bacterial deconjugation of luminal bile salts (decreasing fat digestion), direct mucosal damage by bacterial enzymes, competition for nutrients, and inactivation of luminal lipase. Small intestinal biopsies reveal normal mucosa in nearly all cases. Fortunately, this can be treated with oral antibiotics.

Lactose Intolerance **Disaccharidase deficiency,** commonly known as **lactose intolerance,** is more aptly named **lactase** deficiency. There are two types: the more commonly acquired version affects many African Americans, whereas the severe version is congenital and affects infants with their first exposure to milk. Because lactose is not broken down into components of glucose and galactose, it creates osmotic diarrhea. This condition is diagnosed by increased hydrogen production (bacterial fermentation of lactose) detected by exhaled air in gas chromatography. The acquired form is often mild and treated by avoidance of lactose-containing food or supplementation with the enzyme lactase. The genetic version is more severe with explosive diarrhea, abdominal distension and a colicky baby after the first feeding. Small intestinal biopsy reveals no abnormalities by light or electron microscopy.

Abetalipoproteinemia A rare inborn error of metabolism, abetalipoproteinemia is transmitted in an autosomal recessive manner and causes malabsorption. In this disorder, an infant cannot synthesize **apolipoprotein B** and therefore, when fatty acids and cholesterol meet after transepithelial passage, chylomicrons cannot be formed. In addition, very low density lipoprotein (VLDL), and low density lipoprotein (LDL) cannot be synthesized; there is also defective vitamin E transportation with subsequent deficiency and posterior column abnormalities, pigmented retinopathy as well as skeletal muscle disease. On biopsy, triglycerides are abundant and stored in the mucosal cells creating lipid vacuolation, which is obvious with light microscopy and fat stains. Subsequent essential fatty acid deficiency leads to lipid membrane abnormalities and acanthocytic erythrocytes often termed "burr cells."

Case Conclusion TB suffers from Whipple's syndrome, When appropriately diagnosed, is treated with antibiotics (ceftriaxone and streptomycin) and often resolves with rare exacerbations. TB improved with a long course of antibiotics and is now asymptomatic.

Thumbnail: Malabsorption—Uncommon Etiologies

Cause	Differentiating factors
Whipple's Disease	Malabsorption, joint pain, CNS complaints, abnormal pigmentation, lymphadenopathy; bacteria in intestinal biopsy; Predominantly in white males, age 30–40; Response to antibiotics (ceftriaxone and streptomycin)
Bacterial Overgrowth Syndrome	Small bowel with large numbers of anaerobic and aerobic organisms; seen in patients with (1) intestinal stasis; (2) hypochlorhydria or achlorhydria; (3) immune deficiencies or impaired mucosal immunity; biopsy mucosa normal, jejunal aspiration with increased number of bacteria is diagnostic, response to antibiotics
Disaccharidase Deficiency	Two types of lactase deficiency—acquired >> than congenital; common in African Americans; causes osmotic diarrhea; increased hydrogen on exhaled gas chromatography; inherited—revealed after first feeding—abdominal distension with explosive watery diarrhea; biopsy normal
Abetalipoproteinemia	Autosomal recessive inborn error of metabolism in which infant cannot synthesize apolipoprotein B; no assembly of fatty acid and cholesterol into chylomicrons; biopsy reveals lipid vacuolation, no absorption of essential fatty acids or any chylomicrons, VLDL and LDL; burr cells on hematology smear; vitamin E deficiency

---

Key Points

- Occurs more frequently in males in the 4th or 5th decade
- Presents with chronic diarrhea, malabsorption, weight loss, joint pain, CNS abnormalities, lymphadenopathy, hyperpigmentation

- Diagnosis is confirmed by tissue biopsy with PAS positive macrophages, EM visualization of gram-positive rods
- Caused by the organism *Tropheryma whippelii*
- Treated with antibiotics (ceftriaxone and streptomycin)

Questions

1. A 38-year-old woman, recently diagnosed with malabsorption—most likely celiac sprue (while waiting for the biopsy result, the patient has improved with a gluten-free diet)—is concerned about the long-term consequences of the disease. You discuss with her the increased incidence of gastrointestinal carcinoma, breast carcinoma, and which of the following?
   A. Prostate carcinoma
   B. Acute lymphocytic leukemia
   C. Gastrointestinal T-cell lymphoma
   D. Melanoma
   E. Hairy cell leukemia

2. A 35-year-old man comes to the clinic complaining of chronic diarrhea, joint pains, and weight loss. On physical examination, you note abdominal distension, joint tenderness, and generalized lymphadenopathy. You suspect Whipple's disease and order a small intestinal biopsy. The results reveal a characteristic lesion that confirms your diagnosis. You decide to treat with the appropriate long-term course of antibiotics including streptomycin and ceftriaxone. Streptomycin is known to cause which of the following side effects?
   A. GI (gastrointestinal) distress
   B. Gray baby syndrome
   C. Myositis
   D. Lactic acidosis
   E. Nephrotoxicity and ototoxicity

3. A couple visits the emergency department because of a 1-week history of voluminous foul-smelling stools, increased bloating, and abdominal pain. They both developed symptoms soon after a camping trip. Which of the following is the *most likely* diagnosis?
   A. *Shigella* dysentery from uncooked foods
   B. Giardiasis from contaminated stream water
   C. Amebiasis from contaminated water
   D. Cholera from contaminated stream water
   E. Norwalk virus from uncooked foods

HPI: HW, a 55-year-old male, complains of weakness, lack of appetite, and increasing abdominal girth for a long period of time. He reports that he is a scotch drinker, and has been since he was a young man. HW consumes about one bottle each day. He also notes that he has been losing weight even though his pants are too tight. On questioning, HW states that his stools are black and sticky, his urine is tea-colored, and he is impotent.

PE: HW is 5'7" tall and weighs 139 pounds. HR 100; T 36.8°C; BP 110/75. Gen: appears thin with muscle wasting. HEENT: scleral icterus, yellow under tongue. His skin displays a mild jaundice, he has no chest hair, enlarged breast tissue, palmar erythema, caput medusae, and spider nevi on abdominal wall. The abdomen is positive for bowel sounds, soft, nontender, markedly distended with fluid wave present, no rebound, no guard, liver edge enlarged with irregular, nodular consistency, and nontender splenomegaly. The rectal exam is significant for guaiac positive stool. There is testicular atrophy. The extremities display 2+ pitting edema, and there is mild asterixis of HW's hands.

Labs: WBC 6.5 (4.5–11 × 10³ per μL); hemoglobin 9 (12–16 g/dL); hematocrit 26 (35% to 45%); mean corpuscular 105 (80–100); volume (MCV) platelet 110 (159–450 × 10³ per μL); prothrombin time elevated; bilirubin (tot) 4.5 (0.2–1.0 mg/dL); bilirubin (dir) 2.2 (0–0.2 mg/dL); AST/SGOT 230 (7–40 U/L); ALT/SGPT 120 (7–40 U/L); Alk Phos 450 (70–230 U/L); amylase 34 (25–125 U/L); lipase 65 (10–140 U/L); albumin 2.0 (3.5–5.5g/dL)

You order a CT-guided biopsy of the liver and test for acute hepatitis. The hepatitis panel is negative but the biopsy reveals regenerating nodules of parenchyma with fibrotic changes including perivenular and sinusoidal fibrosis. The nodules represent a micronodular and macronodular pattern. Individual hepatocytes are swollen and some are necrotic with significant neutrophilic infiltrate.

Thought Question

■ What is the *most likely* diagnosis for this patient?

■ What are the key components of the history, physical examination, and lab results that lead to this diagnosis?

■ What is the architecture of the liver; how does the liver follow the dictum "form follows function"?

■ How does the liver respond to injury?

■ What is the pathophysiology of this disorder?

■ What are the common and rare sequelae of this disorder?

Basic Science Review and Discussion

Liver Architecture, Physiology, and Injury In order to understand the pathophysiology of the various disorders of the liver a clear understanding of liver architecture, physiology, and patterns of injury is essential. Unlike the majority of the gastrointestinal (GI) tract, the liver is responsible for the processing nutrients (e.g., amino acids, cholesterol, vitamins), phagocytosis of material in the splanchnic circulation, synthesis of protein, biotransformation of circulating metabolites and detoxification and excretion of pollutants and wastes. How the liver is essential in so many vital processes is inherent in its architecture.

Liver Microanatomy and Physiology The hexagonal lobule is the fundamental unit of liver architecture; it revolves around the terminal hepatic venule with portal triads located at three of the six angles. Each **portal triad** consists of the **portal vein** (60% to 70% of liver flow), **hepatic artery** (30% to 40% of flow), and the outgoing **common bile duct**. Incoming blood is processed by hepatocytes via sinusoids that eventually drain into the central hepatic vein and continues to the inferior vena cava.

The parenchyma of the liver is organized into sheets often referred to as cords because of their cord-like appearance of clusters around a central venule. Between the cords are the vascular sinusoids that arise form the artery, thus uniquely perfusing the hepatocytes from both arterial and venous sources. The sinusoids are lined by endothelial cells that demarcate an extra sinusoidal space called the **"space of Disse"**; this area is important in the pathophysiology of cirrhosis. In addition to hepatocytes, there are *Kupffer* and *Ito* cells that are active in phagocytosis, vitamin A metabolism, and collagen production, respectively. Finally, between the hepatocytes are the bile ducts that drain bile toward the common bile duct.

In relation to the architecture of the liver, exists the metabolic organization in which the parenchyma is subdivided into three zones with relative concentration of oxygen, nutrients, toxins, and other metabolites. Consequently, there is a lobular gradient of enzyme activity for each area. **Zone I,** the periportal, receives the greatest amount of nutrients, toxins, and oxygen. **Zone III** is closest to the terminal venule and receives the least amount of nutrients, metabolites, toxins, and oxygen. **Zone II** is intermediate.

Clearly, injury may exist as a zonal distribution based on what the hepatocytes are exposed to and how they respond.

Liver Injury Liver damage—regardless of the etiologic agent—is classified by five separate stages of injury. **Necrosis** of the liver is characterized by a cellular response of necrosis. In ischemic necrosis, the coagulative pattern dominates with mummified necrotic cells. When the insulting agent is immune related or a toxin, the cells undergo apoptosis with pyknotic cells with intensely eosinophilic **councilman bodies.** Other cells may swell and burst; this is called hydropic degeneration. Necrotic changes are also described according to the extent and the areas involved: focal, zonal, or massive. Typical examples of each include focal (viral damage); zonal, called centrilobular (zone III); secondary to toxins or drugs, and massive damage in response to drug toxicity or extensive viral injury.

Less severe than necrosis, is **degeneration;** hepatocytes have **ballooning degeneration** in which cells become edematous and appear as balloons. In cholestasis, retained biliary material appears foamy. Other cases—such as iron or copper deposition—may appear edematous with swollen cytoplasm.

In contrast to necrosis or degeneration, an inflamed liver has a large influx of inflammatory cells, often lymphocytes or macrophages, in the portal tracts or throughout the parenchyma. **Inflammation** of the liver, regardless of the etiologic agent, is termed hepatitis.

The liver's enormous reserve to insult is characterized by its ability for **regeneration.** Histologically, there is a proliferation of the hepatocytes from the cords. Even when severe necrotic changes occur, if the insult is removed, and the architectural framework remains intact, regeneration can occur.

Finally, when the liver is directly assaulted with a toxin or inflammation, the liver responds with deposition of collage or **fibrosis.** With continuing fibrosis, the liver divides into sections of functioning hepatocytes surrounded by scar tissue termed **cirrhosis.**

Pathophysiology and Biochemistry of Alcohol-Related Liver Disease **Alcohol abuse** and related **alcoholic liver disease** is a staggering global problem; approximately 33% of Americans have had an adverse health outcome related to alcohol abuse. However, not all patients are affected equally by their consumption of alcohol. Of course, the duration and amount of alcohol consumed is a risk factor, but gender, nutritional factors, and genetics also play a considerable role in who suffers most from liver damage. Only 10% to 15% of alcoholics develop cirrhosis. Chronic alcohol consumption results in liver disease in three classifications: **fatty liver disease, alcoholic hepatitis,** and **alcoholic cirrhosis.** **Hepatic steatosis** (fatty liver) may become evident with mild

liver transaminase, bilirubin, and alkaline phosphatase elevations; this stage is not, however, usually symptomatic. **Alcoholic hepatitis,** in contrast, often after a period of binge drinking, presents acutely with malaise, anorexia, abdominal pain, weight loss, and abnormal lab values. In many patients, with cessation of alcohol use the symptoms remit and the liver heals. But even after cessation of alcohol use, a small portion of the population progress to cirrhosis. Alcoholic cirrhosis can result in symptoms and physical manifestations such as portal hypertension, ascites, splenomegaly, hepatic encephalopathy, and liver failure. These are discussed later.

Alcohol is converted to **acetaldehyde** and **nicotine adenine dinucleotide, reduced form (NADH)** by alcohol dehydrogenase. Acetaldehyde interferes with normal hepatocytes secretion of protein by cellular swelling, termed fatty change. Acetaldehyde also disrupts microtubule formation in the hepatocytes and stimulates **Ito** cells in the space of Disse to transform into fibroblast-like cells and secrete collagen. This represents a final pathway to permanent liver damage and distortion of the architecture. Alcohol metabolism also results in elevated levels of NADH. **NADH** reverses the NAD^+ (nicotine adenine dinucleotide, oxidized form)/NADH ratio, which favors the production of lactic acid and triglycerides shunting normal substrates from catabolism to lipid synthesis. There is increased peripheral catabolism of fat and impaired assembly of lipoproteins. NAD^+ is converted to acetate and NADH by aldehyde dehydrogenase. Acetate transforms into **acetyl-CoA,** which leads to ketogenesis.

The cytochrome P_{450} system is induced with increased alcohol use therefore metabolizing other drugs and metabolites at a faster rate. Finally, alcohol induces an immunologic attack on hepatic neoantigens altering hepatic proteins.

Histology of Alcoholic Liver Disease **Alcoholic fatty liver** is the histologic description of the liver even after a moderate amount of alcohol is consumed. Lipid droplets form in hepatocytes; with continued alcohol use all hepatocytes contain large lipid vacuoles. Following this completely reversible stage, alcoholic hepatitis forms. **Alcoholic hepatitis** causes several, sometimes permanent changes. Liver cell necrosis occurs with ballooning of the centrilobular regions. Additionally, **Mallory bodies** are formed that are hepatocytes with eosinophilic cytoplasmic inclusions. Recognizing an alteration, neutrophils and macrophages surround these abnormal cells leading to an inflammatory reaction. Finally, sinusoidal and perivenular fibrosis is observed in **alcoholic hepatitis.**

Irreversible **alcoholic cirrhosis** evolves slowly as the liver shrinks and becomes more nodular in appearance. Collagen is formed in response to continued injury connecting portions of the parenchyma. The fibrous septae initially

77

connect the central portions to the portal regions and finally from central to central and portal to portal. Micronodules are the first to form (< 3mm) and eventually some enlarge into macronodules, resulting in a mixed picture.

Pathophysiology of Cirrhosis HW suffers from alcoholic cirrhosis secondary to his years of alcohol abuse. The other major causes of cirrhosis include chronic hepatitis, biliary disease, iron overload as well as the rarer diseases Wilson's disease and α_1 antitrypsin deficiency. **Cirrhosis** means three distinct things histologically: diffuse fibrosis, an alteration in the parenchymal architecture secondary to fibrosis, and parenchymal nodules regenerated by small foci of hepatocytes. These nodules are termed **micronodular** (< 3mm) or **macronodular** (> 3mm). Cirrhosis begins predominantly with micronodules but, as it progresses, it leads to a mixed histologic picture. The fibrous liver results from relentless diffuse parenchymal injury of different etiologies, in HW's case, the etiology is alcohol. The fibrosis is irreversible. The nodularity reflects the balance between fibrosis and hepatocyte regeneration. Finally, with the fibrosis comes reorganization of the vascular connections.

In a normal liver, collagen is dispersed to provide a framework for the hepatocytes to perform their vital function; but in patients who suffer from cirrhosis, collagen types I and III are dispersed throughout all parts of the lobule. This leads to vascular disruption that impairs blood flow and diffusion of nutrients and solutes through the metabolic zones. Collagen is deposited in the **space of Disse** impairing the movement of proteins such as clotting factors, albumin, and lipoproteins. Chronic inflammation, inflammatory mediators (TNF-α, TNF-β, and IL-1), Kupffer cell mediators, toxin effects, and disruption of the extracellular matrix all are proposed initiators of the Ito cell transformation. The Ito cell abandons its tasks and transforms into a collagen-forming cell, resulting in widespread fibrosis. These histologic changes result in anatomic and physical changes, many of which are present in HW.

The increased resistance of portal blood flow, **portal hypertension,** is a direct result of the abnormal vascular channels secondary to cirrhosis. This portal hypertension results in ascites, formation of portosystemic shunts, congestive splenomegaly, and hepatic encephalopathy. The key to the **ascites** in a cirrhotic patient lies in the starling forces. As described above, the abnormal vascular channels increase the pressure in the sinusoids (sinusoidal hypertension). Additionally, cirrhotic patients have low levels of albumin because of the aforementioned decrease in synthetic function. With the abnormal starling forces the lymphatic channels initially pick up the extra fluid but are soon overwhelmed; the fluid percolates from the liver capsule to the peritoneal cavity. Also, secondary hyperaldosteronism with salt and water retention contributes to ascites. In addition to ascites, the increased portal pressure is shared by all vascular beds that have systemic and portal circulation. Increased pressure causes dilation of the veins in the vasculature of the rectum, cardioesophageal junction, the retroperitoneum, and the falciform ligament leading to **hemorrhoids, varices,** periumbilical and abdominal wall *caput medusae,* respectively. Obviously, the esophageal varices can lead to life-threatening hematemesis in the cirrhotic alcoholic who retches or vomits as a result of drinking. Additionally, the spleen can enlarge secondary to vascular congestion and result in various hematologic manifestations.

Pathophysiology and Sequelae of Liver Failure Regardless of the etiology, when over 80% of liver parenchyma ceases functioning, **liver failure** ensues with severe clinical implications. Indeed, mortality from liver failure is 75% to 90%. HW possesses many of the classic physical and laboratory findings of liver disease. The cause of failure is often grouped according to one of three main categories: **chronic liver disease** (e.g., chronic hepatitis, cirrhosis, inherited, etc.); **ultrastructural lesions** (e.g., tetracycline toxicity, Reye's syndrome, etc.); and rapid **parenchymal necrosis** (e.g., viral hepatitis, acetaminophen toxicity, etc.). Specific problems elucidate the importance of the functioning liver. For instance, HW has jaundice, elevated transaminases and bilirubin reflecting ongoing liver cell necrosis and altered bilirubin metabolism. He has small testicles, increased breast tissue, as well as telangiectasias on his skin and red palms—all related to elevated estrogen levels. In addition to poor hepatic clearance of hormones, HW has poor synthetic function. This includes clotting factors, which leads to increased bleeding. He is also at great risk for a GI bleed from ruptured esophageal varices. HW also has sour pungent breath secondary to sulfur-containing mercaptans that are encephalopathic. **Hepatic encephalopathy** results from shunting the blood around the liver and severe loss of parenchymal cell function. Hepatic encephalopathy often presents with a range of altered consciousness. Common behaviors include confusion, stupor, and coma. These behaviors are often accompanied by hyperreflexia and limb rigidity and asterixis or "liver flap." When HW stretched his arms and dorsiflexed his hands, asterixis was observed; that is, his hands rapidly extend and flex. Patients with severe liver failure also suffer from **hepatorenal syndrome,** which is renal failure in the setting of liver failure with no other obvious source. Patients have elevated blood urea nitrogen (BUN) and creatinine (which resolves if the liver failure is reversed), and decreased urine output. The pathophysiology is not entirely clear, but decreased renal blood flow is suspected as the cause.

Case Conclusion   HW is now in liver failure, is admitted to the hospital, given supportive measures, and improves slightly. However, while on the liver transplant list, he expires secondary to a massive GI bleed.

Thumbnail: GI Pathophysiology—Clinical Implications of Hepatic Failure

Clinical/Laboratory Outcome	Pathophysiology
Elevated AST/ALT	Parenchyma cell death
Jaundice	Altered bilirubin metabolism; conjugated hyperbilirubinemia
Ascites	Decreased albumin (decreased oncotic pressure), increased hepatic lymph formation, secondary hyperaldosteronism
Hypoalbuminemia	Decreased synthetic function of liver
Coagulopathy	Decreased synthetic function of liver, clotting factors (2, 5, 7, 9, 10); could lead to disseminated intravascular coagulation (DIC) poor clearance of activated factors
Fetor Hepaticus (Breath of the dead)	Mercaptan formation in GI tract
Gynecomastia/Testicular atrophy/palmar erythema telangiectasia	Hyperestrogenism (poor liver clearance of estrogen)
Hepatic encephalopathy	Bypass of liver circulation, severe hepatocyte dysfunction
Hepatorenal syndrome	Elevated blood urea nitrogen, creatinine, decreased urine output; pathophysiology theorized to decreased renal blood flow

Key Points

▶ Risk factors include amount and duration of alcohol use/abuse, male gender, genetics

▶ Fatty liver disease; fatty change

▶ Alcoholic hepatitis, which is inflammatory hepatitis with inflammatory infiltrate

▶ Irreversible cirrhosis with collagen deposition

▶ Presents with elevated transaminases, physical findings

▶ Acetaldehyde, which interferes with hepatocyte production of protein; microtubule dysfunction; stimulates collagen synthesis by Ito cell; results in immunologic injury secondary to inflammatory infiltrate

▶ NADH, which favors production of lactic acid and triglycerides

▶ Sequelae: liver failure (above), psychosocial distress (alcoholism)

Questions

1. A 55-year-old male patient presents to the clinic complaining of right upper-quadrant pain, fever, and yellow skin. He has tender hepatomegaly on examination, and you suspect alcoholic hepatitis Which of the following liver function abnormalities will confirm your diagnosis?

   A. Elevated AST > elevated ALT, total bilirubin elevated, direct bilirubin normal

   B. Normal AST, elevated ALT, total bilirubin normal, direct bilirubin normal

   C. Elevated AST, normal ALT, total bilirubin elevated, direct bilirubin elevated

   D. Normal AST, normal ALT, total bilirubin elevated, direct bilirubin normal

   E. Elevated AST > elevated ALT, total bilirubin elevated, direct bilirubin elevated

2. A 40-year-old male suffering from alcoholic liver disease visits your office. He questions you regarding the pathophysiology of his many ailments. Which of the following is the appropriate mechanism for the clinical entity?

   A. Melenic stools with poor clearance of clotting factors

   B. Hematemesis; that is, poor production of clotting factors

   C. Spider angiomas; secondary to, dysfunctional metabolism of hormones

   D. Hemorrhoids with decreased intravenous pressure

   E. Hypogonadism—poor production of testosterone

> **HPI:** BG, a 4-day-old Caucasian girl, is brought in for yellowish hue in her eyes and skin. Her mother, RG, noted the yellow color the day after discharge from the hospital (third day of life) and states that it has worsened. RG reports that BG is feeding well, breast-feeding approximately 12 times a day. The infant is otherwise healthy, with normal bowel movements and urination. No fevers are reported.
>
> **PE:** BG's vital signs are normal, and her development is good. The infant does not appear to be in any distress. HEENT exam shows no cataracts, positive scleral icterus, and a yellow hue of the sublingual mucosa. The baby's skin has an apparent yellow hue. Bowel sounds are positive. The abdomen is soft, nontender, with no masses, no hepatosplenomegaly. The stool is of normal color.
>
> **Labs:** WBC 4 (4.5–11 × 10³ per μL); hemoglobin 16 (12–16 g/dL); hematocrit 45 (35% to 45%); platelet 243 (159–450 × 10³ per μL); bilirubin (tot) 3.5 (0.2–1.0 mg/dL); bilirubin (dir) 0.8 (0–0.2 mg/dL); AST/SGOT 12 (7–40 U/L); ALT/SGPT 23 (7–40 U/L); Alk Phos 100 (70–230 U/L); infant and mother's blood type both B+.

Thought Questions

- What is the *most likely* diagnosis for this infant?

- How is bilirubin metabolized?

- What is the significance of conjugated and unconjugated hyperbilirubinemia?

- What are the key components of the history and lab results that lead to this diagnosis?

- What are the common and rare etiologies of this disorder?

- What is the pathophysiology of jaundice and cholestasis?

Basic Science Review and Discussion

Physiology of Bile and Bilirubin Formation   The patient with yellow skin and mucous membranes suffers from clinical **jaundice**; that is, the retention of bilirubin. BG has physiologic jaundice of the newborn. Neonates can have an **unconjugated hyperbilirubinemia** secondary to decreased hepatic enzyme activity, as well as other reasons, which are discussed below. To understand why BG appears yellow, it is necessary to discuss the physiology of bilirubin. **Bile** consists of **bilirubin, bile acids, cholesterol,** and **phospholipids** and is secreted by hepatocytes. It has two purposes: emulsification of fats for digestion, and elimination of wastes. Bile salts are amphipathic (i.e., hydrophilic and hydrophobic areas) and can therefore serve to solubilize lipids into micelles for absorption. Bile also acts to eliminate cholesterol, bilirubin, and other wastes that are insoluble in water. The removal of these wastes and bilirubin is complex and has many steps in which disruption may occur leading to jaundice or **cholestasis.** Cholestasis is the retention of solutes in addition to bilirubin.

Yellow-colored bilirubin is the end product of heme and hemoprotein (e.g., P_{450} cytochrome) breakdown. At the end of their life span (120 days), immature erythroid cells or red blood cells are taken up by reticuloendothelial cells in the spleen, marrow, or liver and reduced to heme. **Heme** is broken down into **biliverdin** by heme oxygenase and to **bilirubin** by biliverdin reductase. Bilirubin is insoluble in aqueous solutions so it is bound by albumin and transported to the liver where it must undergo several critical steps. It must be taken up by the liver, bound by intracellular proteins (**ligandin**), and transported to the endoplasmic reticulum (ER). In the endoplasmic reticulum, the bilirubin is conjugated by **bilirubin uridine diphosphate (UDP) glucuronosyltransferase (UGT)** resulting in a bilirubin-glucuronic acid conjugate. This water-soluble, nontoxic, conjugated bilirubin is actively secreted into bile ducts and the small intestine. In the small intestine, most of the bilirubin glucuronides are deconjugated by bacterial **β-glucuronidases** into colorless **urobilinogens.** Approximately 20% of the urobilinogens made are reabsorbed via enterohepatic circulation and returned to the liver for reconjugation. Urobilinogen is water soluble and small amounts may be excreted in the urine; however, most urobilinogen is oxidized to urobilins in the colon, which gives stool its characteristic color.

In addition to bilirubin, the liver secretes a substantial amount of **bile acids** into the bile canaliculi. Bile acids (taurine, cholic, and chenodeoxycholic acid) are lost in the feces but are matched by de novo synthesis from cholesterol so that balance is maintained. The enterohepatic circulation allows a large pool of bile acids to be available for digestion and excretion (Figure 23-1).

Pathophysiology of Jaundice and Cholestasis   BG has increased levels of bilirubin in her blood as demonstrated by the laboratory values and physical examination. Bilirubin

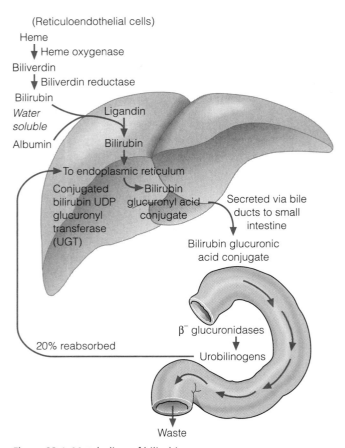

(Reticuloendothelial cells)

Heme
  ↓ Heme oxygenase
Biliverdin
  ↓ Biliverdin reductase
Bilirubin
Water soluble

Albumin

Ligandin

Bilirubin

To endoplasmic reticulum

Conjugated bilirubin UDP glucuronyl transferase (UGT)

Bilirubin glucuronyl acid conjugate

Secreted via bile ducts to small intestine

Bilirubin glucuronic acid conjugate

β⁻ glucuronidases

20% reabsorbed

Urobilinogens

Waste

Figure 23-1. Metabolism of bilirubin.

is deposited in the skin and mucous membranes resulting in jaundice; a level of at least 2.0 mg/dL is necessary for clinical jaundice. **Cholestasis** results from bile secretory failure, which leads to an accumulation of cholesterol bile salts and bilirubin. Severely elevated cholesterol and bile acids can manifest as xanthomas and pruritus, respectively. This discussion is limited to pathologic situations that result in jaundice *without* cholestasis.

Jaundice can be classified as **unconjugated** or **conjugated** depending on the pathophysiologic process. **Unconjugated hyperbilirubinemia** occurs when less than 20% of the bilirubin is conjugated and is circulating in the plasma attached to albumin. Unconjugated bilirubin is insoluble and as such cannot be excreted in the urine. In infants, unconjugated hyperbilirubinemia can be disastrous because the blood-brain barrier is immature, allowing for deposition of bilirubin in the brain, leading to **kernicterus.** Unconjugated hyperbilirubinemia can result from excess production of bilirubin; examples include hemolytic anemia, pernicious anemia, thalassemia, and resorption of a large volume of blood from internal hemorrhage. Additionally, unconjugated hyperbilirubinemia can be caused by decreased hepatic uptake caused by drug interference (e.g., rifampin)

with membrane carrier systems. Finally, impaired hepatocyte bilirubin conjugation secondary to hepatocellular disease (e.g., hepatitis, cirrhosis), immature hepatocytes (physiologic jaundice) or inherited deficiencies (discussed below).

A **conjugated hyperbilirubinemia** results when more than 50% of the bilirubin is conjugated. Conjugated bilirubin is water soluble and nontoxic and may result in bilirubinuria and clay-colored stools (no urobilin). The causes follow the physiologic pathway of bilirubin excretion. Decreased hepatic excretion or obstruction of bile flow after conjugation can result from intrahepatic bile duct disease (e.g., primary biliary cirrhosis, primary sclerosing cholangitis, graft versus host disease) or extrahepatic bile duct disease (e.g., gallstone, obstructive cancer, flukes). Other causes of decreased excretion include hepatocyte disease (e.g., hepatitis, total parenteral nutrition), and medication effects (e.g., oral contraceptives) leading to a conjugated type of jaundice.

Microanatomy of Jaundice　Increased levels of yellow bile pigment in hepatocytes appear wispy with bile pigment and "foamy degeneration"; bile canaliculi are full of bile. Occasionally, these ducts burst and Kupffer cells phagocytose the bile remnants, which are easily observed. In cases of obstruction of the bile tree (intrahepatic or extrahepatic), the pressure leads to swelling ducts and ductal proliferation. Prolonged obstructive cholestasis leads to destruction of the parenchyma causing "bile lakes" of cellular debris and pigment.

Pathophysiology of Hereditary Hyperbilirubinemias　Just as adult hyperbilirubinemias are classified according to the conjugation status of the bilirubin, so are the causes of jaundice in neonates, infants, and children. Severe hereditary disease must be differentiated from asymptomatic and benign disease as well as physiologic jaundice. The most common cause of unconjugated jaundice in a neonate is secondary immaturity of the activity of hepatocyte bilirubin UGT, termed **physiologic jaundice of the newborn.** The enzyme typically reaches normal activity within 2 weeks of life. Of note, infants who are breast-fed are more likely to have physiologic jaundice of the newborn secondary to β-glucuronidases in the breast milk.

There are five main causes of unconjugated hyperbilirubinemia in neonates and infants. Physiologic jaundice of the newborn, which is what BG has (discussed below). **Hemolytic disease of the newborn** caused by blood group (ABO) incompatibility between mother and the child results in jaundice and kernicterus from unconjugated hyperbilirubinemia. In this disease, increased production of heme overwhelms the hepatocyte ability to conjugate the substrate. Additionally, **Crigler-Najjar syndrome, type I** is a rare and lethal cause of severe unconjugated jaundice in which there is *no* bilirubin UGT. Without that enzyme, a severe unconjugated hyperbilirubinemia exists leading to deposition in the neonatal brain resulting in an often fatal ker- nicterus. This disorder is inherited in an autosomal recessive fashion. **Crigler-Najjar syndrome, type II,** is a less severe, nonfatal form with a mild decrease in UGT that is inherited in an autosomal dominant pattern with variable penetrance. **Gilbert's syndrome** is also inherited in the dominant pattern and related to decreased levels of UGT; however, it is common and benign and patients with this disorder present with mild fluctuating levels of unconjugated bilirubin.

There are also several causes of **conjugated hereditary hyperbilirubinemia. Dubin-Johnson syndrome** results from the autosomal recessive inheritance of a defective trans- port in the canalicular membrane of the bile duct. As a consequence, excretion of conjugated bilirubin is impossible. Fortunately, these patients have a normal life expectancy because the conjugated bilirubin is non- toxic to a neonate. Of note, pathologic examination reveals a black liver that distinguishes it from Rotor's syndrome. In **Rotor's syndrome,** patients have an asymp- tomatic conjugated hyperbilirubinemia *without* liver discoloration. Rotor's syndrome is also inherited in an autosomal recessive fashion.

Case Conclusion   BG has physiologic jaundice of the newborn. She is at a higher risk for several reasons. UGT has decreased activity until about 2 weeks of life. Also, neonates have an increased bilirubin load secondary to increased red cell mass and a relatively short half-life of those cells. Additionally, neonates have decreased intestinal bacterial flora with rare conversion of conjugated bilirubin to urobilinogen. Coupled with an increased enterohepatic circulation, neonates less than 2 weeks old are at risk for physiologic jaundice of the newborn. Like most neonates with physiologic jaundice, BG's was not present on the first day, peaked on the fifth, and resolved without complication on day 14.

Thumbnail: Liver Physiology and Pathophysiology—Hyperbilirubinemia

Bilirubin Metabolism	Derangement leads to . . .	Examples
Heme Degradation	unconj. hyperbilirubinemia	Hemolytic anemia, resorption of hematoma or large GI bleed, ineffective erythropoiesis (thalassemia, pernicious anemia)
Reduced Hepatic Uptake (Rifampin)	unconj. hyperbilirubinemia	Drug interference with carrier Gilbert's (rare—usually conjugated)
Decreased Bilirubin Uptake at Level of Hepatocyte	unconj. hyperbilirubinemia	Physiologic jaundice of newborn, Crigler-Najjar, Gilbert's, hepatocyte disease (hepatitis, cirrhosis)
Limited Intrahepatic Excretion of Bilirubin	conj. hyperbilirubinemia	Dubin-Johnson, Rotor's, hepatocyte disease (hepatitis, cirrhosis) intrahepatic bile disease (biliary cirrhosis, sclerosing cholangitis, transplant)
Limited Extrahepatic Excretion of Bilirubin	conj. hyperbilirubinemia	Gallstones, obstructive cancer, fluke

Key Points

Unconjugated Hyperbilirubinemia

▶ Crigler-Najjar type I

Defect/Genetics: No bilirubin UGT, autosomal recessive.

Life Expectancy: Fatal at 18 months kernicterus/jaundice; seizures.

Pathology: Cholestasis

▶ Crigler-Najjar type II

Defect/Genetics: Decreased bilirubin UGT; autosomal dominant, variable penetrance

Life Expectancy: Normal, occasional; mild kernicterus.

Pathology: Usually normal

▶ Gilbert's

Defect/Genetics: Decreased bilirubin UGT, autosomal dominant, heterogeneous

Life Expectancy: Normal, asymptomatic

Pathology: Normal

Conjugated Hyperbilirubinemia

▶ Dubin-Johnson

Defect/Genetics: Defective canalicular membrane; decreased excretion of bilirubin; autosomal recessive

Life Expectancy: Normal; chronic jaundice

Pathology: Black liver

▶ Rotor's

Defect/Genetics: Altered biliary excretion; unknown

Life Expectancy: Normal

Pathology: Normal

Questions

1. A 3-week-old neonate presents with a seizure and on physical examination you note jaundice. You order the appropriate laboratory tests and diagnose the neonate with Crigler-Najjar, type I. You remember that this is an unconjugated hyperbilirubinemia. Which of the following are *both* conjugated types and syndromes of hyperbilirubinemia?

A. Dubin-Johnson and Gilbert's
B. Gilbert's and hemolytic disease
C. Crigler-Najjar and physiologic jaundice
D. Rotor's and Dubin-Johnson
E. Dubin-Johnson and Crigler-Najjar

2. A 45-year-old male presents with jaundice. You order laboratory tests that reveal a total bilirubin of 4.5 and a direct bilirubin of 1.2. You appropriately diagnose an unconjugated disorder. Which of the following pathophysiologic steps is *correctly* matched with the type of hyperbilirubinemia?

A. Decreased excretion of bilirubin glucuronides; unconjugated
B. Decreased bile flow; unconjugated
C. Excess production of bilirubin; conjugated
D. Decreased hepatic uptake; conjugated
E. Hemolysis of red blood cells; unconjugated

3. Which of the following represents appropriately matched hereditary hyperbilirubinemia?

A. Gilbert's; decreased hepatic uptake of bilirubin
B. Crigler-Najjar, type I; absent UDP glucuronyl transferase
C. Rotor's; black pigmented liver
D. Dubin-Johnson; autosomal dominant
E. Rotor's; canalicular transport deficiency

HPI: IM, a 5-year-old boy, presents with a 6-day history of nausea, vomiting, anorexia, fatigue, and fever and chills. His mother notes that many of the children in his day care have similar complaints. When questioned, she reports dark urine.

PE: IM is 35 inches tall and weighs 65 pounds. T 39.4°C; HR 130; BP 95/49. He is thin and his HEENT exam exhibits scleral icterus and jaundice of mucous membranes under tongue; the boy's skin also appears jaundiced. IM's abdomen is positive for bowel sounds, with soft, tender hepatomegaly, and no rebound or guarding.

Labs: WBC 6.5 (4.5–11 × 10^3 per μL); hemoglobin 12 (12–16 g/dL); hematocrit 38 (35% to 45%); platelet 243 (159–450 × 10^3 per μL); bilirubin (tot) 1.5 (0.2–1.0 mg/dL); bilirubin (dir) (0.8 0–0.2 mg/dL); AST/SGOT 536 (7–40 U/L); ALT/SGPT 502 (7–40 U/L); Alk Phos 310 (70–230 U/L); amylase 34 (25–125 U/L); lipase 65 (10–140 U/L); albumin 4.0 (3.5–5.5g/dL); anti-HAV-IgM positive; anti-HAV-IgG negative

Thought Questions

- What is the *most likely* diagnosis for this patient?

- What are the key components of the history and lab results that lead to this diagnosis?

- How are the different types of hepatitis acquired and what are the prognoses?

- What are the sequelae of the varieties of infectious hepatitis?

- What is the importance of serum markers as they pertain to viral hepatitis?

Basic Science Review and Discussion

Pathophysiology, Microanatomy, and Sequelae of Acute and Chronic Hepatitis Hepatitis occurs when there is damage to the liver parenchyma; it has many causes including viral, pharmacologic, toxic, and immune mediated. These and other factors lead to hepatocellular necrosis with similar symptoms, physical examination findings, and laboratory abnormalities. The cellular necrosis may be focal or extensive beginning with inflammatory infiltrate in the portal areas. Cases of hepatitis are marked by transaminasemia with aspartate aminotransferase (AST), often but not always, more elevated than alanine aminotransferase (ALT). This abnormality often accompanies a mixed hyperbilirubinemia. Laboratory abnormalities are accompanied by characteristic pathologic changes.

Acute hepatitis and **chronic hepatitis** refer to the duration of cellular inflammation. Acute duration is less than 6 months regardless of the severity of the illness; chronic indicates that the duration of inflammation duration is greater than 6 months. All cases of hepatitis have distinct stages: a prodrome or incubation period, followed by the symptomatic and icteric phases, and finally the recovery or convalescent period. The **prodrome** differs for all of the viruses and will be discussed individually; however, the end of the prodrome marks the period of greatest infectivity. The **symptomatic** phase is marked by constitutional symptoms such as malaise, anorexia, nausea, headaches, and so on. The symptomatic phase is followed by the **icteric** phase, which is mainly due to a mixed hyperbilirubinemia. The urine turns dark (as in our patient) because of bilirubinuria, stools are light (cholestasis), and the skin becomes itchy (increased bile acids). Finally, **convalescence** ensues with resolution of jaundice and symptoms. The focus of this case will be the viral etiologies of infectious hepatitis, and does not include Epstein-Barr, cytomegalovirus (CMV), or yellow fever.

There are many clinical entities that may result from infection with a hepatitis virus. A "healthy carrier" is an individual who does not exhibit overt symptoms, but who can transmit infection. Another type of carrier may be a patient with chronic hepatitis who unknowingly transmits the virus. These individuals are often immunocompromised, symptom-free, and act as reservoirs of infection.

The histopathology of hepatitis in the healthy carrier state is nearly normal. Much of the tissue is normal; however, there are clusters of hepatocytes with "ground glass" cytoplasm indicating hepatitis B surface antigen (HB_sAg) is present. Others show "sanded" nuclei, which are a sign of plentiful hepatitis B core antigen (HB_cAg) and active viral replication. In acute viral hepatitis, the pathology is more diffuse but still centers around the portal triad with lobular disarray and dense inflammatory infiltrate of lymphocytes leading to focal ballooning degeneration, apoptosis (*Councilman* bodies are often present), and portal tract inflammation. Also, Kupffer cells are characteristically hypertrophied as well as increased in numbers (hyperplastic).

Chronic hepatitis has many causes—all of which may or may not appear indistinguishable pathologically—including infection, alcoholism, drugs (isoniazid, methotrexate), Wilson's disease, and autoimmunity. In chronic hepatitis, the inflammatory infiltrate spills from portal tracts into the surrounding parenchyma. With continued necrosis, fibrous septum formation occurs with hepatocyte regeneration that leads to cirrhosis. The types of hepatitis viruses result in chronic hepatitis in differing proportions. For example, **hepatitis E** virus (HEV) never results in chronic hepatitis, whereas **hepatitis A** virus (HAV) only rarely leads to the chronic form. **Hepatitis B** virus (HBV) becomes chronic in less than 5% of adults but over 90% of neonates. **Hepatitis C** virus (HCV) results in chronic infection in approximately 50% of cases. **Hepatitis D** virus (HDV) will lead to chronic infection in 80% but only when superinfection occurs.

Hepatitis A Virus—Pathophysiology and Pathology of Acute Hepatitis   IM has an **acute HAV** infection with resultant symptoms and physical examination findings. EM reported instances of nausea, vomiting, and fatigue. Other common symptoms of acute hepatitis include pruritis from elevated bile acids, anorexia, weight loss, headaches, muscle and joint aches, abdominal pain, and diarrhea. IM's physical examination illustrated that he was in the icteric phase with jaundice from elevated bilirubin levels and dark urine from bilirubin excretion of the urine. The boy also had tender hepatomegaly and illustrated evidence of cholestasis with pale stools. IM's laboratory abnormalities are consistent with a moderate case as he has a mild mixed hyperbilirubinemia, transaminitis, and IgM antibody to HAV. Other viruses have a prolonged prothrombin time and hyperglobulinemia.

Hepatitis A virus (HAV) is a single-stranded, icosahedral ribonucleic acid (RNA) virus of the picornavirus family that is spread via fecal-oral contamination, certain sexual practices, and shellfish. It does not cause chronic hepatitis or a carrier state. Fulminant hepatitis is rare with HAV so mortality is low—approximately 0.1%. The incubation period is about 2 to 6 weeks; the live virus is shed in stool about 1 week before symptoms appear. Therefore, all the children in IM's class have been exposed and are possibly affected. As in IM's case, after infection the virus is shed and is followed by acute disease (jaundice and symptoms) when IgM anti-HAV peaks. After the immune system responds (several months later) a fourfold increase in IgG anti-HAV is expected. The immunoglobulin persists for life providing immunity against all known strains of HAV to date.

Risk factors associated with acute HAV include intravenous drug abuse, travel to endemic lands (travelers should receive HAV and HAB vaccine prior to departure), those who have anal intercourse, and those exposed to contaminated food or water supplies.

Hepatitis B Virus—Pathophysiology and Serum Markers of Acute Hepatitis   **Hepatitis B virus (HBV)** is transmitted via close contact (blood, breast milk, saliva, sexual intercourse) and is apparent after an incubation period ranging from 2 to 6 months. The virus is present in the bloodstream during late incubation, active, and chronic infection. The virus is resilient and resistant to changes in temperature and humidity yet, unlike HAV, it is not present in stool. Anyone who comes in contact with infected fluids such as intravenous drug users, healthcare workers, vertical transmission in endemic areas (Africa, Southeast Asia), and/or transfusion and dialysis recipients are at risk for HBV. The virus or "Dane" particle is a partially double-stranded DNA virus from the hepadnavirus family that is 3200 nucleotides in length all of which code for proteins. Of importance in diagnosis, infection status, and prognosis is the monitoring of certain components of the virus: hepatitis B core antigen (HBcAg) is the nucleocapsid, hepatitis B surface antigen (HBsAg) is the envelope, and hepatitis B early antigen (HBeAg) is the protein that directs the virus into the blood. The progression of the disease is best monitored by the presence or absence of these so-called serum marker proteins.

After exposure and infection by the virus, there is a long (2 month) incubation period near the end of which, hepatocytes begin to secrete HBsAg. HBsAg is also the last to leave; it declines in 3 to 6 months *if* the infection is cleared. If HBsAg is present after 6 months, then chronic infection ensues. HBeAg and HBV DNA follow and mark active viral replication. HBeAg and HBV DNA are important markers of the infectivity of the virus. The immune response ensues and T-cells (CD8) fight the virus and result in hepatic damage; the virus itself is not cytotoxic. The first marker of immunologic response is finding an anti-HBe antibody. This finding alerts that the virus has been acquired, and is being battled and eliminated. Approximately when the symptoms of HBV appear, the next antibody in one's immune defense becomes detectable: anti-HBc IgM, which always indicates acute infection. HBc IgM is a nonprotective antibody which, along with anti-HBe, are the only markers of infection during the serologic gap, or window, when all the antigens have disappeared. Over time, the HBc IgM is replaced with IgG to the "Dane" (anti-HBc) particle. Upon resolution of the infection, anti-HBs antibody rises about a month after HBsAg is nondetectable. Anti-HBs antibody persists for life and indicates immunity to HBV.

Infection may result in five outcomes: (1) acute infection with recovery, (2) healthy carrier state without progression, (3) acute infection leading to fulminant hepatitis with massive liver necrosis resulting in death, (4) acute hepatitis with subsequent chronic hepatitis—a nonprogressive form in which recovery is common, (5) acute hepatitis with subsequent chronic hepatitis—a progressive form with increased risk of hepatocellular carcinoma, cirrhosis, and death.

Hepatitis C Virus—Pathophysiology and Sequelae   **Hepatitis C virus (HCV)** is transmitted parenterally via blood from transfusions, accidental needle sticks, and/or intravenous drug abuse with needle sharing. It is apparent after about 6 weeks of incubation. The virus is a small RNA virus of the flavivirus family that codes for a single polypeptide. The polypeptide is processed into proteins for the coat, membrane-binding proteins and others necessary for replication. The virus has a highly conserved portion that codes for the nucleocapsid protein and a hypervariable portion that codes for the envelope. This hypervariable region and subsequent differing antigenic expression leads to an unstable virus with resultant immunity challenges.

As in HBV, HCV particles do not destroy hepatocytes and immunologic injury is again postulated as the cause. After incubating, HCV RNA is detectable along with elevations in transaminases. Anti-HCV IgG appears and, despite efforts, is not able to eliminate HCV DNA from the blood. Symptoms in patients with HCV are milder than HAV or HBV and transaminases may rise or fall despite appreciable changes in symptoms. Alternatively, transaminases may be persistently elevated or normal. As mentioned above, 50% of patients have chronic infection that can lead to cirrhosis in as little as 5 years.

Hepatitis D Virus—Pathophysiology, Sequelae, and Superinfection Hepatitis D virus (HDV)— also called "delta agent"—is a unique agent capable of infection only when encapsulated by HBV during coinfection. The delta agent is common in the Middle East and Africa and far less common in the United States. HDV is an RNA virus that is double-shelled and resembles the HBV Dane particle. Infection is detected earliest by HDV RNA in the blood prior to symptoms in patients with known exposure. Hepatitis D results in acute **coinfection** when a patient is exposed to *both particles simultaneously.* Typically (> 90%), coinfection leads to recovery with immunity from both agents: HDV Ag-IgM and HB$_c$Ag-IgM—present in the serum. In 4% of patients, infection leads to fulminant hepatitis and often death. In the remaining patients, chronic hepatitis ensues.

Conversely, if a patient is a carrier of HBV and acquires HDV a state of **superinfection** occurs that is often clinically more severe. In patients with mild disease (HBV) who contract HDV, 10% get fulminant hepatitis and often subsequent liver failure and death. Another 15% have acute severe hepatitis with full recovery. The remaining 75% of patients develop chronic hepatitis with resultant cirrhosis. These patients are also at increased risk for hepatocellular carcinoma. When a patient has chronic superinfection from HDV, HB$_s$Ag and anti-HDV are present.

Hepatitis E Virus—Pathophysiology Hepatitis E virus (HEV) is a single-stranded RNA virus (calcivirus family) that is transmitted via the fecal-oral route (contaminated water) often in young to middle-aged adults. Like HAV, this is a common source of infectious hepatitis in travelers. It is usually self-limiting; however, it can be devastating in pregnant women with a mortality approaching 20%. Patients' symptoms appear 6 weeks after exposure. HEVAg is observed in the cytoplasm of hepatocytes during acute infection and anti-HEV IgM or IgG can be measured. The IgM antibody indicates current infection, whereas IgG indicates that recovery and immunity are present.

Case Conclusion   IM has a moderate case of acute hepatitis A so he is admitted for observation, especially for prompt intervention should the hepatitis worsen. He does quite well. The symptoms and lab abnormalities improve and IM is discharged to home with no long-term complications. It is unnecessary, but an anti-HAV IgG antibody is checked and is positive confirming IM's immunity 6 months after the admission.

Thumbnail: Acute Hepatitis

	Transmission	Incubation	Carrier/Chronic	Type	Fulminant
HAV	Fecal-oral	2 to 6 weeks	No/No	RNA	Rare
HBV	Direct parenteral	2 to 6 months	Yes/Yes	DNA core and surface	Uncommon
HCV	Direct parenteral	6 weeks	Yes/Yes	RNA flavivirus	Uncommon
HDV	Direct parenteral	2 to 6 months	Yes/Yes	DNA hybrid needs HBV coat	Yes
HEV	Fecal-oral	6 weeks	No/No	RNA no envelope	Yes

Key Points

	Serologic Markers	Significance
▶ HAV	Anti-HAV (IgM)	Current or recent infection
	Anti-HAV (IgG)	Current or previous infection; immunity
▶ HBV	HBsAg (surface antigen)	Acute or chronic infection
	HBeAg (E antigen, core component)	Acute infection, persists in chronic infection, high infectivity, active viral replication
	Anti-HBe (antibody to E)	Recovery (transient), chronic (persistent), decreased infectivity
	Anti-HBc (antibody to core)	Acute and chronic infection, past/current infection, IgM suggests viral replication not protective
	Anti-HBs (surface antigen)	Recovery, immunity
▶ HCV	Anti-HCV	3 months after exposure, no protection, chronic infection (persistent)
▶ HDV	Anti-HDV (IgG or M)	Acute or chronic infection; no protection

Questions

1. A patient presents to your office and is unsure of her hepatitis B immunization status. You check for antibodies and find that she was likely infected by HBV and is now immune. Which of the following are the *most likely* antibody results?

   A. (−) anti-HBc IgM antibody, (−) anti-HBc IgG antibody, (−) anti-HBs IgG antibody, (−) anti-HBe IgG

   B. (+) anti-HBc IgM antibody, (−) anti-HBc IgG antibody, (−) anti-HBs IgG antibody, (+) anti-HBe IgG

   C. (+) anti-HBc IgM antibody, (+) anti-HBc IgG antibody, (−) anti-HBs IgG antibody, (+) anti-HBe IgG

   D. (−) anti-HBc IgM antibody, (+) anti-HBc IgG antibody, (+) anti-HBs IgG antibody, (−) anti-HBe IgG

   E. (−) anti-HBc IgM antibody, (−) anti-HBc IgG antibody, (+) anti-HBs IgG antibody, (−) anti-HBe IgG

2. Which of the following *correctly* matches the causative factor?

   A. Hyperbilirubinemia; pale stools

   B. Transaminitis; direct viral attack

   C. Ground glass cytoplasm; presence of HBcAg

   D. Fecal-oral transmission—HDV

   E. Pruritis; elevated bile acids

HPI: VP, a 43-year-old female, presents complaining of several years of fatigue and abdominal discomfort. She notes pruritis that worsens at night as well as the recent development of yellow skin and "elbow pads." VP also reports bulky, greasy, odorous stools but denies any history of gallbladder or liver disease.

PE: VP is 5'4" tall and weighs 134 pounds. She has normal vital signs and in general is thin. HEENT: She has a mild yellow hue to the sclera and mucous membranes. VP's skin appears jaundiced. She has positive bowel sounds; her abdomen is soft, nontender, nondistended, with no rebound, no guarding, or hepatomegaly. Her extremities are non-tender, and there are xanthomas on her elbows bilaterally.

Labs: WBC 3.6 (4.5–11 $\times$ 10^3 per μL); hemoglobin 13 (12–16 g/dL); hematocrit 38 (35% to 45%); platelet 243 (159–450 $\times$ 10^3 per μL); bilirubin (tot) 3.2 (0.2–1.0 mg/dL); bilirubin (dir) 2.1 (0–0.2 mg/dL); AST/SGOT 12 (7–40 U/L); ALT/SGPT 23 (7–40 U/L); Alk Phos 600 (70–230 U/L); amylase 34 (25–125 U/L); lipase 65 (10–140 U/L); total cholesterol 345 (120–220 mg/100ml); antimitochondrial antibodies are positive.

Thought Questions

- What is the *most likely* diagnosis for this patient?
- Which key components of the history and lab results lead to this diagnosis?
- What are the epidemiologic risk factors for this illness?
- What are the sequelae of this disorder?
- What is the pathophysiology of this disorder?

Basic Science Review and Discussion

Clinical Presentation and Epidemiology of Primary Biliary Cirrhosis Primary biliary cirrhosis (PBC) is a chronic, insidious, and occasionally fatal disease of the intrahepatic bile ducts. It often presents with chronic abdominal pain and pruritis, elevated bilirubin and alkaline phosphatase, as well as clinical manifestations of elevated cholesterol levels: xanthomas and hepatomegaly. When an individual with primary biliary cirrhosis presents late in the pathogenesis of the disease—with jaundice—liver decompensation has already occurred.

PBC is a disease more often diagnosed in women in their 40–50s. It is in women six times more often than in men, usually over a prolonged investigation. It is also associated with the **Sjögren's syndrome,** in which patients have dry eyes and mouth. A number of rheumatologic conditions are also associated including the **CREST syndrome** (calcinosis, Raynaud's phenomenon, esophageal dysfunction, sclerodactyly, telangiectasia), scleroderma, thyroiditis, rheumatoid arthritis, membranous glomerulonephritis, and celiac disease. VP presents with elevated laboratory values indicating the progression of her disease. She has elevated cholesterol and alkaline phosphatase and only mild evidence of hyperbilirubinemia and cirrhosis.

Pathophysiology and Microanatomy of Primary Biliary Cirrhosis The specific etiology of the disorder is not yet clear; however, there are several findings that lead to altered immune response as the culprit. PBC is characterized by granulomatous destruction of the interlobular bile ducts. The biliary epithelium expresses an antigen with resultant accumulation of T-cells around and inside of the bile ducts. PBC leads to small-duct fibrosis in a focal and variable pattern with differing degrees of severity in different portions of the liver. Early in the disease, granulomatous destruction occurs only in the portal tracts but, as the years pass, the parenchyma becomes involved. Early on, lymphocytes, histiocytes, and plasma cells form granulomas and destroy the interlobular area. Over time, fibrosis occurs with hepatocyte death and typical nodular regeneration. The gradual descent to cirrhosis and liver function decline is pathologically similar to that of chronic active hepatitis. Of note, more than 90% of patients have antimitochondrial antibodies to the bile duct epithelium, but the role these antibodies play is not yet clear.

Clinical Presentation, Epidemiology, and Pathophysiology of Primary Sclerosing Cholangitis Primary sclerosing cholangitis (PSC) is similar in many respects to PBC: presentation, associations, and etiology all draw many parallels. Focusing on the differences between the two is therefore important. PSC is often diagnosed in males (2:1), in their 30s to 50s and is characterized by inflammation and fibrosis of the intrahepatic and extrahepatic bile ducts. These undergo fibrosis and dilation and are described as "beading" on radiographs illustrating the patchy strictures of the bile ducts.

In contrast to patients with PBC, 70% of patients with PSC have coexisting ulcerative colitis (UC), but only 4% of patients with chronic UC have PSC. Despite the association, the cause of PSC is unknown. There are several theories including, direct immunologic attack secondary to toxins released by the inflamed gastrointestinal (GI) tract, as well as fibrosis secondary to patchy ischemia. However, there is no hard data to neither confirm nor deny these theories; further studies are needed.

The microanatomy of PSC is the appearance of patchy fibrosis with lymphocytic infiltrate leading to progressive atrophy of the duct lumen. The ductal fibrosis is termed "onion skinning" due to its layered appearance that obliterates the lumen. As this condition heals, a fibrotic closed bile duct remains that first leads to increases in liver enzymes, then later to cholestasis.

Like persons who suffer from PBC, individuals with PSC may complain of fatigue, pruritis, and jaundice. Alternatively, they may be asymptomatic and elevated bilirubin is noted on routine screening. PSC is best diagnosed with endoscopic retrograde cholangiopancreatography (ERCP). Sequelae include those associated with liver failure (e.g., ascites, encephalopathy, coagulopathy, etc.). Liver transplant is the only cure.

Case Conclusion   VP presented late in the course of PBC and has a few early signs and symptoms of liver failure. Her jaundice and xanthomas will worsen as her hepatic function degrades. Unfortunately, there is no curative treatment. But, while awaiting liver transplantation, VP's symptoms are relieved and the clinical progression is slowed by use of ursodeoxycholic acids, which replace endogenous toxic bile acids.

Thumbnail: Primary Biliary Cirrhosis

Epidemiology

Female to male, 6:1, middle age

Presents with pruritis, abdominal pain, steatorrhea with hepatomegaly, elevated direct bilirubin, elevated alkaline phosphatase, elevated cholesterol, xanthoma, late jaundice (with cirrhosis)

Pathogenesis

Progressive autoimmune destruction with patchy destruction of interlobular bile ducts, portal inflammation, late cirrhosis

Etiology

Likely autoimmune

Associated with Sjögren's, CREST syndrome, elevated serum IgM, antimitochondrial antibodies (> 90%), scleroderma, thyroiditis, rheumatoid arthritis

Sequelae

Liver failure

Key Points

Primary Sclerosis Cholangitis

▶ Features of primary sclerosis cholangitis include male to female ratio of 2:1

▶ Presents with pruritis, abdominal pain, light stools, dark urine, hepatomegaly, elevated bilirubin (direct), alkaline phosphatase, and cholesterol

▶ Pathogenesis is characteristic for periductal fibrosis, segmental stenosis of extrahepatic and intrahepatic biliary ducts

▶ The etiology of the disease is unknown; hypothesized that toxin release from diseased GI tract damages ducts; immune-mediated attack; ischemia

▶ Liver failure

▶ UC is associated in 70% of cases; elevated IgM; hypergamma-globulinemia

Questions

1. A 45-year-old man with years of abdominal pain, pruritis, and a long history of UC presents with new jaundice. You suspect PSC and would expect to see which of the following on biopsy?
   A. Antimitochondrial antibodies to bile duct epithelium
   B. Perivenular fibrosis of the terminal hepatic venule
   C. Ballooning degeneration and apoptosis
   D. Patchy extraductal and intraductal inflammatory fibrosis
   E. Chronic hepatic congestion

2. Which of the following are *correctly* matched?
   A. PBC—more common in males
   B. PSC—associated with antimitochondrial antibodies
   C. PSC—patients are also likely to have UC
   D. PBC—patchy stenosis of extrahepatic ducts
   E. PSC—pathology significant for septal fibrosis

HPI: SP, a 43-year-old Native American female, presents to the emergency department complaining of right upper-quadrant pain. The pain began approximately 8 hours ago and became worse after a meal (within 30 minutes) at a fast-food restaurant. SP reports that the pain "shoots up" to the right shoulder and back (points to her scapula). She took acetaminophen without relief; following that she experienced three episodes of nausea and vomiting. SP remembers one other episode of this pain that resolved with over-the-counter (OTC) pain remedies and a bland diet. She has lost 30 pounds over the past month and this was the first fast-food or fatty food she has eaten in 2 months. SP believes that what she's now experiencing may be a reaction to this food. She has not taken her temperature but has felt a bit warm.

SP has a history of type 2 diabetes mellitus, Crohn's disease, and hypercholesterolemia for which she is treated with glucophage and clofibrate. She is also taking oral contraceptive pills (OCPs) to prevent conception.

PE: SP is 5'4" tall, weighs 254 pounds, and is obese. Her temperature is elevated at 38.6°C; her other vital signs are normal. She has no scleral icterus or jaundice of her skin or under her tongue. Her abdominal exam reveals epigastric and right upper quadrant tenderness, voluntary guarding, and rapid inspiratory arrest with deep palpation of the right upper quadrant.

Labs: WBC 17 (4.5–11 × 10^3 per μL); diff-neutrophil 88% (57% to 67%); seg 60% (54% to 62%); bands 18% (3% to 5%); hemoglobin 13 (12–16 g/dL); hematocrit 36 (35% to 45%); platelet 322 (159–450 × 10^3 per μL); bilirubin (tot) 1.0 (0.2–1.0 mg/dL); bilirubin (dir) 0.2 (0–0.2 mg/dL); AST/SGOT 25 (7–40 U/L); ALT/SGPT 34 (7–40 U/L); GGT 102 (8–40 U/L); Alk Phos 455 (70–230 U/L); amylase 90 (25–125 U/L); lipase 56 (10–140 U/L); ESR 56 (< 20 mm/hr); right upper quadrant ultrasound reveals thickened gallbladder wall with sludging and several gallstones, one of which appears at the junction of the cystic duct.

Thought Question

- What is the *most likely* diagnosis for this patient?

- Which key laboratory results lead to this diagnosis?

- What is the relevant anatomy; that is, the liver, gallbladder, ducts, adjacent organs, and so on?

- How is a cholesterol gallstone formed?

- How is a pigment gallstone formed?

Basic Science Review and Discussion

The most likely diagnosis is **acute cholecystitis,** which is an acute inflammation of the gallbladder. The symptoms of right upper quadrant pain with referred pain, nausea, and emesis following a meal with high fat content along with the patient's risk factors place her at greater risk of acute cholecystitis. The physical examination, laboratory, and ultrasound findings confirm the diagnosis. To better understand this patient's condition, the physiology and pathophysiology of the gallbladder and the sequelae that can result from having gallstones is discussed below.

Anatomy and Physiology of the Gallbladder   The gallbladder is inferior and flush against the liver typically at the anatomic division of the right and left lobes. In preparation of digesting fatty meals, 500 to 1000 cc of **bile** is secreted each day by the liver (exocrine secretion); in between meals, bile is stored in the gallbladder (approximately 50 cc capacity) and concentrated by active absorption of electrolytes and passive H_2O movement. Bile is a fluid that is composed of **bile salts, phospholipids, cholesterol,** and **bilirubin.** Bile facilitates the emulsification, digestion, and absorption of fatty acids and cholesterol, minerals and the fat soluble **vitamins A, D, E,** and **K.** Hepatocytes secrete the bile through the right and left hepatic ducts that meet to form the (common) hepatic duct. The hepatic duct joins with the cystic duct, which leaves the gallbladder at the **spiral valves of Heister** to form the common bile duct. The common bile duct courses to the duodenum through the head of the pancreas and releases bile into the duodenum via the **ampulla of Vater.**

Formation of Gallstones   In the gallbladder, **cholesterol** is solubilized by water soluble **bile salts** and insoluble **lecithin.** When there is an excess of cholesterol such that the detergent capacity of bile salts and lecithin are overwhelmed cholesterol stones may form. More specifically, there are three conditions that must occur for cholesterol stones to form: Bile salts and lecithin must be confronted with too much cholesterol. Along with this state of "supersaturation" there must be stasis in order for the cholesterol crystals to have time to aggregate (form) into the stones. Stasis occurs in pregnancy or in rapid weight loss; the latter is what affects SP. The third criterion is that nucleation of the cholesterol monohydrate must be chemically favorable. Other promoters of stone formation include biliary sludge, mucins, and calcium salts.

Pigment stones are formed by complex mixtures of insoluble calcium salts. Although patients may not possess any identifiable risk factors, details from a patient's past medical history may indicate that the stones are likely pigmented. For instance, the presence of high levels of unconjugated bilirubin secondary to hemolysis can predispose to pigmented stones. Additionally, the risk of pigmented stones increases with infection of the biliary tract by *Escherichia coli* or *Ascaris lumbricoides*. Of note, pigmented stones are often (50% to 75%) radiopaque.

Cholelithiasis There are two types of stones: **cholesterol** and **pigment gallstones.** In the United States, approximately 80% of stones are cholesterol gallstones that contain more than 50% of crystalline cholesterol monohydrate. Cholesterol stones are more common in patients with a positive family history, and those from native American, Mexican American, Northern European, and North and South American populations. Additional risk factors including hyperlipidemia, obesity, recent rapid weight loss, gender, pregnancy, and medications such as OCPs and clofibrate are associated with excess estrogen and increased secretion of biliary cholesterol and thus cholesterol stones. Risk factors associated with the less common pigment gallstones include Asian ancestry, rural living, chronic hemolytic syndromes, biliary infection; also in patients with ileal diseases such as Crohn's or cystic fibrosis with concomitant pancreatic insufficiency. Patients with gallstones are deemed to have **cholelithiasis.**

Choledocholithiasis If a patient also presents with jaundice and elevated direct bilirubin with the clinical and laboratory picture described above, the obstruction is likely in the common bile duct (and is mild). This is termed **choledocholithiasis.** These patients may present with acholic (no bile = pale) stools or biliuria (bile in urine). Also of note, these patients may present with fluctuating jaundice differentiating it from jaundice of intrahepatic origin. Finally, an increase in amylase and/or lipase indicates involvement of the pancreas where the distal common bile duct courses through the pancreas. Commonly termed **gallstone pancreatitis,** these patients suffer midepigastric with right upper quadrant pain.

Acute Cholecystitis In acute cholecystitis, the stone often becomes impacted in the gallbladder neck where it narrows or in Hartmann's pouch, which is a nearby outpouching. Pain is often intense and occurs when the gallbladder contracts in response to **cholecystokinin** that is released by the I cells of the duodenum and jejunum after a fatty meal. In SP, this is the most likely scenario with elevated **alkaline phosphatase** and **GGT** (both specific to duct cells) and mild or absent transaminitis (**AST/ALT**). **Hyperbilirubinemia,** if present is typically very mild. As is the case with our patient, fever, and **leukocytosis** indicate infection of the gallbladder.

With the stone impacted, the gallbladder becomes more distended, inflamed, and edematous. Blockage is followed by chemical irritation and inflammation of the gallbladder wall. Enzymes produce lysolecithin, which is toxic to the mucosa. If hyperbilirubinemia is present, it is commonly due to the inflamed and edematous gallbladder that obstructs the adjacent common hepatic duct. When infection is present, the most common organisms include *Escherichia coli, Enterobacteriaceae, Clostridium welchii* or *perfringens* or *Bacteroides.*

Case Conclusion The diagnosis of acute cholecystitis with the stone location most likely in the gallbladder neck is made based on history and includes risk factors, physical exam, laboratory, and imaging data. All patients with acute cholecystitis should be admitted to the hospital, administered IV fluids, and treated with antibiotics. Approximately, two in three cases of acute cholecystitis will resolve spontaneously; therefore, expectant management is ideal in patients with many medical issues. Serious consideration of a surgical solution should be entertained for any patient who deteriorates during the hospital stay, to avoid the complications of acute cholecystitis such as perforation, empyema, or ascending **cholangitis.** However, many patients choose to have an early or interval cholecystectomy. SP chose an interval laparoscopic cholecystectomy, which proceeded without complications.

Thumbnail: Cholesterol versus Pigment Gallstones

	Cholesterol	**Pigment**
Composition	Cholesterol monohydrate	Insoluble calcium salts
Pathogenesis	Cholesterol supersaturation nucleation; time to allow formation (stasis)	Presence of (abnormal) calcium salt, bilirubin calcium salts, infection
Frequency	> 80%	Up to 20%
High-Risk Groups (Ethnicity)	Northern European, Native American, Hispanic, African American	Asian, rural
High-Risk Comorbidity	Estrogen (female gender, oral contraceptive, pregnancy), obesity, gallbladder stasis, hyperlipidemia, inborn errors of bile acid metabolism	Chronic hemolytic syndrome, biliary infection, ileal disease, Crohn's, cystic fibrosis
Appearance on X-ray	10% to 20% radiopaque	50% to 75% radiopaque

Key Points

- Patients present with right upper quadrant pain, fever
- Often diagnosed in obese women around age 40, with high levels of estrogen due to pregnancy or OCPs.
- Persons at high risk include those of African, native American, and Mexican American heritage; other risk factors include diabetes, chronic extravascular hemolysis
- Cholelithiasis is differentiated by biliary colic, risk factors

- Acute cholecystitis is associated with fever; elevated white blood cells, alkaline phosphatase, GGT; transaminases (AST/ALT) and bilirubin with normal to mild elevation
- Signs of choledocholithiasis include fever; elevated white blood cells; jaundice elevated direct bilirubin, alkaline phosphatase GGT; transaminases (AST/ALT) mild elevation or normal
- Pancreatitis presents with elevated amylase, lipase; pain may be in midepigastrium

Questions

1. A patient presents to the emergency department with acute right upper quadrant pain, fever, nausea, and vomiting after consuming a meal with high fat content. You suspect acute cholecystitis and consider the pathophysiology of the illness. Which of the following is the *inciting event* of cholecystitis?
   A. Obstruction
   B. Increased production of cholesterol stones
   C. Bacterial infection with gram-negative gut flora
   D. Enzyme degradation of mucosal wall
   E. Schistosomes

2. Which of the following is deemed the most efficacious antibiotic to use against bacterial organisms that are *most likely* causing acute cholecystitis?
   A. Tetracycline
   B. Azithromycin
   C. Piperacillin-tazobactam or ampicillin-sulbactam or ticarcillin-clavulanate
   D. Trimethoprim-sulfamethoxazole
   E. Third-generation cephalosporin plus metronidazole or clindamycin

3. A patient with a history of acute cholecystitis presents with abdominal pain, nausea, and vomiting. On examination you note distension and absent bowel sounds. The *most likely* diagnosis is
   A. acute cholecystitis.
   B. choledocholithiasis.
   C. ascending cholangitis.
   D. gallstone ileus.
   E. cystic fibrosis.

4. Which of the following is *not* included in the layers of the gallbladder?
   A. Mucosal lining (single layer of columnar epithelial cells)
   B. Muscularis mucosa
   C. Peritoneal covering (except where the gallbladder is directly adjacent to the liver)
   D. Subserosal fat
   E. Fibromuscular layer

HPI: LL, a 43-year-old man, complains of epigastric pain, nausea, and vomiting for 4 days. He is a frequent recipient of emergency room treatment for alcohol withdrawal and injuries secondary to his alcoholic binge drinking. LL consumed his last drink about 40 hours ago. He describes pain that has worsened and radiates toward his back like a knife. He has had nothing to eat since the pain began. Past medical history is significant for alcohol dependence, alcohol withdrawal, acute pancreatitis.

PE: LL is 6′1″ tall and weighs 178 pounds. Vital signs: T 36.8°C; HR 110; BP 134/78; RR 16. LL appears thin, is shaking, and smells of alcohol. There is no ecchymosis on his skin. His abdominal examination reveals normoactive bowel sounds, midepigastric tenderness to light palpation, with no masses or distension. LL does, however, have rebound tenderness and guarding.

Labs: WBC 11 (4.5–11 × 10³ per μL); hemoglobin 12 (12–16 g/dL); hematocrit 36 (35% to 45%); platelet 243 (159–450 × 10³ per μL); bilirubin (tot) 0.2 (0.2–1.0 mg/dL); bilirubin (dir) 0.1 (0–0.2 mg/dL); AST/SGOT 245 (7–40 U/L); ALT/SGPT 248 (7–40 U/L); Alk Phos 100 (70–230 U/L); amylase 780 (25–125 U/L); lipase 945 (10–140 U/L); albumin 4.0 (3.5–5.5g/dL); blood glucose 104 (70–110 mg/100 ml with fasting); lactic dehydrogenase (LDH) 230 (45–90 U/L).

Upright abdominal and chest x-rays, and an abdominal CT are helpful. The x-rays reveal a few dilated loops of small bowel with two discrete air-fluid levels, no pleural effusion, and no intra-abdominal free air. The CT shows slight pancreatic edema and some soft tissue stranding. There is no evidence of necrosis.

Thought Questions

- What is the *most likely* diagnosis for this patient?

- How does the exocrine pancreas aid in digestion of foodstuffs?

- Which key components of the history, physical examination, laboratory results, and imaging lead to this diagnosis?

- What are the sequelae of this disorder?

- What is the etiology of this disorder?

Basic Science Review and Discussion

It is clear from the history, physical examination, edematous pancreas on CT and elevated amylase and lipase that LL has **acute pancreatitis.** In order to understand the inflammation of the pancreas it is essential to review the form and function of the exocrine pancreas. Without its digestive prowess, foodstuffs are not broken down into usable energy; this is well illustrated by **cystic fibrosis.**

The pancreas is a small organ in the posterior upper abdomen derived from the fusion of the dorsal and ventral bud (of the duodenum) that drains its products into the common bile duct or duodenum via the duct of Wirsung. The purpose of the pancreas is to release digestive enzymes to break down foodstuffs. The organ is organized into acini that are lined with columnar epithelial cells. Their form

follows function; they are radially oriented secretory cells with basophilic staining secondary to extensive rough endoplasmic reticulum and an extensive Golgi apparatus. These epithelial cells produce **zymogen** granules that, when activated, contribute to digestion.

Physiology of Digestion and Protection—Exocrine Pancreas
The pancreas secretes two to three liters of alkaline fluid and zymogens in response to humoral and neural stimulation. The phrase "rest and digest" aptly describes the pancreatic response to **acetylcholine,** which is a major stimulant for zymogen release and, to a lesser extent, bicarbonate flow. Additionally, when the duodenum is exposed to fatty foods and amino acids, **cholecystokinin (CCK)** and **secretin** are released, both of which are major stimulants to zymogen and fluid (bicarbonate alkaline) flow into the duodenum. The pH must be reduced in the duodenum in order for the enzymes to work.

Zymogens are pro-drugs or inactive forms of enzymes; there are several categories of enzymes active in protein, starch, and fat digestion. These enzymes are to some extent governed by **trypsinogen,** main function of which is to activate other pre-enzymes. Trypsinogen is activated on the duodenal brush border to its active form **trypsin,** which in turn activates other pro-enzymes and creates a positive feedback loop activating trypsinogen as well. Fat is split into fatty acids and glycerol in the presence of bile acids by a host of pro-enzymes that are activated by trypsin including **colipase** and **phospholipase A;** lipase is secreted in active form. Proteins are broken down into peptides by trypsin, **chymotrypsin, elastase,** and **carboxypeptidases.** There are a few secretory products from the exocrine pancreas that are secreted in the active form and include **α-amylase,** which cleaves starch into dextrins and disaccharides.

The pancreas protects itself from auto digestion in several ways. As already discussed, the enzymes are mostly secreted as pro-enzymes and are sequestered in membrane-bound granules. Additionally, trypsin is activated by enterokinase, which is present only on the brush border of the duodenum. There are also inhibitors of enzymes within the acini to protect the pancreas from auto digestion; presence of trypsin activates different enzymes that degrade other pro-enzymes. Finally, the acini are resistant to trypsin and lipase.

Pathophysiology of Acute Pancreatitis LL represents the mild end of the clinical spectrum for acute pancreatitis. Patients have variable amounts of epigastric pain that radiates toward the back with elevated blood or urine pancreatic enzymes. LL suffers from alcohol dependence and an acute inflammation of the pancreas. In addition to alcohol as a predisposing factor, gallstones are the other major etiologic factor; together these factors account for 80% of acute pancreatitis. Other rare causes include mumps, coxsackievirus, and *Mycoplasma* infections, as well as *Ascaris lumbricoides* and *Clonorchis sinensis.* Some types of familial hyperlipoproteinemia, trauma (especially in children), medications (e.g., azathioprine), trauma and vascular ischemia or thrombosis (e.g., shock, lupus) have been associated with acute pancreatitis. Men are more commonly afflicted if the etiology is alcohol; it is more common in women if gallstones are the causal factor.

The pathophysiology is not entirely clear; however, there are several leading hypotheses. In one leading theory, there is duct obstruction (either from a stone or an alcoholic's thick protein secretions) with increased pressure resulting in rupture of smaller ductules within the pancreas. Following acinar damage, extravasation of excretions and zymogens occur leading to activation of trypsin and further destruction. Other concomitant theories relate to direct acinar cell injury by alcohol, viruses, or deranged activity of the zymogen transport system. Whatever the etiology of the inciting events, inflammation, proteolysis, lipolysis, and hemorrhage occurs—with activation of trypsin as the initial event. With proteolysis, proteins are degraded; when lipolysis occurs, membrane phospholipids are destroyed; with elastase release the elastic tissue in blood vessels is destroyed. Coupled with the activity of elastase, is the activation of the kinin system (trypsin) resulting in hemorrhage.

Histology and Sequelae of Acute Pancreatitis Histologically, the pancreas has several obvious alterations secondary to the autolytic processes. There is clear proteolytic destruction of the pancreas as well as necrosis of the blood vessels and subsequent hemorrhage. In addition, there is an inflammatory reaction of neutrophils and fat necrosis. In severe disease, the pancreas becomes necrotic.

Depending on the severity of the process, the sequelae can be locally and systemically severe. Locally, a pseudocyst, abscess, or duodenal obstruction may result. Systemically, there may be hypocalcemia, organ failure with disseminated intravascular coagulation (DIC), fluid sequestration and shock, acute respiratory distress syndrome (ARDS), peripheral vascular collapse with acute tubular necrosis (ATN), and diffuse fat necrosis. The severity of this illness is underscored by the fact that 5% of patients with severe acute pancreatitis die during the first week of therapy.

Case Conclusion LL is admitted to the hospital, given IV fluid resuscitation, and allowed nothing by mouth while his pancreas rests. He requires analgesia and nasogastric decompression secondary to intractable vomiting. LL is followed clinically with serial abdominal examinations and demonstrates improved pain over the course of 2 days. His diet is advanced and his pain medication tapered down by the third day of his hospital stay. LL also receives extensive counseling regarding his alcohol dependence and is discharged to a rehabilitation program.

Thumbnail: Acute Pancreatitis

Epidemiology

Middle-aged; males more often if alcohol is etiologic agent; female if gallstone

Presentation

Severe boring epigastric pain, radiates to back; nausea, vomiting, anorexia with elevated amylase and lipase (serum or urinary)

Etiology

80% of cases secondary to gallstones or alcohol. Rare cases include:

drugs, viral, bacterial, nematodes, trematodes, hyperlipoproteinemia, or vascular ischemia/thrombosis

Pathogenesis

Obstruction (thick protein secretions of alcoholic or stone) leading to increased pressure within duct; leads to increased permeability and eventual activation of zymogens within the pancreas by trypsin; direct toxic effect on acini or transport mechanism

Sequelae

Pseudocyst, abscess, hypovolemic shock, DIC, ARDS, ATN

Key Points

▶ Secretin is released by duodenum in response to fatty acid and low pH; this stimulates pancreas to release alkaline fluid (enzymes cannot function in acidic pH)

▶ CCK is released by duodenum in response to fatty acids and low pH; this stimulates zymogen release and HCO_3.

▶ Lipase is secreted in active form; fat is split into fatty acids and glycerol

▶ α-amylase is secreted in active form, which cleaves starch into dextrins and disaccharides

▶ Digestion is initiated by trypsin, cleaved from trypsinogen by enterokinase in brush border of duodenum, which activates other pro-enzymes

▶ colipase and phospholipase A cleave fat into fatty acids and glycerol in the presence of bile acids

▶ trypsin, chymotrypsin, elastase, and carboxypeptidase split proteins into peptides

Questions

1. Your patient is in the hospital receiving treatment for pancreatitis. This patient describes numbness and tingling around his mouth and, during your physical examination, you note facial twitching after you tap over the area of cranial nerve VII. Additionally, you note carpal spasm when you take your patient's blood pressure. You order an ionized calcium level and an EKG because you assume hypocalcemia. Which of the following will *most likely* show in the results?

   A. Short QT interval
   B. ST segment depression
   C. Peaked T-waves
   D. Prolonged QT interval
   E. Diffuse ST segment elevations

2. Which of the following *correctly* matches the subsequent action?

   A. CCK: cleaves proteins to amino acids
   B. Colipase: splits fat into amino acids in the absence of bile acids
   C. Trypsin: activates α-amylase into cleaving starch
   D. Enterokinase: cleaves trypsin from chymotrypsin
   E. Elastase: destroys vessel elastase in acute pancreatitis

HPI: EZ, a 22-year-old male, complains of 1-day history of sharp abdominal pain. He first noted the pain around his belly button, but now is pointing to the right lower quadrant. EZ also complains of nausea and vomiting, which began after his pain; he also notes fever and chills and has no appetite. Otherwise he is healthy.

PE: EZ is 5'7" tall and weighs 145 pounds. Vital signs: T 38.3°C; HR 102; BP 129/66; RR 18. Gen: discomfort, diaphoretic. EZ's abdomen has positive bowel sounds but is hypoactive and soft, with marked tenderness in the right lower quadrant at McBurney's point. There is distension, positive rebound, and involuntary guarding

Labs: WBC 12.5 (4.5–11 $\times$ 10^3 per μL); diff-neutrophil 88% (57% to 67%); Seg 60% (54% to 62%); bands 18% (3% to 5%); hemoglobin 14 (12–16 g/dL); hematocrit 44 (35% to 45%); platelet 243 (159–450 $\times$ 10^3 per μL).

An x-ray and a CT of the abdomen are ordered. The kidney ureter bladder radiograph reveals a normal gas pattern with no free or intraperitoneal air. The CT reveals fat stranding and an oval appendicolith.

Thought Questions

- What is the *most likely* diagnosis for this patient?

- Which key components of the history and lab results lead to this diagnosis?

- What are the common and/or rare sequelae of this disorder?

- What is the etiology of this disorder?

- What is the differential diagnosis of abdominal pain?

Basic Science Review and Discussion

From the history, physical examination, laboratory, and imaging findings it is clear that EZ has **appendicitis,** which is often diagnosed in adolescents and young adults who were previously well. Classically, but not always, the presentation is as follows: Peri-umbilical pain followed by right lower quadrant pain at McBurney's point (between the umbilicus and the anterior superior iliac spine); then nausea and vomiting. Tenderness and possibly rebound and guarding (indications of peritoneal irritation) are elicited during a physical examination. Next, a low-grade fever followed by an elevation in the white blood cell count is observed. This sequence does not apply to patients who are pregnant, have a retrocecal appendix, or a malrotated gut. In pregnant patients, the pain may be right lower, middle, or upper quadrant; whereas in those patients with a retrocecal appendix the pain may be in the flank; in those with a malrotated gut the pain would be in the right upper quadrant. Additionally, the presentation may differ in the very young and the very old.

Pathophysiology of Acute Appendicitis Appendicitis is associated with obstruction of the appendix in over 50% of the cases. Often, the obstruction is caused by lymphoid hyperplasia, a fecalith or less commonly a tumor, gallstone, or

even worms. The obstruction leads to increased pressure secondary to continual secretion of mucinous fluid (physiologic), which results in the collapse of the lymphatics and veins; this collapse leads to ischemia. Afterward, secondary bacterial invasion occurs, in which secretion of an exudate results in more edema and inflammation. With ischemia and invasion, gangrene results secondary to venous thrombosis. The bowel wall may rupture secondary to ulceration, bacterial infection, and ischemia.

Morphology of Appendicitis Initially, in appendicitis, there is a neutrophilic invasion of the mucosa and submucosa. The neutrophils secrete an exudate that is apparent on the serosa as it grossly changes from pink and normal to granular and red. As the neutrophilic invasion expands to include the muscularis the gross appearance is a fibrinous purulent serosal reaction. As bacterial invasion ensues, an abscess can form followed by ulceration and necrosis. Finally—in the final step prior to rupture—grangrene sets in with a green or green-black appearance. Major sequelae of appendicitis in addition to rupture include peritonitis, pylephlebitis with thrombosis of the portal vein, liver abscess, peri appendiceal abscess, or bacteremia.

Differential Diagnosis of Acute Abdominal Pain There are several causes of acute abdominal pain that can often be diagnosed based on history, physical examination, laboratory tests, and imaging studies. Epigastric pain from a **perforated ulcer** classically presents as severe epigastric pain with rapid progression to the entire abdomen in conjunction with the history of an ulcer. The pain is often accompanied by signs of peritoneal irritation (e.g., rebound and guarding). Free air is observed on radiograph. **Peptic ulcer disease** (PUD) is more common in men and associated with *Helicobacter pylori* infection as well as chronic obstructive pulmonary disease (COPD), chronic nonsteroidal anti-inflammatory drug (NSAID) use, as well as tobacco and alcohol use/abuse.

Biliary tract disease presents in middle-aged female patients (age 35 to 55) with right upper quadrant crampiness. History of multiparity, obesity, and oral contraceptive pill (OCP) use are risk factors. On laboratory and imaging evaluation, patients have elevated γ-glutamyl transferase (GGT) and alkaline phosphatase; and stones in the gallbladder as well as ductal dilation. With elevated white blood cell (WBC) count and fever, patient may have cholecystitis or cholangitis. Acute epigastric pain with radiation toward the back accompanied with nausea, vomiting, and low-grade temperature in a patient with a history of alcohol abuse is often diagnosed with **pancreatitis.** On physical examination, the pain seems out of proportion to the findings and only in the most severe cases does the examiner find rebound or guarding because the organ is in the retroperitoneum.

Kidney stones or ureteral colic (**nephrolithiasis**) often afflicts men in their 30s with risk factors that can lead to stone formation such as family history, gout, *Proteus* genitourinary tract infection, cystinuria or renal tubular acidosis. Upon presentation, these patients are writhing in bed with an acute onset of flank pain that radiates toward the groin. Ureteral colic is often associated with nausea and vomiting and patients have costovertebral angle tenderness, a benign abdominal exam, and hematuria. Spiral CT or intravenous pyelography is the mainstay of diagnosis. Any age

patient—infants to adults—may have periumbilical pain with vomiting and a tender, distended abdomen with hyperactive bowel sounds leading to the diagnosis of intestinal **obstruction.** Abdominal films are a good way to diagnose; obstruction is more common in at-risk patients (those with cancer, adhesions, hernias, abscess, intussusception or volvulus).

Patients with **diverticulitis** complain of lower left quadrant pain and changing stool consistency. They may have fever, left lower quadrant tenderness without rebound, a heme positive stool or even a palpable mass. Risk factors include age greater than 50 and high fat, low fiber "Western" diet. The diagnosis is made by CT.

Additional causes of lower abdominal pain in women patients include **pelvic inflammatory disease** (PID) and **ovarian torsion.** PID occurs in young, often sexually active women. They present with lower abdominal pain, fever, elevated WBC count, cervical motion, adnexal and uterine tenderness on bimanual examination. These patients are diagnosed on a clinical basis only. Young women with adnexal masses who present with an acute onset of severe unilateral pain may have had torsion of an ovary. In torsion, the size of the mass allows the ovary to twist cutting off the vascular supply. Emergent ultrasound can indicate presence of a mass, as well as absence of blood flow.

Case Conclusion   EZ is admitted to the hospital for surgical management of the appendicitis. He undergoes an uncomplicated laparoscopic appendectomy and stays in the hospital for 3 days. EZ is released when his pain is controlled and he is tolerating a regular diet.

Thumbnail: Differential Diagnosis of Acute Abdominal Pain

Diagnosis	Epidemiology/ Etiology	Presentation/PE	Studies
PUD	Men, 50s, bacteria, COPD, NSAID, ETOH, tobacco	Epigastric pain, often relieved by food/antacid, diffuse abdominal pain; when perforates, peritoneal irritation	Endoscopy, urease breath test
Biliary Colic	Female, obese, 40s, OCPs, multiparous	Right upper quadrant pain, radiates to scapula, Murphy's sign, fever in cholecystitis	Alk phos, WBC, ultrasound
Pancreatitis	Males, EtOH abuse, gallstones, hyperlipidemia, history of ERCP, hypercalcemia	Acute onset, epigastric, nausea/vomiting, radiates toward back, pain out of proportion of PE, fever, no rebound/guarding (retroperitoneal)	Amylase, lipase, CT, ultrasound
Appendicitis	Young adults; appendix obstruction ischemia, infection, perforation	Epigastric/peri-umbilical then right lower quadrant pain, fever, anorexia, rebound, guarding	WBC, CT
Ureteral Colic	Male, 30s, gout, family history, *Proteus* infection, stone in ureter	Acute flank pain, radiates to groin, CVAT, abdomen is benign	CT, IV pyelogram
Obstruction	Infants to adults, history of surgery (adhesion), cancer, volvulus, intussusception	Crampy, diffuse abdominal pain, vomiting, hyperactive bowel sound, distension, tenderness, peritoneal signs if strangulated	Abdominal radiograph, CT
Diverticulitis	Male, elderly, low fiber diet, colonic diverticula	Left lower quadrant pain, N/V, stool abnormalities, fever, rectal bleeding, no rebound	WBC, CT
PID	Female, sexually active, high-risk behavior	Low abdominal pain, nausea, vomiting, fever, uterine and adnexal tenderness, cervical motion tenderness, cervical discharge	Clinical exam
Ovarian Torsion	Female, adnexal mass twists stops blood supply	Acute onset unilateral low abdominal pain, nausea, vomiting, tenderness	Ultrasound with vascular evaluation

Key Points

▶ Presents with pain, cramping, inability to pass flatus/stool, nausea, vomiting, distension, hyperactive bowel sounds with rushes, rectal bleeding (currant jelly stool); infarction

▶ Usually seen in young adults and adolescents; however, persons of any age can be affected; slightly more common in males

▶ Classic peri-umbilical pain followed by right lower quadrant pain

▶ Progresses from quadrant pain, then nausea/vomiting; after which patients have fever and leukocytes

▶ Obstruction followed by increased intraluminal pressure; collapsed lymph drainage and veins leads to bacterial invasion, pus, and ulceration; compromised arterial blood supply leading to gangrenous necrosis; rupture

▶ Caused by luminal obstruction secondary to: (1) lymphoid hyperplasia, (2) fecolith, (3) foreign body, (4) tumor, (5) gallstone, (6) worms

▶ KUB x-ray and CT should reveal oval calcified appendocolith and gas-filled appendix with air fluid levels are pathognomonic; nearby gas fluid levels or evidence of inflammation—fat streaking or obliteration of the right peritoneal fat line

▶ Perforation, liver or peri-appendiceal abscess, peritonitis, pylephlebitis with thrombosis of portal vein, bacteremia

Questions

1. A 23-year-old woman presents to the emergency department. She complains of 3 to 4 days of low abdominal pain, fever, nausea and vomiting. She has normal bowel movements. The patient reports a history of an ectopic pregnancy, several sexual partners, as well as a chlamydial infection 3 months ago. Her last menstrual period was 9 days ago. Her examination is notable for cervical motion tenderness and right lower abdominal pain. What of the following is the likely diagnosis?

    A. Right ectopic pregnancy
    B. PID
    C. Gastroenteritis
    D. Renal calculi
    E. Crohn's disease

2. In which of the following is the pathogenesis of acute appendicitis and diverticulitis similar?

    A. Lymphoid hyperplasia
    B. Increased bulk of stool
    C. Western diet
    D. Primary bacterial invasion
    E. Obstruction by a fecalith

HPI: LC, a 23-year-old woman, presents with 9 months of low abdominal pain and intermittent diarrhea. The pain has intensified over the past few months greater on the right side. She characterizes it as crampy and constant; nothing worsens or relieves the pain. LC's bowel movements have become looser but do not contain any mucus or blood. She also notes weight loss, malaise, fatigue, and intermittent fevers.

PE: LC is 5'8" tall and weighs 115 pounds. She has normal vital signs and is afebrile. She is thin and appears ill. Her abdomen has positive bowel sounds, is soft, nontender, and slightly distended, with no rebound, no guard, a slight right lower quadrant fullness. Her rectum has normal tone, guaiac (+).

Labs: WBC 15 (4.5–11 $\times$ 10^3 per μL); hemoglobin 11 (12–16 g/dL); hematocrit 32 (35% to 45%); platelet 243 (159–450 $\times$ 10^3 per μL); bilirubin (tot) 0.2 (0.2–1.0 mg/dL); bilirubin (dir) 0.1 (0.0–0.2 mg/dL); AST/SGOT 12 (7–40 U/L); ALT/SGPT 23 (7–40 U/L); alk phos 100 (70–230 U/L); amylase 34 (25–125 U/L); lipase 5 (10–140 U/L); albumin 2.7 (3.5–5.5g/dL); ESR 60 (< 20mm/hour)

LC undergoes several diagnostic examinations to better elucidate the source of her symptoms. An abdominal radiograph reveals dilated loops of small bowel with air-fluid levels and moderate air in the colon. Next, she undergoes a barium enema, which is significant for a normal colon and a stricture is noted in the distal ileum with proximal dilation. Finally, endoscopy is performed that is diagnostic. The findings include a granular mucosal surface with nodules and areas of friability as well as erosions and aphthous ulcers. A serpiginous linear ulceration is observed with sharply demarcated areas of normal mucosa. Mucosal biopsy of the affected areas reveals transmural involvement with non-caseating granulomas and significant inflammatory infiltrate.

Thought Questions

- What is the *most likely* diagnosis for this patient?

- Which key components of the history, physical exam, lab and study results lead to and confirm this diagnosis?

- How do you differentiate between the two main causes of this disorder?

- What are the common and rare sequelae of this disorder?

- What are the proposed etiologies of these disorders?

Basic Science Review and Discussion

LC has a chronic relapsing disorder broadly termed **inflammatory bowel disease** (IBD) and specifically, **Crohn's** disease. There are two types of IBD: Crohn's and **ulcerative colitis.** Each possesses a unique presentation, sequelae, and gross and histologic findings; however, they share in common an elusive etiologic process that results in a final common pathway of inflammatory damage. IBD runs in families as there is a tenfold increase in first-degree relatives as well as concordance in twin studies. Normally, the physiologic state of the intestine is one of balance between immune activation and down-regulation. It is unclear what tips the scales in favor of activation in cases of Crohn's

disease and ulcerative colitis (UC); many theories exist but none adequately explains the pathogenesis. Proposed infectious etiologies are ambiguous at best with culprits including viruses, bacteria, atypical bacteria, and even food antigens, but the data are unclear; another theory stems from the observation of increased mucosal permeability and abnormal mucosal glycoproteins in patients with IBD; other theories point to psychological associations. The most plausible theory stems from altered immune system functioning. Possible causes include abnormal proliferation of cytokines, abnormal antigen-presenting cells or lymphocytes, or antiepithelial antibodies. Regardless of the exact mechanism, the immune system is activated and mucosal injury occurs.

Pathophysiology of Crohn's Disease LC suffers from **Crohn's disease**—a chronic inflammatory condition affecting mostly young women in their late teens and twenties (a second peak incidence occurs among women in their 50s and 60s). Crohn's affects all layers of the tract wall (i.e., **transmural**) most commonly in the small bowel and colon (40%), the terminal ileum alone (30%), or the colon alone (20%), but may affect any place in the alimentary tract. Patients present with chronic colicky pain often in the area where the disease is first active. LC's pain is the right lower quadrant, which is the area where the stricture was discovered. Another hallmark of Crohn's disease is the discontinuous nature of the lesions or "skip" areas (**skip lesions**) that are sharply contrasted with areas of normal mucosa. There are several hallmarks that help differentiate Crohn's disease from UC. Initially, the shallow ulcerations resemble canker sores. As these lesions grow, the ulcerations coalesce into linear lesions, contrasted with nearby normal mucosa; the classic description is a **"cobblestone"** appearance. These linear lesions are at danger of becoming fistulae into any nearby structures (e.g., bowel, skin, bladder, vagina etc.). On gross inspection, the mucosal wall is noted to be rubbery, thick, and erythematous secondary to edema, inflammatory infiltration, fibrosis, and hypertrophy of the muscularis propria. This results in a narrowed lumen seen as a **"string sign"** on barium enema. Histologically, there is mucosal ulceration and inflammation characterized by neutrophils that invade the crypts and result in crypt abscesses. The destructive process continues with crypt atrophy. As in our patient, the inflammation and ulcerative destruction occurs through all layers; hence, the pathognomonic, **transmural** involvement. Finally, Crohn's disease is commonly accompanied by noncaseating granulomas.

The course of Crohn's is of relapsing and remitting symptoms, occasionally worsened by physical or psychological stress. **Microcytic anemia** is common with nearly perpetual loss of red blood cells. Other associations and sequelae help describe the disease, direct treatment, and differentiate Chron's disease from UC. As discussed earlier, strictures can complicate affected regions often in the small intestine as can fistulas to the bowel or other organs. If the small bowel has significant disease, the patient can suffer from malabsorption, protein loss, and various vitamin deficiencies (e.g., B_{12}). Additionally, sufferers of Crohn's can have a multitude of extra-intestinal manifestations including arthritis, ankylosing spondylitis, erythema nodosum, clubbing of the nails,

perihepatic cholangitis, or uveitis. There is a five- to six-fold increased risk of GI cancers in patients with long-standing Crohn's disease.

Pathophysiology of Ulcerative Colitis   UC is also a chronic ulcero-inflammatory condition of unknown etiology affecting only the colon. UC is rare but has a slightly higher incidence than Crohn's disease. In the United States, whites and females are more often affected than their counterparts and the onset of disease often occurs in the 20s. Patients complain of crampy pain, rectal bleeding, tenesmus and chronic diarrhea with blood and mucus. UC only affects the colon and the diseased tissues extend only into the submucosa; the anus is not involved. The disease begins at the rectum and extends proximally leaving behind a friable red mucosa. Characteristically, the diseased mucosa progresses to ulcerations with pseudopolyps that progress histologically into **crypt abscesses** with eventual atrophy. In only the most severe cases does the illness progress past the submucosa into the muscularis propria; in these severe cases there is a higher risk of toxic megacolon (complete cessation of bowel function). Histologically, there is mucosal damage and ulceration in affected areas with a mononuclear infiltrate in the propria with neutrophils and mast cells. Like Crohn's disease, there is an increased incidence in adenocarcinoma of the colon, which is proportional to the duration of the illness. Dysplasia can arise in different sites increasing a patient's risk of adenocarcinoma by almost 30 times. Clearly, surveillance is important. Common associations include sclerosing pericholangitis and ankylosing spondylitis (with HLA B-27).

Case Conclusion   LC was treated with immunosuppressive medications and her symptoms improved greatly. She also noted the importance of limiting her psychological stressors because her number of exacerbations appeared to be related to the stress level of her job and personal life. LC's anemia and hypoalbuminemia also improved with immunosuppressive therapy. She has not had any extra-intestinal manifestations of her illness.

Thumbnail: Inflammatory Bowel Disease—Ulcerative Colitis versus Crohn's Disease

	Ulcerative Colitis	Crohn's Disease
Location	Begins at rectum, extends to colon commonly; rarely affects the anus	Small intestine, colon commonly, but any part of alimentary tract
Depth	Mucosa, submucosa	Transmural
Gross	Diffuse ulceration, pseudopolyps, no strictures, thin wall, dilated lumen	Skip lesions with strictures, thick or thin wall (thick in small bowel), cobblestone appearance
Histology	Crypt atrophy and abscess, many pseudopolyps, mild lymphocytes and PMNs	Deep linear ulcers, noncaseating granulomas, marked inflammatory infiltrate (lympho, polymorphonuclear [PMN]), fistulas
Sequelae	Increased risk for adenocarcinoma (30 to 35 years after diagnosis), sclerosing pericholangitis, toxic megacolon	Increased risk for GI malignancy (not as high as UC) extra-intestinal manifestations (polyarthritis, uveitis clubbing of the nails, ankylosing spondylitis), strictures, fistulas, malabsorption, protein-losing enteropathy, fat-soluble vitamin deficiency

Key Points

Ulcerative Colitis
▶ Presents with relapsing attack of bloody diarrhea, tenesmus, mucus in stool, pain
▶ Labs: may have no abnormalities, rarely microcytic anemia
▶ Etiology: ultimately idiopathic, several theories exist: infections, genetics, intestinal mucosal structural abnormalities, abnormal immunoreactivity
▶ Treatment: immunosuppression, surgery

Crohn's Disease
▶ Presents with intermittent colickly abdominal pain, diarrhea, fever

▶ Labs: Fat and vitamin malabsorption (low albumin, deficiency of fat soluble vitamins A, D, E, and K) abnormal liver function tests (cholangitis), elevated creatinine (strictures obstructing the ureters) electrolytes
▶ Etiology: ultimately idiopathic, several theories exist: infections, genetics, intestinal mucosal structural abnormalities, abnormal immunoreactivity
▶ Treatment: immunosuppression

Questions

1. A 28-year-old female presents with an 8-month history of bloody diarrhea, intermittent crampy abdominal pain, persistent spasms of the bowel, and stringy mucus in her stools. You suspect IBD, with the likely diagnosis of UC. Which of the following will allow you to differentiate it from Crohn's disease?
   A. areas of affected and unaffected mucosa, "skip" lesions
   B. Transmural involvement on biopsy
   C. Involvement of the small bowel
   D. Pseudopolyps
   E. Fistula formation

2. A 33-year-old white female presents with colicky right lower quadrant abdominal pain, diarrhea, and rectal bleeding for over 10 years. You perform the appropriate work-up. Her biopsy reveals colon and small bowel involvement with characteristic transmural skip lesions, a cobblestone appearance, and a narrow lumen in the distal small bowel. She presents 3 months later with electrolyte abnormalities and complains of tingling and numbness in her hands and feet. Which of the following laboratory abnormalities would you expect to receive?
   A. Decreased hemoglobin and hematocrit, macrocytosis
   B. Low albumin
   C. Decreased hemoglobin and hematocrit and microcytosis
   D. Abnormal clotting profile
   E. Decreased bone mineral density

3. A 55-year-old white female with a 30-year history of UC returns for a follow-up visit. She recently recovered from an acute exacerbation for which she was hospitalized and given immunosuppressive therapy, to which she responded. She knows about her increased risk for adenocarcinoma of the colon. Which of the following is *more common* in patients who suffer from UC than Crohn's disease?
   A. Fistula formation
   B. Aphthous ulcers
   C. Toxic megacolon
   D. Granulomas
   E. Malabsorption

HPI: KJ, a 67-year-old male, presents with a 2-day history of crampy abdominal pain. He reports that the pain is in the left lower quadrant and is associated with nausea and a loss of appetite. Initially, the pain was only intermittent, but is now constant and more severe. KJ also feels flushed. Although he is normally constipated, over the past 2 days KJ has had bouts of constipation and diarrhea.

PE: He is 6′ tall and weighs 215 pounds. Vital signs: T 38.1°C; HR 92; BP 135/81; RR 16. In general, KJ is flushed; his abdomen is obese and soft, with notable left lower quadrant tenderness; he has no rebound, guarding, bowel sounds are present. There is no distension and the rectal is normal without traces of heme.

Labs: WBC 17.5 (4.5–11 × 10^3 per μL); diff-neutrophil 88% (57% to 67%); seg 60% (54% to 62%); bands 18% (3% to 5%); hemoglobin 13 (12–16 g/dL); hematocrit 40 (35% to 45%); platelet 243 (159–450 × 10^3 per μL).

You order an abdominal x-ray followed by a CT of the abdomen. The x-ray series is normal and shows no free air but the CT reveals colonic wall thickening and stranding of pericoloic fat. There are no areas suspicious for abscess. Again, no air is noted in the abdominal cavity.

Thought Questions

- What is the diagnosis for this patient?

- What is the physiology of the colon?

- What is the difference between a "true" and "false" diverticula?

- What is the proposed etiology and the sequelae of this disorder?

Basic Science Review and Discussion

Pathophysiology of Diverticulum, Diverticulosis, and Diverticulitis A **diverticulum** is a mucosal herniation leading off of the alimentary tract that is contiguous with the lumen of the gut. Most **diverticula** are acquired; that is, "false" in that they have an attenuated or absent muscularis propria. "True" diverticula have all three layers of the gastrointestinal (GI) tract included; an example, **Meckel's**, will be discussed below. **Diverticulosis** is many diverticula in a single patient. Colonic diverticula are common in older (> age 50) patients who eat a Western diet that is commonly low in fiber. As many as 50% of Americans over age 60 have been diagnosed with diverticulosis. The theorized etiology is based on the physiology of peristalsis. In a Western diet, low fiber increases intestinal transit time, which necessitates increased intraluminal pressure to propel stool. The colon is lined with three longitudinal bands of muscle called **taeniae coli.** Diverticula often form along the taeniae coli where the wall is penetrated by the blood vessels and nerves forming weak spots. These weak spots are susceptible to increased intraluminal pressure. The propulsive activity results in painful cramps, often in the left lower quadrant. Indeed, the sigmoid is the most commonly affected portion of the colon, but fortunately only 20% of those patients with diverticula become symptomatic. Many cases of diverticulosis resolve with little intervention. KJ has diverticulitis, a limited infection of the diverticula; this occurs when a fecalith obstructs the neck of the diverticulum leading to a microperforation and swelling of the adjacent tissues. This diagnosis is based on KJ's history, physical exam, fever, and elevated white blood cell count. The CT scan illustrates the local infection with stranding and colonic wall thickening. Sequelae from diverticulosis include hematochezia, diverticulitis, perforation, abscess formation, bowel stenosis, and fistula formation.

Physiology of the Colon The main function of the colon is to reabsorb water and electrolytes. Just as in the small intestine, the colon wall is made up of similar layers: the mucosa, submucosa, muscularis propria (inner circular and outer longitudinal layers) and adventitia. The mucosa is composed of columnar absorptive cells that have numerous **goblet cells** and microvilli. The mucosa is predominantly flat, lacking villi but is interspersed with finger-like crypts that extend through the level of the mucosa to the muscularis mucosa. The crypts contain goblet and endocrine cells. The colon regenerates from the crypts as proliferation and differentiation of cells is followed by migration from the depths of the crypts that replenishes the surface every 3 to 8 days. Colonic peristalsis increases contact of the luminal contents with the mucosa maximizing absorption. As described in the Hirschprung's case, peristalsis is mediated both intrinsically (via the myenteric plexus) and extrinsically (via autonomic innervation).

Gross and Histologic Appearance of Diverticulosis The appearance of a diverticula is a flask-like circular out-pouching, often 0.5 to 1 cm in diameter, commonly in the sigmoid colon. In fact, 95% of those diagnosed with diverticulosis have disease in the sigmoid along the taeniae coli. These defects are compressible and easily empty of luminal contents. Histologically, these appear as a tissue under increased pressure with atrophic mucosa and a weakened or even absent muscularis propria. The taeniae coli are unusually prominent and hypertrophy of nearby layers of the circular layer of the muscularis propria is also observed.

Pathophysiology of Meckel's Diverticulum Meckel's diverticulum is a "true" congenital diverticulum often located in the terminal ileum from a remnant of the **vitelline duct.** The vitelline duct connects the lumen of the developing GI tract to the yolk sac and usually involutes in utero. When it does not, Meckel's diverticulum results. Meckel's diverticulum is usually located within 30 cm of the ileocecal valve and contains mucosa, submucosa, and muscularis propria. Fortunately, most persons are asymptomatic because it affects approximately 2% of the population; however, many who are symptomatic have GI bleeding. Additionally, 50% of the patient population have heterotopic nests of gastric mucosa that may ulcerate and present with symptoms that mimic appendicitis. Patients with Meckel's are at an increased risk for intussusception, incarceration, or perforation and may present with symptoms characteristic of these complications.

Case Conclusion KJ is admitted to the hospital, given intravenous fluids and antibiotics, and is not allowed to eat or drink. His pain is also controlled. He improves quite rapidly and is pain free by the third hospital day. KJ tolerates a regular diet and leaves with continuation of his antibiotics by mouth.

Thumbnail: Diverticulosis

Epidemiology

Occurs in 50% of those over age 60 who eat a Western diet

Presentation

Left lower quadrant crampy pain, change in bowel habits (constipation, diarrhea, alternating diarrhea and constipation), distension, sensation of never completely emptying rectum, rectal bleeding (5% to 10%)

Pathogenesis

Diet low in fiber, increasing intestinal transit time, increased intraluminal pressure, weak spot where vessels traverse colonic wall, out-pouching of colonic mucosa, "false" diverticula

Sequelae

Microperforation (diverticulitis with fever, WBC count), perforation, abscess, fistula, massive bleeding

---

Key Points

▶ Meckel's diverticulum is/has: a congenital abnormality as vitelline duct that does not involute, which creates a "true" diverticulum of all three layers (mucosa, submucosa, and muscularis propria)

▶ Present in 2% of population

▶ Often asymptomatic, but most commonly presents with bleeding

▶ Sequelae include intussusception, incarceration, hernia, ulcer formation, and bleeding

▶ Usually located within 30 cm of the ileocecal valve, often in the distal ileum

Questions

1. A 65-year-old woman presents to the emergency department with obvious diaphoresis and shortness of breath. You quickly ascertain that she has had a large amount of bright red blood from her rectum (hematochezia). What is the *most likely* cause of this bleeding?
   A. Diverticulosis
   B. Diverticulitis
   C. Angiodysplasia
   D. Adenocarcinoma of the colon
   E. Appendicitis

2. You have just diagnosed diverticulitis in a 63-year-old woman and are trying to determine which intravenous antibiotic to administer. You choose an aminoglycoside for gram-negative aerobic organisms and another drug to cover which of the following important bacteria?
   A. Anaerobic gram-positive bacteria
   B. Protozoa
   C. Aerobic gram-positive bacteria
   D. Anaerobic gram-negative bacteria
   E. Obligate intracellular parasites

3. A 67-year-old woman who has had three previous attacks of diverticulitis returns to your clinic and reports that she loathes eating the high-fiber diet you have restricted her to. She asks why this diet prevents a recurrence of her disease. Which of the following is *not* a reason why a high-fiber diet prevents attacks of diverticulosis?
   A. Fiber decreases gut transit time
   B. Fiber increases stool weight
   C. Fiber lowers intraluminal pressure
   D. Fiber decreases muscle hypertrophy
   E. Fiber strengthens the mucosa

HPI: JS, a 48-year-old male, complains of three days of nausea, vomiting, and abdominal pain. He describes the pain as crampy in nature without localization or relief. Three days ago, soon after the pain began, JS had a bowel movement, which afforded him some relief. Yesterday he began vomiting green material. He reports no meals for 4 days and no bowel movements for 3 days. On direct questioning he reports that the emesis also relieves his pain. He reports a history of two abdominal surgeries: "gallbladder" removal and an exploratory laparotomy following a car accident.

PE: JS is 5'7" tall and weighs 145 pounds. Vital signs: T 37.3°C; HR 90; BP 133/86; RR 18. He is in obvious discomfort. His abdomen shows two well-healed scars—one in the right upper quadrant, the other vertical from pubic bone to xiphoid; + bowel sounds but hyperactive with occasional rushes, soft, tender to soft palpation over the entire abdomen, marked distension, no rebound or guarding; rectal, heme (−).

Labs: WBC 12.5 (4.5–11 × 10³ per μL); diff-neutrophil 55% (57% to 67%); seg 40% (54% to 62%); hemoglobin 16 (12–16 g/dL); hematocrit 48 (35% to 45%); platelet 243 (159–450 × 10³ per μL); sodium 135 (135–145 mmol/L); potassium 3.8 (3.5–5.0 mmol/L); chloride 98 (98–108 mmol/L); bicarbonate 24 (24–32 mmol/L); BUN 12 (7–18 mg/dL); creatinine 1.0 (0.6–1.2 mg/dL).

You order an x-ray of the abdomen. The kidney ureter bladder and upright abdominal radiograph reveals multiple loops of distended small bowel that have air-fluid levels (layering) and a "stepladder" pattern, with no gas in the colon. There is no free air under the diaphragm.

Thought Questions

- What is the *most likely* diagnosis for this patient?

- Which key components of the history and lab results lead to this diagnosis?

- What are the common and rare sequelae of this disorder?

- What is the etiology of this disorder?

Basic Science Review and Discussion

Presentation of Intestinal Obstruction The gastrointestinal (GI) tract may become obstructed at any level; however, the most common site is the small intestine because it has the narrowest lumen. The differential diagnosis of intestinal **obstruction** is great. In this discussion, a congenital cause—Hirschsprung's disease—is omitted. The most common causes of intestinal obstruction and their presentations are discussed here. Like JS, patients with obstruction complain of diffuse pain, nausea, vomiting, inability to pass flatus, and obstipation. They are often markedly distended on examination, tender to light palpation yet have no masses or specific tender areas; they also have hyperactive bowel sounds with rushes.

On laboratory examination, these individuals may evidence dehydration (edematous bowel with decreased oral intake) with elevated hematocrit, as well as electrolyte abnormalities indicating renal compromise (increased blood urea nitrogen [BUN] and creatinine with a ratio often > 20:1).

Some patients have evidence of hypochloremic hypokalemic metabolic acidosis from prolonged emesis of acidic gastric contents. In JS, the abdominal imaging is classic for small bowel obstruction with distended loops of small bowel, air-fluid levels in the absence of colonic gas.

Common Etiologies and Pathophysiology of Obstruction JS has had two abdominal surgeries and this is likely related to the cause of his small bowel obstruction. **Adhesions** are the most common cause of obstruction and are commonly acquired after peritonitis from a previous surgery, intra-abdominal infection (e.g., pelvic inflammatory disease [PID]), or endometriosis. Regardless of the cause, as the inflammation heals, adhesions develop between the anterior and lateral abdominal wall and loops of small bowel. These fibrous adhesions can cause closed loops through which other viscera can slide increasing pressure that may impair venous drainage. Resultant stasis and edema increase the size of the stuck loop and lead to **incarceration** or permanent trapping. Following incarceration, the arterial blood supply becomes compromised (**strangulation**), which leads to infarction of the trapped segment.

Indirect and direct **inguinal hernias** (as well as umbilical and ventral) are the second most common cause of obstruction when these incarcerate. A **hernia** is a weakness or defect in the abdominal wall that allows the protrusion of a pouch-like sac of peritoneum. The small or large bowel or even the omentum may become stuck. The pathway to infarction is similar to that in adhesions. More specifically, in **indirect inguinal hernias** the small bowel passes laterally to the triangle of Hesselbach, through the deep and superficial inguinal rings, and into the scrotum. This defect is secondary to failure of closure of the processus vaginalis during embryonic development and is discovered in young boys. When a patient suffers from a **direct inguinal hernia,** the bowel protrudes through the posterior wall of the canal— the center of the triangle of Hesselbach; direct inguinal hernias are often observed in older men. There are many types of hernias. An **umbilical hernia** is common in pregnant women, children, and individuals with ascites; a **ventral hernia** occurs through an incisional site.

Another cause of obstruction—**intussusception**—occurs when one segment of proximal bowel, which is constricted during peristalsis, telescopes into the immediate distal segment of bowel. The proximal portion is often the termi-

nal ileum and the distal is the cecum. Once it is trapped, the bowel is pushed farther with peristalsis, which pulls the mesentery along with it. These patients are usually infants or children who present with colicky abdominal pain and rectal bleeding ("currant-jelly stools") from infarction. In adults, intussusception signifies a tumor, polyps, or intraluminal mass as the nidus of initiation.

Volvulus is a complete twisting of the bowel around the base of attachment that occurs most commonly in large redundant loops of sigmoid. The twisting along the mesentery causes obstruction and subsequent infarction. Other causes, not discussed here, include tumor, inflammatory strictures, foreign bodies, congenital strictures, cystic fibrosis, imperforate anus, and obstructive gallstones.

Case Conclusion   JS is given aggressive fluid replacement and reluctantly agrees to placement of a nasogastric tube that is placed on suction. This allows for decompression of the small bowel. He improves quickly and avoids surgery to lyse the adhesions. JS develops no electrolyte abnormalities and has no evidence of permanent bowel injury (fever, leukocytosis, acidosis, or peritoneal signs). He begins a regular diet on hospital day two after a small bowel movement.

Thumbnail: GI Pathophysiology—Small Bowel Obstruction

Presents with diffuse abdominal pain, nausea, vomiting of stomach contents; tender abdomen with hyperactive bowel sounds, distension, no focal pain

Risk factors include a history of surgery, adhesions, hernia, cancer

Kinking of bowel wall secondary to some anatomical disruption or compression of lumen by fibrous adhesions or the incarceration of

bowel through a hernia sac pressure results in decreased venous drainage followed by stasis and edema

Without release infarction or strangulation may ensue

Abdominal imaging reveals (1) loops of distended small bowel, (2) air-fluid levels, and (3) usually no gas in colon

Dehydration, electrolyte abnormalities, prerenal acute renal failure, hypochloremic metabolic acidosis, bowel ischemia, and infarction

---

Key Points

▶ Pressure is exerted on loop of bowel with decreased venous drainage; stasis and edema follow increasing pressure leading to permanence (incarceration); with time the arterial supply is compromised (strangulation); infarction ensues

▶ Causes and risks include adhesions from previous surgery, peritonitis, endometriosis

In order of relative frequency

▶ Indirect inguinal hernia (protrudes lateral to triangle) a congenital defect; processus vaginalis does not close, usually found in young boys

▶ Direct inguinal hernia (through Hesselbach), usually occurs in elderly men

▶ Umbilical hernia is found in children and adults with ascites or pregnancy
Ventral hernia is caused by a previous surgery
Intussusception is found in children, adults with tumors, polyps, or mass
Volvulus are large redundant loops of bowel

Questions

1. A 56-year-old woman with newly diagnosed colon cancer presents to the emergency room with 4 days of abdominal pain, nausea, vomiting, and distension. She has a temperature of 38.7°C, peritoneal signs, and her laboratory values are suggestive of infection, acidosis, dehydration, and acute renal failure. Which of the following is the *most appropriate* management choice?

   A. Surgery because her bowel has no blood supply
   B. Fluid management that will correct her acidosis and prerenal failure
   C. Nasogastric decompression to improve her symptoms
   D. Imaging because you need a definitive diagnosis
   E. Admit for observation

2. Which of the following risks is *appropriately matched* with the resultant type of obstruction?

   A. Indirect inguinal hernia—usually elderly men
   B. Ventral hernia—pregnancy
   C. Intussusception—cancer
   D. Direct inguinal hernia—ascites
   E. Adhesion—congenital defect

Case 14

1. B
2. C
3. A
4. C

Case 15

1. A
2. D
3. E

Case 16

1. D
2. E
3. B
4. A

Case 17

1. C
2. B
3. E
4. D

Case 18

1. D
2. A
3. E

Case 19

1. A
2. E
3. B

Case 20

1. D
2. A

Case 21

1. C
2. E
3. B

Case 22

1. E
2. C

Case 23

1. D
2. E
3. B

Case 24

1. D
2. E

Case 25

1. D
2. C

Case 26

1. A
2. C
3. D
4. B

Case 27

1. D
2. E

Case 28

1. B
2. E

Case 29

1. D
2. A
3. C

Case 30

1. A
2. D
3. E

Case 31

1. A
2. C

Part III

Rheumatology

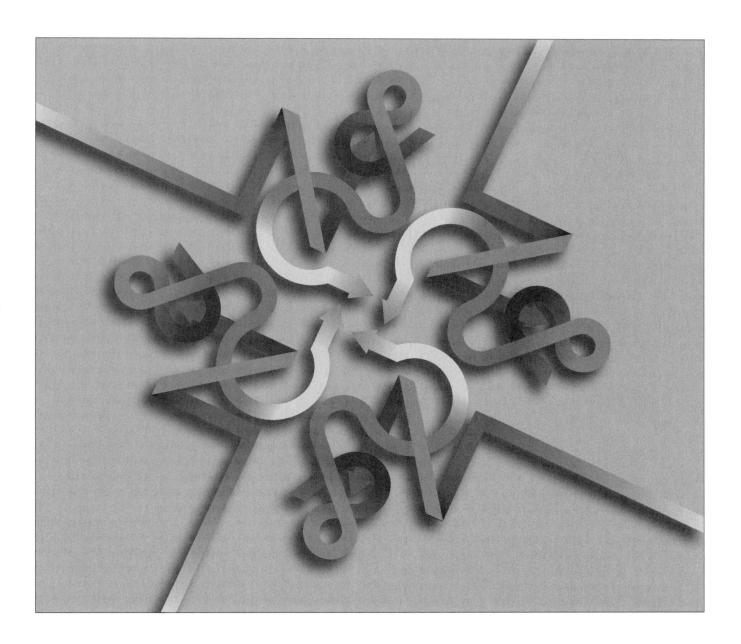

HPI: BH, a 30-year-old African American woman, presents to her primary care physician complaining of joint pain in her fingers for the past 2 months. The patient also reports associated fatigue, loss of appetite, and weight loss. Initially, BH felt it could be related to increased stress from her job at an Internet start-up company. However, her symptoms have persisted despite a recent 2-week vacation in Hawaii. She states that she felt even worse after her lazy days at the beach. Activities such as body surfing and snorkeling were less enjoyable because she found herself sensitive to the bright sunshine. Moreover, BH complains of an unusual "sunburn" that has continued to bother her since her return. The patient is concerned and feels that now she has turned 30 everything in her body is going awry. "My hair seems to be falling out and even brushing my teeth seems to give me trouble as my gums are always seeming to bleed!" she exclaims. She recalls her mother having arthritis and always being sickly and fears that soon she will be the same way. The patient denies any past medical history. She has no drug allergies, and is currently taking birth control pills and multivitamins. Both of her parents have hypertension and, in addition to arthritis, BH's mother is currently receiving dialysis for renal failure.

PE: The patient is noted to have a low grade fever of 38.1°C. Her vital signs are otherwise within normal limits. She is noted to be a thin, athletically built woman who is anxious but in no acute distress. A butterfly rash with scaling is noted on her face, and discrete macular lesions are observed on her arms and legs. Ocular exam reveals acute sensitivity to having a light shined into her eyes. Oral ulcers are seen on the hard palate. The patient has no lymphadenopathy and her thyroid is noted to be normal. Cardiac, pulmonary, and abdominal exams are unremarkable. Extremity exam reveals swelling and tenderness of her distal interphalangeal (DIP) joints in both hands.

Labs: WBC 5.0; RBC 38.0; platelets 75,000; creatinine 0.9; ESR 120; rheumatoid factor positive; ANA positive; urinalysis 1.012, negative protein, negative ketones, no WBC, no RBC.

Thought Questions

■ What is the *most likely* diagnosis for this patient?

■ What is *immunologic tolerance* and how is it achieved?

■ How would you describe the proposed mechanisms for autoimmunity?

■ If BH's mother's renal failure was caused by SLE what would you expect to see on a biopsy of her kidney and how would you follow her disease?

■ What is the mechanism underlying this patient's thrombocytopenia?

Basic Science Review and Discussion

Clinical Features and Epidemiology This young woman most likely has **systemic lupus erythematosus (SLE),** an autoimmune disorder. This disease is seen predominantly in women with a 9:1 female to male ratio. There is also a higher prevalence in black women 1:250 versus 1:1000 for Caucasian women. The onset is typically between age 16 and 55. SLE can affect nearly every organ system in the body and is therefore a disease with varying presentations. BH has a typical presentation with vague constitutional symptoms of fatigue, anorexia, weight loss, and fever in conjunction with arthritis (seen in 95%) and abnormalities of the skin, hair, and mucous membranes (seen in 85%).

The **arthritis** associated with this disorder is usually symmetric and involves the small joints of the hands and feet. The two most common skin manifestations of SLE are (1) a classic malar butterfly rash that is an erythematous, confluent macular rash with fine scaling covering both cheeks and the bridge of the nose and frequently sensitive to sunlight; and (2) discrete discoid erythematous plaques on the face, scalp, forearms, fingers and toes. Diffuse alopecia and painless mucosal ulcers are also commonly seen. Other organs that can be affected include the kidneys, lung pleura, pericardium, cardiac valves, and central nervous system (CNS). These patients are also noted to have hematologic disorders including hemolytic anemia, thrombocytopenia, lymphopenia, and leukocytopenia.

Because this disease can vary widely in its presentation, criteria for diagnosis were established in 1982 and are outlined in Box 32-1.

Tolerance and Autoimmunity **Immunologic tolerance** is unresponsiveness of a functioning immune system to certain antigens. It prevents the immune system from attacking self tissues and allows a fetus to develop in the womb without being rejected by the maternal immune system. Immunosuppressive drugs given following organ transplantation enhance tolerance preventing rejection of

---

Box 32-1 Criteria for the Classification of SLE*

1. Malar rash
2. Discoid rash
3. Photosensitivity
4. Oral ulcers
5. Arthritis
6. Serositis
7. Renal disease
   a. > 0.5 gm/day proteinuria or
   b. ≥ 3+ proteinuria on dipstick or
   c. cellular casts
8. Neurologic disease
   a. seizures or
   b. psychosis (without other cause)
9. Hematologic disorders
   a. hemolytic anemia, or
   b. leukopenia (< 4000/μl), or
   c. lymphopenia (< 1500/μl), or
   d. thrombocytopenia (< 100,000/μl)
10. Immunologic abnormalities
    a. positive LE cell preparation, or
    b. antibody to native DNA, or
    c. antibody to Sm, or
    d. false-positive serologic test for syphylis
11. Positive ANA

*To meet the diagnosis, a patient needs to have any four of the 11 criteria listed.

---

the foreign organs. **Clonal deletion** is the main process by which self-reactive **T-cells** are eliminated. During fetal development T-lymphocytes are exposed to self antigens, primarily self major histocompatibility proteins (MHC). Those **T-lymphocytes** that react with self antigens are "negatively selected" and die via programmed cell death. In the thymus, tolerance acquired in this way is termed **central tolerance**. The exact molecular mechanisms of this process are not as yet known or documented. **Clonal anergy** is tolerance that is acquired outside of the thymus. This process involves functional inactivation of T-cells. Tolerance acquired in this fashion may be transient and change over time. Like clonal deletion, the exact mechanism of clonal anergy is unknown. It is, however, suspected to be related to suppressor cells or inappropriate presentation of antigen and thus a failure of costimulatory signals. **B-cell** tolerance likely develops in a similar fashion with clonal deletion occurring in the bone marrow and clonal anergy in the periphery. However, B-cell tolerance is less complete and shorter lasting than that in T-cells as evidenced by the fact that most autoimmune diseases are mediated by antibodies.

Autoimmune disorders such as SLE occur when tolerance is lost. These diseases can involve humoral or cell-mediated reactions. However, most are **antibody mediated**. Three general mechanisms of autoimmunity have been suggested. The first involves release of sequestered antigens. According to this theory, the body possesses immunologically privi-

leged sites that contain tissues that are not exposed to the immune system. When these antigens are accidentally released into the circulation an immune response is triggered. A second possible mechanism underlying autoimmunity involves T-cell loss of tolerance. T-cell tolerance is maintained by continued presence of self antigen as well as the presence of suppressor T-cells that provide important constimulatory signals. Exposure to foreign antigens that are similar to self antigens may terminate tolerance and lead to an autoimmune response. Also, decreased suppressor T-cell function may lead to loss of T-cell tolerance. A third general mechanism of autoimmunity involves a loss of B-cell tolerance. This type of tolerance is far more readily lost than that of T-cells. Activated T-cells can produce interleukins and costimulatory proteins like CD 28, which in turn stimulate anergic B-cells to produce antibodies against self antigens.

Pathophysiology of SLE SLE is a multisystem autoimmune disease that varies widely in presentation. Almost every organ in the body can be affected. The disease itself is characterized by the production of auto-antibodies. Auto-antibodies directed at components of the cell nucleus, known as anti-nuclear antibodies (ANA), are most commonly seen. However, at this time the exact pathophysiology of all the various manifestations is not clearly understood. Examination of affected tissues at autopsy reveals minimal pathologic changes including nonspecific inflammation, vessel abnormalities, or no changes at all. The best characterized pathology is that observed in the kidney because biopsies of this organ are often performed in the course of the disease.

The renal damage caused by SLE is mediated by **immune complexes**. Auto-antibodies, primarily antinuclear antibodies and antidouble-stranded DNA antibodies react with antigens in the circulation and are deposited in the glomerulus. These complexes subsequently set off the complement cascade leading to the release of inflammatory mediators from circulating leukocytes. The resulting inflammation causes damage to the glomerular structure and glomerulonephritis results. Lupus patients with renal disease therefore have proteinuria, casts and white blood cells in their urine. On renal biopsy five histologic patterns have been described (Table 32-1).

Given that BH's mother has renal failure, the most likely lesion found on this patient's renal biopsy would be class 4. Patients with this lesion on biopsy are usually symptomatic with microscopic or gross hematuria, proteinuria severe enough to cause nephritic syndrome, hypertension, and mild to severe renal insufficiency. Once a biopsy is performed and the baseline level of disease is determined, serum complement and anti-DNA antibodies are followed serially. Decreasing complement and or increasing anti-DNA antibodies can thus be used as early indicators of disease

Table 32-1. Renal Disease in SLE

Class 1	Normal	Rare	* No abnormalities
Class 2	Mesangial lupus glomerulonephritis	25%	* Mildest
			* Slight to moderate increase in the intercapillary mesangial matrix
			* Granular mesangial deposits of immunoglobulin and complement are present
Class 3	Focal proliferative glomerulonephritis	20%	* Focal lesion affects < 50% of glomeruli
			* Swelling and proliferation of endothelial and mesangial cells
			* Infiltration with neutrophils ± fibrinoid deposits and intracapillary thrombi
Class 4	Diffuse proliferative glomerulonephritis	35%–40%	* Most serious
			* Most or all glomeruli involved
			* Proliferation of endothelial, mesangial, and sometimes epithelial cells; crescents filling Bowman's space
			* + Fibrinoid necrosis and hyaline thrombi
Class 5	Membranous glomerulonephritis	15%	* Widespread thickening of capillary walls

exacerbation or progression. Treatment consists of corticosteroids or immunosuppressive agents such as cyclophosphamide depending on the severity of the lesions and progression. Such therapy can be effective. However, it is important to realize that opportunistic infections as well as lupus nephritis are the leading causes of death in SLE patients.

In addition to forming antinuclear antibodies, patients with lupus form auto-antibodies against red cells, white cells, and platelets. Cell destruction is the result of type II hypersensitivity in which auto-antibodies bind antigens on the blood cell or platelet and the cell is either lysed through activation of the complement cascade and membrane attack complex or more commonly becomes susceptible to phagocytosis via fixation of the antibody or C3b to the cell surface.

Case Conclusion   The differential diagnosis is SLE, rheumatoid arthritis, discoid lupus. One month after diagnosing this patient with SLE and starting her on nonsteroidal anti-inflammatory drugs (NSAIDs) to relieve her joint pain and having her avoid sun exposure BH returns for follow-up. She reports that her skin rash is much improved and that she has less joint pain.

Thumbnail: Autoantibodies and Associations with Connective Tissue Diseases

Auto-Antibody	Main Disease Association	Other Disease Associations	Comments
Antinuclear antibody (ANA)	SLE	- Rheumatoid arthritis - Scleroderma - Sjögren's syndrome - Discoid and drug-induced lupus	Screening test for SLE, high sensitivity (95%), low specificity, titers do not correlate with disease severity
Anti-double-stranded DNA antibody (anti-ds-DNA)	SLE	- Rheumatoid arthritis - Connective tissue disease (low titers)	Good confirmatory test for SLE, high positive predictive value if high titers
Anti-Smith antibody (anti-Sm)	SLE	None	Low sensitivity, high specificity
Rheumatoid factor	Rheumatoid arthritis	SLE, chronic infections, elderly patients, some healthy patients	Low sensitivity, titers do not correlate with disease severity
Anti-ribonucleoprotein (RNP) antibody	Scleroderma, mixed connective tissue disease	SLE, Sjögren's syndrome, rheumatoid arthritis, discoid lupus	High sensitivity for MCTD (> 95%)
Anti-SS-A*/Ro antibody	Sjögren's syndrome	SLE, rheumatoid arthritis, vasculitis	Positive test associated with neonatal SLE and congenital heart block
Anticentromere antibody	CREST syndrome	Scleroderma, Raynaud's disease	High positive predictive value for scleroderma
Antineutrophil cytoplasmic antibody (ANCA)	Wegener's granulomatosis	Polyarteritis nodosa	Titers do not correlate with disease activity

MCTD, mixed connective-tissue disease
* SS-A, Sjögren's substance A = anti RO antibody

Key Points

▶ Immunologic tolerance occurs when the immune system fails to mount an immune response to a specific antigen. Loss of this immunologic tolerance can result in autoimmune disease.

▶ The two primary mechanisms of self-tolerance are **clonal deletion** and **clonal anergy. Clonal deletion** is the loss of self-reactive T- and B-lymphocytes that occurs in the process of maturation. **Clonal**

anergy is functional inactivation of lymphocytes that occurs in the periphery after encountering specific antigens.

▶ SLE is a multisystem autoimmune disease with multiple clinical presentations. The primary effect of this disease is a failure to process regulating self-tolerance, which results in the production of numerous auto-antibodies.

Questions

1. BH's younger sister now presents 3 weeks postpartum with fevers, arthritis, and fatigue. She denies any health problems except for some elevated blood pressures noted at the time of delivery that have been treated with hydralazine. What is the *most likely* diagnosis?
   - A. Postpartum arthritis
   - B. Rheumatoid arthritis
   - C. Lupus
   - D. Discoid lupus
   - E. Drug-induced lupus-like syndrome

2. You suspect that one of your patients has SLE. Which of the following is the *most specific* laboratory test that will help confirm your diagnosis?
   - A. Erythrocyte sedimentation rate (ESR)
   - B. Rheumatoid factor
   - C. ANA
   - D. Antidouble-stranded DNA antibody
   - E. Lupus anticoagulant

3. A patient presents with a malar rash, oral ulcers, pleuritis and psychosis. ANA titers are notably elevated. Which of the following *best* describes the mechanism underlying her disease?
   - A. Clonal deletion of self-reactive T-cells
   - B. Release of a sequestered antigen
   - C. Primary enzyme deficiency
   - D. Failed clonal anergy
   - E. Molecular mimicry

4. A patient with severe long-standing SLE dies of renal failure. On autopsy which of the following is *unlikely* to be observed?
   - A. Erosive changes in joints
   - B. Pleural effusion
   - C. Verrucous lesions on the mitral valve
   - D. "Onion skin lesions" in the central arteries of the spleen
   - E. Fibrinoid necrosis and hyaline thrombi affecting more than 50% of glomeruli

HPI: RS, a 38-year-old man, presents with a chief complaint of pain and stiffness of his hands, wrists, and knees that is most pronounced in the morning. He reports he hasn't really felt right for the past year following his divorce. Initially, he thought the fatigue, malaise, anorexia, and weight loss were all related to the lifestyle adjustments he had to make. However, now that his life is in order and he is enjoying himself more he continues to be bothered by his symptoms. Moreover, the problem with his hands and knees is starting to impair his ability to work as a plumber.

RH states that he has been healthy without any history of prior medical problems. He has never been hospitalized, has no drug allergies, and is currently taking no medications. RH is active and enjoys the outdoors. However, he admits that it has been increasingly difficult to hike and fish due to the pain in his joints. He denies tobacco use but does report consuming one or two beers after work and on the weekends.

PE: T 37.0°C; BP 132/78; HR 88; RR 18; SaO$_2$ 99%; Gen, thin. NAD CVR: RRR, chest CTA bilaterally. Abdomen, soft, non tender, +BS; extremities, + swelling, tenderness, and warmth over proximal interphalangeal joints of both hands and knees.

Labs: WBC 7.5; Hct 42; plt 360; ESR 98; ANA 1:250; rheumatoid factor 1:400.

Thought Questions

■ Who is most likely to get rheumatoid arthritis? What are the most common clinical manifestations?

■ How would you describe the changes that occur in the joints with rheumatoid arthritis? Which characteristic joint deformities develop after progressive joint destruction?

■ How would you describe the autoimmune reaction that occurs in the joints in rheumatoid arthritis? What are the key mediators of joint damage?

■ What is rheumatoid factor? What is the general structure of immunoglobulins? What are the different classes of immunoglobulins and what roles do they play in the immune response?

Basic Science Review and Discussion

Clinical Features   Rheumatoid arthritis is a chronic, inflammatory disease that can affect multiple organ systems including skin, blood vessels, heart, lungs, and muscles. The most common manifestation is destruction of articular cartilage. Rheumatoid arthritis's global prevalence is approximately 1% to 2% in the general population. This disease is more common in women with a 3:1 female to male predominance. The typical age of onset is the 20s and 30s. Initial symptoms are usually insidious with vague prodromal symptoms of malaise, weight loss, and joint stiffness. The stiffness is most pronounced in the morning and after periods of inactivity. Symmetric joint swelling, warmth, tenderness, and pain are noted. The most com-

monly affected joints include the proximal interphalangeal and metacarpophalangeal joints as well as the wrists, knees, ankles, and toes. Subcutaneous "rheumatoid" nodules located over bony prominences are seen in approximately 20% of patients with rheumatoid arthritis. Other less common extra-articular manifestations include pericarditis, pleural disease, and vasculitis.

Histopathology of the Joint in Rheumatoid Arthritis   In rheumatoid arthritis the joint undergoes characteristic changes as the disease progresses. Initially, the synovium becomes edematous, thickened and hyperplastic. An inflammatory infiltrate made up of CD4 cells, plasma cells, and macrophages fills the synovial stroma and increased vascularity is noted. This inflamed synovium assumes a polypoid form producing a pannus that then erodes into the underlying articular cartilage. Inflammatory cells release mediators that increase osteoclastic activity thereby allowing the synovium to further erode into the subchondral bone. The result is juxta-articular erosions and subchondral cysts. Over time, the articular cartilage is totally destroyed, the pannus expands bridging the distance between the opposing bones of the joint and forms a fibrous ankylosis that eventually ossifies. This process correlates with the clinical joint symptoms. Initially, joints are inflamed and painful. With time, the inflammation resolves as the normal anatomy of the joint is completely destroyed. This progressive joint destruction leads to characteristic deformities, including radial deviation of the wrist, ulnar deviation of the fingers, **boutonniere** deformity of the fingers (hyperextension of the distal interphalangeal joint with flexion of the proximal interphalangeal joint), and **swan-neck** deformity of the fingers (flexion of the distal interphalangeal joint with extension of the proximal interphalangeal joint).

Pathophysiology The exact initiating event for the synovitis characteristic of rheumatoid arthritis is currently unknown. However, it is postulated that this disease is triggered by an exposure of an immunogenetically susceptible host to an arthritogenic microbial antigen. A majority of patients with this disease have class II MHC molecules alleles HLA-DR4 and/or HLA-DR1 and thus have a shared binding site that predisposes them to development of synovial inflammation. Initiation of this inflammation is thought to occur with exposure to a microbial agent that has not yet been identified. This exposure triggers an autoimmune reaction within the synovial membranes. It is the inflammatory mediators of this reaction that ultimately cause joint destruction. T-cells play the primary role in the immune reaction in rheumatoid arthritis; in particular, CD4 memory T-cells. Shortly after the onset of joint symptoms large numbers of these cells are seen in the synovial fluid of the affected joints. The endothelial cells of the synovial vessels are subsequently activated and there is an increase in the expression of intracellular adhesion molecules-1 (ICAM-1). As a result other inflammatory cells such as neutrophils, plasma cells and macrophages are recruited to the joint. Activated T-cells, B-cells and macrophages then release numerous cytokines including **TNF-alpha** and **IL-1,** which stimulates the release of **collagenases** from synovial cells and inhibits synthesis of proteoglycans in cartilage thus leading to destruction of cartilage. Neutrophils release **proteases** and **elastases** that further contribute to the alteration of the normal structure of the joint.

Rheumatoid factor is an IgM autoantibody that reacts with the Fc portion of autologous IgG molecules. It is found in about 3% of healthy persons and its incidence increases with age. More than 75% of persons with rheumatoid arthritis will have this autoantibody present in their serum. High levels of the antibody are commonly associated with severe disease. However, this auto-antibody is not unique to rheumatoid arthritis; it is also observed in other conditions including sarcoiditis, tuberculosis, leprosy, parasitic infections, sarcoidosis and other autoimmune disease such as systemic lupus erythematosus (SLE). In rheumatoid arthritis, these autoantibodies form immune complexes with autologous IgG molecules. These immune complexes are found in the serum, synovial fluid, and synovial membranes. Those found in the serum are believed to be responsible for the extra-articular manifestations of rheumatoid arthritis.

Antibodies Antibodies are proteins that react with specific antigens and thus play an important role in humoral immunity. They make up 20% of serum proteins and are produced by plasma cells. Structurally, these globular proteins are composed of four polypeptide chains, two identical heavy chains and two identical light chains that form a "Y" shape. The variable regions of the light and heavy chains are located at the tips of the Y and are where antigen binding occurs. In contrast, the constant regions of these chains are responsible for complement activation and binding to cells' surface receptors. If treated with proteolytic enzymes antibodies are broken into three pieces: two identical **Fab fragments** containing the antigen binding sites, and one Fc fragment that is made up of the constant regions of the heavy chains. It is this **Fc fragment** that rheumatoid factor binds to.

There are five classes of antibodies: IgG, IgM, IgA, IgE, and IgD. **IgG** is the predominant class and is made up of immunoglobulin monomers (two heavy chains/two light chains). This antibody class plays an important role in the secondary host defense response against bacteria and viruses through opsonization and complement fixation. It is the only antibody that can cross the placenta. **IgM** is the antibody produced in a primary immune response. It is a pentamer made up of five immunoglobulin monomers connected by a J (joining) chain. This class of antibody has a total of 10 antigen binding sites and is the most efficient immunoglobulin in agglutination and complement fixation and therefore plays a key role in host defenses against bacterial and viral infections. **IgA** is the primary antibody found in secretions including saliva, tears, intestinal/GI/genital secretions, and colostrum. IgA molecules are made up of two immunoglobulin monomers connected by one J chain. This class of antibodies prevents attachment of microorganisms to mucus membranes. **IgE** antibodies are found in only trace amounts in the serum. These are made up of immunoglobulin monomers. Their primary roles are (1) in the host defenses against parasitic infections, and (2) in mediating type I (anaphylactic) hypersensitivity reactions. **IgD** is an antibody found bound to the surface of B-cells as well as in serum. It exists as an immunoglobulin monomer. The function of this class of antibodies is not presently well understood.

Case Conclusion Differential diagnosis: rheumatoid arthritis, ankylosing spondylitis, Reiter's syndrome, SLE, osteoarthritis, gout, chronic Lyme disease, polymyalgia rheumatica.

The patient is diagnosed with rheumatoid arthritis and counseled extensively on the chronic nature and likely course of the disease. A program of physical and occupational therapy combined with stretching, exercise, and rest is initiated. Nonsteroidal anti-inflammatory drugs (NSAIDs) are prescribed for symptomatic relief. Despite this treatment regimen, RH's symptoms continue to worsen and, after 7 months, he is started on gold salts.

Thumbnail: Immunoglobulin Classes

	Percent of Ig in Serum	Structure	Crosses Placenta	Main Functions
IgG	75%	Monomer	YES	* Main antibody in secondary response against bacteria and bacterial toxins • Opsonizes bacteria • Fixes complement • Crosses the placenta
IgA	15%	Monomer or dimer	No	Found in secretions • Prevents attachment of microorganisms to mucus membranes
IgM	9%	Monomer or pentamer	No	• Main antibody in primary response to antigen • Fixes complement • Antigen receptor on surface of B-cells
IgD	0.2%	Monomer	??	* Unknown function * Found on surface of B-cells as well as in serum
IgE	0.004%	Monomer	No	* Mediates immediate hypersensitivity reactions by causing degranulation of mast cells and basophils * Important in host defenses against helminthic infection through triggering the release of enzymes from eosinophils

Key Points

▶ Rheumatoid arthritis is a chronic, inflammatory disease that primarily affects the proximal inter-phalangeal and metacarpophalangeal joints bilaterally

▶ Inflammation in the joint is characterized by a synovitis that is progressive and eventually leads to joint destruction and deformities

▶ Rheumatoid arthritis is more common in women (3:1 female:male); age of onset is the 20s and 30s

▶ Patients with rheumatoid arthritis often have HLA-DR4 and/or HLA-DR1 alleles and have rheumatoid factor in their serum

▶ Rheumatoid factor is an IgM autoantibody to the Fc portion of autologous antibodies.

Questions

1. Analysis of fluid removed from one of this patient's affected joints would reveal
   A. fragments of *Chlamydia trachomatis.*
   B. turbid fluid with high levels of WBCs.
   C. birefringent crystals seen with polarized light microscopy.
   D. bloody fluid.
   E. high levels of rheumatoid factor.

2. After failing treatment with NSAIDs and gold salts the patient is started on a new medication. Three weeks later he notes oral ulcers and nausea. He is seen again in your office and you send him to the lab to have blood tests drawn. Which of the following abnormalities is *most likely* to be found?
   A. Decreased levels of rheumatoid factor
   B. Decreased red blood cells
   C. Decreased white blood cells
   D. Increased red blood cells
   E. Increased white blood cells
   F. Elevated creatinine
   G. Elevated AST

3. Despite treatment this patient's disease progresses. He develops joint deformities and has increasing difficulties at work secondary to limited range of motion and pain. X-rays are done and reveal

   A. global demineralization of ulnar and radius.
   B. increased bony cortex, with increased bone density.
   C. joint space narrowing, osteophytes, and dense subchondral bone.
   D. calcification of the anterior and lateral spinal ligaments with squaring and demineralization of the vertebral bodies.
   E. multiple lytic lesions.
   F. joint space narrowing and erosions.

4. A 30-year-old woman presents to the office complaining of facial swelling and urticaria that developed after eating barbequed shrimp for the first time. This reaction is *most likely* caused by which of the following?

   A. IgG-mediated immune complexes deposited in the skin
   B. IgG-mediated complement lysis
   C. IgE-induced mast cell degranulation
   D. IgA-mediated histamine release
   E. IgD-mediated histamine release

> **HPI:** FR, a 31-year-old Caucasian male, presents to the acute care clinic complaining of urinary frequency and burning. He states that he hasn't felt right since returning from a vacation in Thailand a couple of weeks ago. Initially, FR thought he was merely experiencing some jet lag with fatigue and general malaise. However, over the past 2 weeks he has developed pain in his right heel and knee as well as in his back. Overnight he noted the onset of urinary symptoms. The patient denies any prior medical problems. However, he does describe having a week of bloody diarrhea while in Thailand.
>
> **PE:** The patient is afebrile. He is mildly ill appearing, with red itchy eyes. Painless oral ulcers are noted on his buccal mucosa and palate. Extremity exam reveals sausage-shaped toes, tenderness of the heels and low back, and swelling of the right knee. The remainder of the exam is unremarkable.
>
> **Labs:** First void urine is positive for white blood cells; however, it is negative for both gonorrhea and chlamydia.

Thought Questions

- What is the most likely diagnosis? Who is at most risk for this disease?
- Which infectious agents are associated with this disorder?
- Describe the concept of molecular mimicry and how it could explain the mechanism of Reiter's syndrome.
- Which gene is associated with this form of arthritis? What are the two classes of HLA or MHC molecules and what role do they play in the immune system?
- Which other spondyloarthropathies are associated with HLA-B27 and how do they compare to Reiter's syndrome?

Basic Science Review and Discussion

Clinical Features The combination of arthritis, conjunctivitis, urethritis, and mucocutaneous lesions is classic for Reiter's syndrome, which most commonly affects young men in their 20s and 30s. The arthritis is characteristically polyarticular and asymmetric. The most common joints affected are knees, ankles, feet, wrists, and spine. Inflammation of the tendinous insertions on the bone is unique to Reiter's syndrome and the associated spondylopathies. In the fingers and toes this inflammation leads to a "sausage digit" appearance, whereas in the ankles it is seen as heel pain.

The onset of Reiter's syndrome typically follows a genitourinary tract infection with *Chlamydia trachomatis,* or a gastrointestinal (GI) infection with *Salmonella, Shigella, Yersinia,* or *Campylobacter.* Synovial fluid cultures are negative for these organisms. However, fragments of these bacteria have been identified in synovial tissues.

Pathophysiology The exact pathophysiology of this disease is not clearly understood at this time. However, the association of Reiter's syndrome with specific infections suggests that **molecular mimicry** may be a mechanism underlying this autoimmune disorder. Normally, the immune system exhibits tolerance toward self tissues. When this tolerance is lost, the immune system mounts an attack against native tissues resulting in autoimmune disease. Molecular mimicry is one proposed mechanism used to explain how tolerance is lost. According to this theory, an environmental trigger—in this case *Chlamydia, Salmonella, Shigella, Yersinia* or *Campylobacter*—resembles or "mimics" self antigens. These self antigens are therefore viewed as "foreign" and are subject to immune attack. The result is inflammation of tissues in the joints, urethra, and mucus membranes.

Genetics of Reiter's Syndrome There is a genetic predisposition to Reiter's syndrome. Most affected individuals carry the gene for **human leukocyte antigen B27 (HLA-B27).** HLA molecules were initially identified as antigens that triggered rejection of transplanted organs and so were named **major histocompatibility complex** molecules (MHC). There are tremendous within-species variations in these proteins; therefore, these molecules play an important role in the recognition of self and non-self. The genes coding for these proteins are found on chromosomes 6 and 15. Three of these genes—HLA-A, HLA-B, and HLA-C—code for class I MHC proteins, whereas the HLA-D genes code for class II MHC proteins. These genes contain hypervariable regions that lead to a high degree of polymorphism in the proteins that are produced thereby accounting for the vast differences between individuals within the same species.

Major Histocompatibility Molecules In addition to their role in recognition between self and non-self, HLA molecules play an important role in shaping the body's immune response. The primary function of these molecules is to bind peptide fragments of foreign proteins and present them to the appropriate T-cells, leading to a T-cell mediated immune response. **Class I MHC** molecules are found on all cells and are composed of a long alpha (α) chain and a short beta (β) chain. These MHC molecules present peptides from proteins synthesized within the cell and are therefore important in immune surveillance and destruction of virus infected or otherwise altered body cells such as tumor cells. The antigen/MHC complexes of these abnormal cells are recognized and killed by CD8 T-cells. **Class II MHC** molecules, on the other hand, are only found on specific cells of the immune system such as B-cells, macrophages, Langerhans cells, and dendritic cells. These molecules are made up of two intrinsic membrane proteins that are approximately equal in length. Exogenous foreign peptides that are phagocytosed by cells expressing these molecules are digested and then presented by class II MHC molecules. These complexes are in turn recognized by CD4 T-cells leading to either a type II delayed hypersensitivity reaction or production of antibodies through a T-cell-dependent humoral response.

It has recently been learned that certain HLA types are associated with specific diseases. Even though the exact pathophysiology underlying these disorders has not yet been elucidated, the HLA associations have led to speculation on possible disease mechanisms. Diseases related to class I MHC include ankylosing spondylitis and Reiter's syndrome; those diseases related to class II MHC include rheumatoid arthritis, Graves' disease, and systemic lupus erythematosus (SLE) (Table 34-1).

Table 34-1. Spondylopathies associated with HLA-B27

	Reiter's Syndrome	**Ankylosing Spondylitis**	**Psoriatic Arthritis**	**Enteropathic Arthritis**
Age at onset	Young to middle-aged adult	Young adult < age 40	Young to middle-aged adult	Young to middle-aged adult
Sex ratio	Males:Female 3:1	Male:Female 10–15:1	Male:Female 1:1	Male:Female 1:1
Arthritis	Peripheral arthritis > sacroiliitis/spondylitis	Sarcoiliitis > spondylitis >> peripheral arthritis	Peripheral arthritis >> sacroiliitis/spondylitis	Peripheral arthritis > spondylitis > sacroiliitis
Disease associations	*Chlamydia* infection, dysentery (*Shigella/Salmonella*)	None	Psoriasis	Crohn's disease, ulcerative colitis
Extra-articular manifestations	GU, oral/GI, eye	Eye, heart	Skin, eye	GI, eye
Clinical course	Acute > chronic	Chronic	Chronic	Acute or chronic
Triggered by infection	Yes	No	No	No

Case Conclusion Differential diagnosis: Reiter's syndrome, enteropathic arthritis, ankylosing spondylitis, rheumatoid arthritis. FR is diagnosed with Reiter's syndrome and is treated with nonsteroidal anti-inflammatory drugs (NSAIDs). Over the following few weeks his symptoms gradually resolve.

Thumbnail: Differences between Class I and II MHC

	Class I MHC	Class II MHC
Genes	HLA-A, HLA-B, HLA-C	HLA-D
Type of cells on which they are located	All nucleated cells	Macrophages B-cells Dendritic cells of the spleen Langerhans cells of the skin
Structure	α chain, which is an intrinsic membrane protein and a short β chain	α and β chains are intrinsic membrane proteins of approximately the same length
Site of the genes	α chromosome 6 β chromosome 15	α chromosome 6 β chromosome 6
Antigen-binding domain	Composed of the α1 and α2 two domains of the α chain	Composed of the α1 domain of the α chain and the β domain of the β chain
Antigens presented	Peptides from proteins synthesized within the cell	Exogenous proteins that are ingested and degraded in lysosomes
Type of T-cell involved in recognition of antigens presented	CD 8	CD4
Consequences of T-cell recognition	Cytotoxic T-cell killing of antigen presenting cell	Induction of T helper cells and antibody production or delayed hypersensitivity reactions
Disease associations	HLA-B27; ankylosing spondylitis and Reiter's syndrome	HLA-DR4; rheumatoid arthritis, insulin-dependent diabetes HLA-DR3; Sjögren's syndrome

Key Points

▶ Reiter's syndrome is a reactive arthritis that is seen following urethritis or dysentery. Symptoms include arthritis, urethritis, conjunctivitis, and mucocutaneous lesions.

▶ Reiter's syndrome is just one of a group of interrelated disorders including ankylosing spondylitis, psoriatic arthritis, and enteropathic arthritis. These disorders are characterized by (1) arthritis affecting the spine, sacroiliac joints and peripheral joints; (2) extra-articular inflammation involving the eye, intestines, urethra, skin, or heart; (3) association with HLA-B27.

▶ Molecular mimcry is one proposed mechanism explaining autoimmune disease. According to this theory there may be homology between certain infectious agents and host proteins. Thus infection with these microorganisms generates an immune response that cross-reacts with autologous body constituents.

Questions

1. Which of the following is *not* typically seen in Reiter's syndrome?
   - A. Diarrhea
   - B. Arthritis
   - C. Macular papular rash with scaling
   - D. Urethritis
   - E. Conjunctivitis

2. Which of the following findings is associated with Reiter's syndrome?
   - A. HLA-DR4 positive
   - B. Urethral culture positive for *Chlamydia*
   - C. Urethral culture positive for gonorrhea
   - D. Synovial fluid culture positive for *Chlamydia*
   - E. Synovial fluid culture positive for gonorrhea

3. Class I MHC molecules
   A. are found only on B-cells and macrophages.
   B. present antigen to CD4 cells.
   C. such as HLA-DR4 are associated with autoimmune disorders,
   D. play an important role in cytotoxic T-cell killing of abnormal host cells.
   E. trigger the complement cascade.

HPI: MA, a 50-year-old woman, presents to her primary care physician complaining of pain and swelling in her hands and feet that has progressively worsened over the past few months. The pain is located in the finger joints and increases later in the day after activity. The swelling is most pronounced in her fingertips and worsens when MA is under stress and after working in her garden. The patient reports that she has always had poor circulation and difficulty keeping her fingers and toes warm. However, MA now wonders if she could have frostbite because, at times, the tips of her fingers and toes appear blue after exposure to the cold. Review of systems reveals some problems with heartburn for which the patient takes antacids. Lately, her digestive problems have worsened and MA has had to take her antacids daily. Moreover, she has recently experienced difficulty swallowing solid foods and finds that she needs to consume large amounts of liquids with meals in order to get everything to go down smoothly.

MA is otherwise healthy and has no other medical problems. She has no drug allergies and is currently only taking her hormone replacement therapy (HRT) and over-the-counter antacids.

PE: The patient is noted to be a mildly obese woman in no acute distress. She is afebrile and normotensive. HEENT exam reveals moist mucus membranes and no oral ulcers or dental caries. Cardiac, pulmonary, and abdominal exams are unremarkable. Examination of the patient's extremities reveals tightened, thickened skin on the fingers and toes. Loss of the normal skin folds in these areas is noted. Moreover, there is ulceration at the fingertips of the second and third digits of the right hand. Joint examination is within normal limits.

Labs: You reassure MA that she does not have frostbite but order lab tests.

Thought Questions

▶ What is the *most likely* diagnosis for this patient?

▶ How would you describe the clinical spectrum of connective tissue diseases?

▶ What are the key laboratory and pathologic findings in this disease?

▶ Which autoantibodies are unique to this disease?

▶ How would you describe the structure and function of collagen? What are the different types?

▶ What is the normal process of wound healing?

Basic Science Review and Discussion

The differential diagnosis of this patient's disease includes systemic lupus erythematosus (SLE), rheumatoid arthritis, polymyositis, and **scleroderma**. MA's arthritis and polymyalgias could be explained by any of these disorders. However, what distinguishes her disease are the skin changes that she has experienced. The swelling and episodic vasoconstriction seen in her fingers and toes is characteristic of **Raynaud's phenomenon**, which is the initial presenting symptom in 70% of patients with scleroderma. Thickened skin and dysphasia due to esophageal fibrosis are other hallmarks of this disease. Scleroderma is a disorder that affects the connective tissues of the skin and other organs. It is **characterized by fibrosis, microvascular changes, and the presence of auto-antibodies.** This disease covers a spectrum

from mild localized disease (morphea) to limited systemic sclerosis otherwise known as the CREST syndrome (calcinosis, *R*aynaud's phenomenon, *e*sophageal disease, *s*clerodactyly, *t*elangectasia), to diffuse rapidly progressive disease that affects the internal organs as well as the skin of the extremities.

Scleroderma is most commonly seen in adults in their 40s and 50s. Females are more commonly affected than males. Unlike other autoimmune diseases, familial cases are rare. The most common initial symptoms include Raynaud's phenomenon, swelling and puffiness of the fingers or hands, polyarthralgias or polyarteritis. Occasionally, as observed in this patient, gastrointestinal (GI) or pulmonary problems may be presenting symptoms. Skin changes are the hallmark of this disease. Initially, patients experience painless pitting edema which, over time, evolves to thickened indurated tight skin. Normal skin folds are lost. At later stages of disease atrophy may develop, especially over joints at sites of flexion. These areas are also prone to ulceration. Subcutaneous calcification and telangiectasias may also be seen. Esophageal dysfunction and fibrosis can lead to dysphagia and reflux esophagitis. If left untreated, stricture and ulceration may develop. Similar dysmotility can be observed in the large small intestine where it leads to intermittent diarrhea, bloating, cramping, and malabsorption. Large-mouth diverticula may develop. If this disease affects the lungs, it manifests as diffuse pulmonary fibrosis and pulmonary vascular disease that results in low diffusing capacity and decreased lung compliance. Pulmonary hypertension can lead to right heart failure. Direct heart involvement causes pericarditis, heart block, and/or myocardial fibrosis. Obstruction of small renal vessels can lead to hypertensive uremic syndrome.

Laboratory findings in patients with scleroderma include mild hemolytic anemia, which results from the mechanical damage that occurs in diseased small vessels; elevated sedimentation rate; and hypergammaglobulinemia. These patients are also noted to have antinuclear antibodies. The two auto-antibodies, unique to scleroderma, are **anti-DNA topoisomerase I (anti Scl 70)** and **anticentromere antibody.** Anti Scl 70 is more often seen in patients with systemic sclerosis, whereas anticentromere antibody is more common in patients with CREST syndrome.

Pathogenesis The exact etiology of scleroderma is unknown. However, evidence suggests that the excessive fibrosis and microvascular changes are related to abnormalities in the immune system. One hypothesis attributes the problem to **abnormal activation of the immune system.** According to this hypothesis, in response to an as of yet unidentified antigen or auto-antigen located in the skin T-cells release cytokines that recruit inflammatory cells. These cells include mast cells and macrophages, which in return produce inflammatory mediators such as histamine, heparin, IL-1, TNF-α, PDGF, and TGF-β. In response to these mediators fibroblast growth and collagen synthesis is enhanced. Findings of activated CD4+ cells as well as the accumulation of mast cells and activated monocytes in the skin of patients with this disease support this hypothesis. A second hypothesis proposes that **early microvascular disease** is responsible for the fibrosis. According to this hypothesis, the endothelium of the microvasculature is injured in some undetermined fashion. This injury then leads to platelet aggregation and the release of platelet factors such as PDGF and TGF-β, which in turn triggers fibrosis. The damaged endothelium itself may also release these factors as well as fibroblast chemotactic substances. The subsequent narrowing and thickening of the small blood vessels then leads to ischemic tissue injury, which in turn triggers fibrosis. The finding of microvascular disease in early systemic sclerosis as well as increased platelet activation appear to support this hypothesis.

Pathologic Findings The characteristic pathologic finding in systemic sclerosis is fibrosis of the skin and other organs, including the blood vessels. Early in the disease, affected areas of the skin are noted to be edematous with perivascular infiltrates containing CD4+ T-cells as well as swelling and degeneration of collagen fibers. As the disease progresses a marked increase in collagen and other extracellular matrix is noted. This thickening of the dermis is accompanied by thinning of the epidermis and loss of the retia pegs. Capillaries and small arteries in these affected areas show thickening of the basal lamina, damaged

endothelial cells, and are oftentimes partially occluded. With further progression, calcification of the affected areas may be seen as well as cutaneous ulcerations and atrophy secondary to loss of blood flow.

Collagen Structure and Function **Collagen** is the most common protein and most abundant fiber in connective tissue. It is produced primarily by fibroblasts. There are at least 14 different kinds of collagen, all of which share the same basic structural unit: tropocollagen. **Tropocollagen** consists of three polypeptide chains with high glycine, proline, hydroxyproline, and hydroxylysine content. These chains are arranged in a triple helix. The ability of the triple helices to aggregate and cross-link determines the structural properties and type of collagen. In skin and fascia, collagen is arranged as woven sheets that serve to hold these tissues together. When arranged in rope and strands (as in tendons and ligaments) it provides tensile strength. The numerous types of collagen can be subdivided into fibrillar collagens (types I, II, and III) that are found in cartilage, bone, and skin and nonfibrillar; or amorphous collagens (types IV, V, and VI) that make up basement membranes and interstitial tissue. The four most common types include type I found in skin, bone, tendon, and cornea; type II, which makes up cartilage, and the vitreous body of the eye; type III, which is the primary component of the reticular network found in lymphoid organs, blood vessels, and skin; and type IV collagens that take the form of sheets and make up the basal lamina. Collagen is synthesized by a number of different cells, fibroblasts (I, II, III), chondrocytes (II), osteocytes (I), smooth muscle (I, III, IV), and epithelial cells (type IV).

Collagen Synthesis and Wound Healing Wound healing is a complex process whereby damaged tissue is replaced by connective tissue. There are four key steps to this process: angiogenesis, fibroblast migration and proliferation, deposition of extracellular matrix, and remodeling.

Wound healing and tissue repair begins as early as 24 hours following an injury. **Granulation tissue** is the hallmark of early healing. Grossly, this type of tissue appears pink, soft, and granular. Histologically, this granulation tissue is characterized by the proliferation of new small blood vessels, a predominance of fibroblasts, and edema.

Angiogenesis is the process whereby new blood vessels are formed that expand an existing vascular network. This process begins with the degradation of the basement membrane of the existing vessel by proteolytic enzymes. Once this degradation has occurred it is possible for new capillaries to form. Endothelial cells then migrate toward this area and proliferate. As these endothelial cells mature, further growth is inhibited and the capillaries are remodeled into a new network. Finally periendothelial cells and smooth muscle cells are recruited to provide support for the new vessels. This process is regulated by the interaction between vascular endothelial cells, extracellular matrix proteins, and growth factors like **vascular endothelial growth factor (VEGF)** and angiopoiesis. VEGF is the key growth factor in angiogenesis. It functions to: promote angiogenesis; increase vascular permeability; stimulate endothelial cell migration and proliferation; and upregulate endothelial expression of plasminogen activator, plasminogen activator inhibitor-1, tissue factor and interstitial collagenase all of which have a role in remodeling the extracellular matrix. Expression of VEGF is stimulated by specific cytokines and growth factors such as TGF-β, PDGF, TGF-alpha as well as by tissue hypoxia. Proteases such as plasminogen activators and matrix metalloprotease play a key role in altering the extracellular matrix to permit endothelial cell invasion and vascular remodeling. Integrins are important in directing endothelial cell migration and invasion.

Following the formation of new capillary networks in areas of tissue damage, **fibroblasts migrate to the area and proliferate.** VEGF causes an increase in vascular permeability resulting in increased deposition of fibrinogen and fibronectin. These proteins in turn provide a framework for fibroblast invasion. This process of migration and proliferation is triggered by cytokines such as interleukin-1 and TNF-α, and growth factors, including TGF-β PDGF, EGF, and FGF. Platelets, endothelial cells and inflammatory cells such as macrophages produce these factors and cytokines. **TGF-β** is the key player in this step of wound healing. It is produced by most cells in granulation tissue. In addition to triggering fibroblast migration and proliferation, this

growth factor causes an increase in collagen and fibronectins synthesis as well as inhibits the breakdown of the extracellular matrix by metalloproteinase. Of note increased expression of this growth factor is seen in chronic fibrotic diseases such as scleroderma.

Once fibroblasts have established themselves in areas of tissue injury, they mature and begin to produce increasing amounts of collagen and other extracellular matrix proteins. Growth factors like TGF-β, FGF, and PDGF as well as cytokines like IL-1 and IL-4 stimulate the production of collagen. These factors are secreted by leukocytes and fibroblasts. As more and more collagen is deposited, vascular regression occurs and granulation tissue is replaced with a dense avascular scar.

Throughout this process of extracellular matrix deposition, collagen and other proteins are being degraded. **Tissue remodeling** is the result of extracellular matrix synthesis and degradation. Matrix metalloproteinase are zinc-dependent enzymes responsible for the breakdown of extracellular matrix proteins. Collagenases break down collagen types I, II, and III. Gelatinases degrade amorphous collagen and fibronectin. Stomelysins cleave other extracellular matrix proteins such as proteoglycans and fibronectin. These enzymes are produced by fibroblasts, macrophages, neutrophils, and epithelial cells in response to growth factor (PDGE, FGF), cytokines (IL-1, TNF-α), and physical stress. TGF-β and steroids inhibit the secretion of these enzymes. Tissue inhibitors of metalloproteinase are proteins produced by mesenchymal cells which limit the action of these degradative enzymes.

Case Conclusion Laboratory results reveal a positive ANA and mildly elevated sedimentation rate. Further testing indicates that the patient has anticentromere antibodies. The patient is started on nifedipine to help relieve her Raynaud's symptoms, and omeprazole to aid her digestion. MA is also instructed to protect her extremities by avoiding cold exposure, and wearing gloves while gardening. To help with her esophageal dysmotility and reflux she is advised to avoid late-night meals, elevate the head of her bed, and take her medications in liquid or crushed form.

Thumbnail: Rheumatology

Types and Function of Collagen

Type	Form	Source	Tissues
I	Fibers composed of broad fibrils	Fibroblasts, osteocytes, smooth muscle cells	Skin, bone, tendon, cornea
II	Thin fibrils	Fibroblasts, chondrocytes	Cartilage, vitreous body
III	Thin fibrils	Fibroblasts, smooth muscle cells	Lymphoid organs, blood vessels, skin
IV	Sheets	Smooth muscle cells, epithelial cells	Basal lamina

Growth Factors and Wound Healing

Stage of wound healing	Growth Factors	Cytokines
Angiogenesis	VEGF, angioproteins, FGF	
Fibroblast migration and proliferation	PDGF, EGF, FGF, TGF-β, TNF	IL-1, TGF-α
Collagen synthesis	TGF-β, PDGF, TNF	IL-1, IL-4
Collagenase secretion	PDGF, FGF, EGF, TNF	IL-1, TGF-α
Inhibition of collagenase secretion	TGF-β	

Key Points

▶ Scleroderma is an autoimmune disease characterized by excessive fibrosis. It may be limited to the skin or be widespread affecting various organ systems including the GI system, kidneys, heart, muscles, and lungs.

▶ The exact pathogenesis of scleroderma is uncertain; however, it is clear that the underlying defect involves an abnormal immune response to an as of yet unidentified antigen resulting in excessive fibrosis and microvascular disease.

▶ **Antitopoisomerase I (anti Scl-70)** and **anticentromere antibody** are auto-antibodies unique to scleroderma.

▶ **Vascular endothelial growth factor (VEGF)** is a key mediator of angiogenesis. It promotes this process by increasing vascular permeability, stimulating fibroblast migration and proliferation, and triggering the upregulation of enzymes and factors important in extracellular matrix remodeling.

▶ **TGF-β** is the key growth factor involved in the process of fibrosis. It stimulates fibroblast migration and proliferation, increases the synthesis of collagen and fibronectin, and decreases the degradation of newly deposited collagen and fibrin by metalloproteinase.

Questions

1. A 17-year-old male presents to the urgent care clinic 24 hours after cutting his palm with a piece of shattered glass. Inspection of the wound reveals soft, pink, debris-free granular tissue. No signs or symptoms of infection are noted. At this point, which of the following growth factors is *most important* for wound healing?

A. IFN-gamma
B. PDGF
C. VEGF
D. IL-1
E. TNF-β

2. An otherwise healthy couple gives birth to a male infant with severe skeletal deformities, extremely fragile bones, and blue sclera. The baby dies shortly after birth. The patient's doctors inform the couple that their infant's condition was likely due to a genetic abnormality in gene coding. Which of the following proteins would be abnormal?

A. Elastin
B. Type I collagen
C. Type II collagen
D. Type IIII collagen
E. Type IV collagen

HPI: JE, a 54-year-old woman, presents to your office for her annual exam. She has been menopausal for 5 years and is currently doing well without any hormone replacement therapy (HRT). She has no specific complaints but does have some questions about seasonal allergies. JE has been healthy her entire life and has never experienced allergies. However, over the past 9 months JE's eyes have become increasingly dry and itchy. Initially, she believed it was due to the time she was spending outside in her garden under a hot sun. JE is now experiencing a gritty sensation, as though she has sand in her eyes. Moreover, she doesn't seem to be able to produce enough tears to clear the "dust" in her eyes. JE's good friend has pollen allergies and has the same symptoms every spring. Your patient now wonders whether or not she should get prescription medication to treat these allergies.

On further questioning JE reveals that she has also had a decrease in her appetite. "Food just doesn't taste the same lately," she says. Also, JE is finding it increasingly difficult to chew and swallow dry foods like breads and crackers. She feels as though she has to drink four or five glasses of water with her meals just to get everything to go down. And, if that is not enough, JE states that she has also recently had three cavities filled. She denies any problems with joint pains or muscle aches. The patient is otherwise healthy without any major health problems except depression for which she takes amitriptyline.

PE: The patient is noted to be a thin woman in no acute distress. She is noted to have mildly erythematous eyes that do not tear when touched lightly with cotton. Oral examination reveals dry buccal mucosa with some ulcerations. On neck examination, a mildly enlarged, nontender, submandibular gland is palpated. There is no lymphadenopathy. Cardiac, pulmonary, and abdominal examinations are normal. Pelvic examination reveals dry vaginal mucosa, without evidence of atrophy. Extremity and skin examinations are unremarkable.

Thought Questions

- What is the *most likely* diagnosis for this patient?
- What other diseases are associated with this condition?
- How is this disease diagnosed?
- What are the key pathologic findings?
- What are the different types of lymphocytes and what role do they play in the immune response?
- Which auto-antibodies are associated with Sjögren's syndrome? What are the potential implications for women with anti-SS-A (Ro) antibodies?
- What accounts for the diversity of antibodies?

Basic Science Review and Discussion

Sjögren's syndrome is an **autoimmune disorder** that is characterized by chronic inflammation of the exocrine glands. It may be primary and seen in the absence of other diseases, or may be secondary and associated with rheumatoid arthritis, systemic lupus erythematosus (SLE), systemic sclerosis, myositis, biliary cirrhosis, chronic hepatitis, cryoglobulinemia, vasculitis, or thyroiditis. The disease progresses slowly and can be limited to lacrimal and salivary glands, or may involve multiple organs including the lungs, kidneys, blood vessels, and muscles. It is most commonly seen in middle-aged women but can occur in all ages and in both sexes.

Presentation of the Disease The signs and symptoms are often subtle and progress slowly over time. Patients typically complain of dry eyes, which are described as feeling "sandy" or "gritty." This symptom is associated with decreased tearing, increased redness, itching, and sensitivity to light. Over time, with continued dryness, the corneal and conjunctival epithelium of the eye becomes eroded and eventually destroyed. These erosions can be seen with slit lamp examination of eyes stained with rose Bengal. Xerostomia is another common symptom in Sjögren's disease. Patients complain of oral dryness and describe having difficulty chewing and swallowing dry foods. They also note an increase in dental caries secondary to decreased saliva with its antibacterial properties. In addition to these two exocrine glands, other mucosal surfaces may be affected. When the respiratory tract is involved, epistaxis, dry throat with hoarseness, bronchitis, or pneumonia may result. Mucus gland involvement in the gastrointestinal (GI) tract is manifested as dysphagia, reduced gastric acid output, constipation and pancreatic insufficiency. When the mucosal glands of the external genitalia are involved vaginal dryness is observed.

Systemic manifestations can develop slowly over time. However, these are more commonly seen in primary rather than secondary Sjögren's syndrome. Sites that are affected include the lungs, kidneys, blood vessels, muscles, and reticuloendothelial system. In the lungs, lymphocytic infiltration leads to a diffuse interstitial pneumonitis. Renal involvement includes interstitial nephritis and renal tubular acidosis. Sjögren's vasculitis is most commonly seen as palpable purpura. However, if it involves the vessels of the central nervous system (CNS) peripheral and cranial, neuropathies can be observed. Finally, lymphoproliferation, particularly of the B-cell lineages, may be seen. These abnormalities are manifested as lymphoma or Waldenström's macroglobulinemia.

Diagnosis The differential diagnosis of Sjögren's syndrome includes other conditions that lead to dry mouth, dry eyes, and parotid gland enlargement: bacterial infection of the salivary glands; viral infections, such as mumps, Epstein-Barr, coxsackievirus, Cytomegalovirus (CMV), or human immunodeficiency virus (HIV); salivary gland neoplasm; sarcoidosis; amyloidosis; or drugs with anticholinergic effects. The diagnosis of Sjögren's syndrome is made on the basis of oral and ocular symptoms, objective evidence of ocular and salivary gland involvement, histopathologic findings and the presence of auto-antibodies. Sjögren's syndrome is the *probable* diagnosis if three of the above six are present and the diagnosis can be considered *definite* if four of the six criteria are met. Objective evidence of ocular involvement is determined by a positive Schirmer test in which filter paper is applied to an unanesthetized eye and wetting of less than 5 millimeters is noted in 5 minutes, or by demonstration of corneal erosions and sloughing of the corneal epithelium through slit lamp examination with rose Bengal staining. Xerostomia can be documented by salivary flow measurements, parotid sialography and salivary scintigraphy. Biopsy of the lower lip reveals lymphocytic infiltrates with acinar atrophy and hypertrophy of ductal epithelial and myoepithelial cells. The majority of the cells in the lymphocytic infiltrate are T-helper cells. **Auto-antibodies** are common in Sjögren's syndrome, the most specific being those directed against RNA, **anti-SS-A (Ro)**, and **anti-SS-B (La)**. However, elevated levels of antinuclear antibodies as well as rheumatoid factor can also be seen.

Lymphocytes and the Immune System The body's ability to mount a specific immune response is due primarily to the functions of **lymphocytes,** which are the smallest white blood cells. There are two main types of lymphocytes: B- and T-lymphocytes. These two types differ in their immune function, where they mature, how they interact with antigen, and their specific surface markers. Although both types have their origin in the bone marrow, **B-cells** develop and become immunocompetent in the bone marrow, whereas **T-cells** develop and become immunocompetent in the thymus. In the initial stages of development, a population of lymphocytes forms that is capable of responding to a wide variety of antigens. Individual cells in this population each develop a unique antigen receptor. This development

is antigen-independent and occurs in the absence of antigen. Self reactive lymphocytes are eliminated through clonal deletion during this process of development. The next stage of development occurs in peripheral lyphoid regions, lymph nodes, the spleen, and lymphoid aggregates such as Peyer patches and tonsils. During this stage of development, immunocompetent lymphocytes are exposed to foreign antigens that trigger division and differentiation. Division results in the formation of a clone of lymphocytes with the same antigen specificity. Differentiation leads to the development of effector cells that perform the actual immune function and memory cells that circulate for years and maintain the ability to respond rapidly to reexposure to antigen.

T-lymphocytes play a primary role in **cell-mediated immunity.** There are two main populations of T-cells: **helper T-cells,** which are distinguished by the cell surface marker **CD4;** and **cytotoxic T-cells,** which are distinguished by the cell surface marker **CD8.** Both types have CD3 and T-cell receptors as characteristic cell surface molecules. CD4 helper T-cells (1) assist in B-cell development and differentiation into antibody-producing plasma cells; (2) help CD8 T-cells become activated cytotoxic T-cells; and (3) enhance macrophage action in delayed hypersensitivity reactions. This type of T-cell can be further subdivided into Th-1 cells and Th-2 cells. Th-1 cells produce IL-2 and gamma interferon, both of which enhance the delayed hypersensitivity response. Th-2 cells produce IL-4 and IL-5, both of which assist in B-cell activation. CD8 cytotoxic T-cells kill virus-infected cells, tumor cells, and allograft cells via the release of perforins that damage cell membranes or via induction of programmed cell death. T-cells are activated by recognition of polypeptide antigens associated with major histocompatibility molecules on antigen-presenting cells. CD4 T-cells interact with MHC class II associated antigen, and CD8 T-cells interact with MHC class I associated antigen. Both cell types interact with MHC molecules through T-cell receptor molecules. T-lymphocytes are subsequently activated by signals transmitted by CD3.

B lymphocytes play a key role in **humoral immunity.** These cells are distinguished by the cell surface markers CD19, CD20, and surface IgM and/or IgD. The two primary functions of these cells are antibody production and antigen presentation. Once exposed to antigen, these cells differentiate into plasma and memory cells. Plasma cells secrete antibodies specific to the antigen responsible for its activation. B-cell activation is enhanced by helper T-cell interaction with antigen presented by activated B-cells on MHC class II molecules. This interaction leads to the production of stimulating cytokines IL-2, IL-4, and IL-5 by these helper T-cells.

Auto-antibodies in Sjögren's Syndrome Sjögren's syndrome is characterized by the presence of **auto-antibodies,** most commonly antiribonucleoprotein anti-SS A (Ro), and anti-SS B

(La) antibodies. However, other auto-antibodies such as ANA as well as rheumatoid factor may be seen. Additionally, auto-antibodies directed against specific tissues such as gastric parenchyma, thyroid, smooth muscle, and salivary duct can be found. The exact pathogenesis underlying the production of these auto-antibodies is not clearly understood but has been postulated to be related to overall immune dysregulation. The presence and levels of these auto-antibodies have not been found to correlate with disease severity or activity. However, the presence of anti-SS A (Ro) antibodies has been associated with the development of neonatal SLE and congenital heart block or arrhythmias in babies of mothers who have these antibodies.

The Genetics of Immunoglobulins   Each individual person possesses a wide variety of unique immunoglobulin molecules on the order of 10^6 to 10^9. However, there are only seven immunoglobulin genes, one for each of the **light chains** (kappa and lambda), and five **heavy chain** genes. How is such diversity generated given the limited number of genes? The answer lies in the structure of the immunoglobulin molecule, the structure of the genes, the rearrangement of the genes in the process of transcription, and finally mutations.

Basic immunoglobulin molecules are made up of **two light** and **two heavy polypeptide chains** that are connected by disulfide bonds forming a Y shape. Each light and heavy chain is subdivided into variable and constant regions. The variable regions are where antigen binds and the constant regions are responsible for binding cell surface receptors for phagocytoses or activating compliment. In the formation of an immunoglobulin monomer different heavy and light chains come together. The numerous permutations by which the different chains can join is one factor contributing to the diversity of immunoglobulins. Each chain is coded for by a different gene and is made up of various segments: a variable (V) segment, a diversity (D) segment in heavy chains, a joining (J) segment, and a constant (C) segment. The germline genes for each chain are located on different chromosomes, chromosome 2 for kappa light chain, chromosome 22 for lambda light chain and chromosome 14 for the heavy chains. These germ line genes are made up of multiple V, D, and J segments. Therefore in the process of producing a gene for each chain the germ line gene undergoes DNA rearrangement in which only one V, D, and J segment for a heavy chain gene; or only one V and J segment for a light chain gene are combined. The multiple gene segments as well as this process of DNA rearrangement are other mechanisms by which diversity in the antibody pool is created. Yet another way that diversity is created is through additions of new nucleotides at the splice junctions between the V-D and D-J segments. Finally, mutations can lead to variation in antigen binding specificity.

Case Conclusion   Labs are drawn and the patient is noted to have elevated anti-SS-A titers, as well as +ANA. A salivary gland biopsy is obtained. Based on the findings, the patient is diagnosed with Sjögren's syndrome. JE is treated with artificial tears and instructed to discontinue her amitryptiline. JE is also advised to avoid drugs such as decongestants because these would further decrease exocrine gland secretions. On a return visit 6 months later the patient reports improvement.

Thumbnail: B- and T-Lymphocytes

	T-cells	B-cells
Primary Immune function	Cell-mediated immunity Host defense against fungal, viral, and TB infections Regulate the immune response (CD4 cells) Kill virus-infected cells, tumor cells, and allografts (CD8 cells)	Humoral immunity Host defense against bacterial, viral, and parasitic infections Production of antibodies Antigen presenting-cells
Site of maturation	Thymus	Bone marrow
Cell surface markers	CD4, CD8, CD3, TCR (T-cell receptor)	CD19, CD20, IgM
Antigen recognition	T-cell receptor + CD3 recognize antigen bound to MHC molecules on antigen-presenting cells CD4 cells—class II MHC CD8 cells—class I MHC	Surface IgM binds free-floating antigen

Response to antigen activation	CD4 cells:
	  Th1—production of gamma interferon and IL-2
	  Th2—production of IL-4 and IL-5
	CD8 cells kill infected/abnormal cells
		Production of antibodies
		Antibody presentation

Key Points

▸ Sjögren's syndrome is an autoimmune disorder that primarily affects the exocrine glands.

▸ Clinical features of the disease include keratoconjunctivitis sicca, xerostomia

▸ Key findings include the presence of auto-antibodies in particular antiribonuclear protein anti-SS A (Ro) and anti-SS B (La) antibodies,

and salivary gland biopsy revealing lymphocytic infiltrates

▸ The broad diversity of antibodies found in the human repertoire is the result of the organization of the immunoglobulin genes and the mechanisms by which they are rearranged and combined into immunoglobulin molecules

Questions

1. Which of the following are characteristic findings on a salivary gland biopsy in Sjögren's syndrome?
   A. High levels of anti-SS-A(Ro) antibodies
   B. Collagen deposition and fibrosis of the interglandular tissue
   C. Lymphocytic infiltrates
   D. Proliferation of glandular cells that distort the normal architecture
   E. Increased numbers of neutrophils in the glands

2. The primary immune function of the predominant cell type seen in a salivary biopsy of a patient with Sjögren's syndrome is
   A. immunoglobulin production.
   B. opsonization of foreign bacteria.
   C. activation of the compliment cascade.
   D. secretion of cytokines that enhance the immune response.
   E. rapid activation of memory cells after reexposure to antigen.

3. A 37-year-old nulliparous woman with rheumatoid arthritis presents to your office at 7 weeks gestation for her first prenatal visit. She and her husband are very excited about the pregnancy. However, they are concerned about the potential affects of her rheumatoid arthritis on the pregnancy. The patient's disease is currently well controlled on NSAIDs alone. Which test should be obtained at this visit to help counsel your patient?
   A. Amniocentesis
   B. ANA
   C. AFP
   D. Rheumatoid factor
   E. Anti-SS A (Ro)

HPI: MA, a 3-year-old Filipino boy, presents to your office with an 8-day history of high-fevers and rashes. His mother reports that at first they thought it was the flu and gave him ibuprofen and soup but then he developed a rash on his chest and hands. Normally quite a calm boy, MA has been unusually fussy according to his grandmother. He is refusing to eat and cries saying that his mouth hurts. MA's mother denies vomiting, headaches, vision changes, bowel, or bladder changes. He has a 5-year-old sister who has a cold. The patient has no known drug allergies. He is taking ibuprofen and traditional herbal remedies. The patient has a normal developmental history and his vaccines are up to date except for second hepatitis A vaccine.

PE: T 39.3°C; RR 32; HR 174; BP 120/60. Gen: screaming loudly in his mother's arms. HEENT: bilateral injected conjunctivae, erythematous oropharynx and tongue with dry, cracked lips. Neck: 2 anterior cervical lymph nodes of 1–2 cms each on right side. Chest: CTA B no signs of respiratory distress. Cor: hyperactive precordium; II/VI SEM at LUSM, nl S1 but extra S2 sound. Abd: + BS, soft, nontender, nondistended, no hepatosplenomegaly. Ext: warm, well perfused. Skin: fine maculopapular rash on chest, hands, and feet. Neuro: very agitated but grossly intact.

Labs: WBC 14.8; Hgb 12.2; Plt 605; ESR 84; Monospot negative, Rapid Strep Antigen negative.

Thought Questions

- What is the differential diagnosis of this child's ailment?
- What is the epidemiology of this disease?
- What tissue types seem to be specifically targeted in this disease?
- Why is early recognition so vital?
- Which other disorders are characterized by inflammation of the blood vessel? What is the typical epidemiology of these related disorders?

Basic Science Review and Discussion

Kawasaki's disease (KD; also known as mucocutaneous lymph node syndrome) is an **autoimmune** vasculitis characterized by inflammation of the mucous membranes, lymph nodes, lining of the blood vessels (vascular endothelium), and the heart. This acute self-limited disease is the most common cause of acquired heart disease in the pediatric population. At least 3000 cases are diagnosed annually in the United States with an incidence of 6–11 cases per 100,000. The disease is most prevalent in Japan, where it was first described. Most children who acquire the disease are under age 2 and 80% are under age 5. It occurs somewhat more frequently in boys than girls (ratio 1.5:1). Approximately 20% of children with Kawasaki's disease (KD) will develop coronary artery abnormalities resulting in aneurysm, thrombosis, and myocardial infarction if left untreated.

The exact etiology of Kawasaki's disease remains unclear but epidemiologic evidence and clinical presentation both point to an infectious cause. Although a direct infectious- or antigen-mediated response has not been clearly characterized, an exaggerated inflammatory response is mostly responsible for its pathophysiology. It is postulated that secreted cytokines somehow target vascular endothelial cells producing cell-surface neo-antigens. Kawasaki's disease associated vasculitis is most severe in medium-sized arteries, and is pathologically indistinct from **infantile periarteritis nodosa.** Inflammatory cells of the blood vessels are initially neutrophils and later monocytes and possibly T-cells. These cells produce the numerous cytokines responsible for the clinical manifestations of the illness. Of these, **IL-6** has been associated with the acute febrile illness and increased acute phase reactants. IL-2, TNF-α, IL-1a appear to be responsible for the acute cutaneous responses. The presence of **IgA**-producing cells in the vascular wall suggests an antigen-driven immune response to an etiologic agent with either a respiratory or gastrointestinal (GI) port of entry.

Diagnosis and Treatment The differential diagnosis of Kawasaki's disease includes: scarlet fever, staphylococcal toxic shock syndrome (TSS), Stevens-Johnson syndrome (erythema multiforme), leptospirosis, EBV, juvenile rheumatoid arthritis, measles, acrodynia, polyarteritis nodosa, Rocky Mountain spotted fever, drug reaction, and scalded skin syndrome. Classically, Kawasaki's disease is diagnosed after at least 5 days of fever plus four out of five of the following clinical criteria.

1. Rash primarily on the trunk (maculopapular, erythema multiforme, or scarlitiniform; but not vesicular)
2. Changes in the hands and feet (swelling and redness in the acute phase, periungual desquamation in the subacute phase)
3. Bilateral conjunctival injection

4. Changes in the oral mucosa (may be irritation or inflammation of mouth mucous membranes, lips, and throat with erythematous dry, fissured lips, erythema of the pharynx and the so-called strawberry tongue

5. Cervical lymphadenopathy (node diameter > 1.5 cm).

Fever usually subsides within 1 to 2 weeks and subacute disease may follow with arthritis, arthralgias, and thrombocytosis. Atypical disease is more common among younger children and may only involve two or three of clinical criteria. The cardiac findings in Kawasaki's disease include pericardial effusion, myocardial inflammation (with nonspecific ECG changes), coronary artery abnormalities, and signs of ischemia. Approximately 25% of children present with an aseptic meningitis during the acute phase of Kawasaki's disease.

Laboratory abnormalities typically involve an elevated erythrocyte sedimentation rate (ESR), neutrophil count, and platelet count but are otherwise highly variable and nonspecific. Treatment for Kawasaki's disease involves early recognition, supportive care, and initiation of aspirin and intravenous immunoglobulin. Clinical suspicion should be followed by rapid ascertainment via two-dimensional echocardiogram to rule out coronary aneurysms.

Other Vasculitides There is a heterogenous group of disorders characterized by inflammation of the blood vessel wall. Vessels of any size in any location may be affected. The affected vessels determine the symptoms of each of these syndromes. There are a number of pathologic mechanisms underlying the various vasculitides. The two most common are direct injury to vessels by infectious pathogens, and physical or chemical injury or immune-mediated inflammation. Immune-mediated vascular inflammation may be caused by immune complexes, or direct antibody attack. Some of the vasculitides are associated with **antineutrophil cytoplasmic antibodies (ANCA).** Cytoplasmic or **C-ANCA** is seen in Wegener's granulomatosis and microscopic polyangitis. Perinuclear or **P-ANCA** are seen in polyarteritis nodosa. The exact role of these antibodies in the pathogenesis of these disorders is as yet unclear. However, it is clear that the levels of the antibodies are associated with disease activity. Both C-ANCA and P-ANCA are directed against myeloperoxidase in the primary granules of neutrophils. One proposed mechanism is that these antibodies activate neutrophils, causing a respiratory burst and degranulation and release of toxic oxygen-free radicals and lytic enzymes. This results in endothelial cell damage. The etiology of some vasculitides is still undetermined (Box 37-1).

Blood Vessel Structure All blood vessels—regardless of size—share the same basic structure: they are made up into three layers. The innermost **tunica intima** is made up of the endothelium, the basal lamina, and subendothelial connective tissue. An arterial internal elastic lamina is included in

---

Box 37-1 Vasculitides by Pathogenesis

Infectious
Bacterial (*Neisseria*)
Rickettsial (Rocky Mountain spotted fever)
Spirochetal (syphilis)
Fungal (herpes)

Direct Vascular Injury
Mechanical trauma (iatrogenic)
Radiation

Immunologic Immune Complex-mediated
Henoch-Schönlein purpura
Essential cryoglobulinemic vasculitis
Lupus vasculitis

Direct Antibody Attack-mediated
Kawasaki's disease
Goodpasture's syndrome

ANCA* associated
Wegener's granulomatosis
Microscopic polyangitis
Churg-Strauss syndrome
Polyarteritis nodosa

Unknown
Giant-cell arteritis
Takayasu's arteritis

*Unclear whether or not ANCA directly involved in pathogenesis.

---

this layer. The next layer is the **tunica media,** which is made up of connective tissue elements including elastic fibers, collagen fibers, and proteoglycans as well as a varying number of smooth muscle cells layered in a circular fashion. The outer layer is the **tunica adventitia** that is made up primarily of connective tissue, which functions to stabilize the blood vessel in its surrounding connective tissue environment. In larger vessels, smooth muscle fibers and the **vasa vasorum** or vessels of the vessel are included in this layer. These three layers are best developed and most distinct in arteries. These are less prominent in veins and capillaries.

Classification of Vasculitides by Type of Vessel Affected
Systemic vasculitis may be classified by the size of the vessels affected as well as the histologic characteristics of the lesions. There is considerable overlap among these disorders. Those affecting large vessels include giant cell (temporal) arteritis and Takayasu's arteritis. Medium-sized vessels are the primary target in polyarteritis nodosa and Kawasaki's disease. Disorders affecting the small vessels include Wegener's granulomatosis, Churg-Strauss syndrome, microscopic polyangiitis, and Henoch-Schönlein purpura. Both medium and small arteries and veins are affected in thromboangiitis obliterans (Winiwarter-Buerger's disease).

Case Conclusion After admitting MA and starting him on high-dose aspirin and intravenous immunoglobulin an electrocardiogram (ECG) reveals mild ST segment depression. An echocardiogram reveals multiple large coronary aneurysms along the left anterior descending (LAD) coronary artery and the boy was started on antithrombotic therapy.

Thumbnail: The Vasculitides

Vasculitides	Vessels Involved	Pathogenesis	Histopathology of Lesions	Other Organs Affected	Incidence	Age at Onset
Giant cell (temporal) arteritis	Large and medium muscular arteries **Temporal arteries**	Unknown	Granulomatous arteritis or aorta and branches	Renal ischemia related to renal artery involvement, granulomatous hepatitis	15–30 per 100,000	60s
Takayasu's arteritis	Large elastic and some muscular arteries including **aorta**	Unknown, but immune complex mediated occlusion of vessels	Granulomatous inflammation with decreased tunica media leading to dissection and aneurysms	Ocular disturbances and weakened pulses of the upper extremities secondary to fibrous changes and narrowing of the aortic arch and origin of great vessels	0.26 per 100,000	20s
Polyarteritis nodosa	Small and medium muscular arteries	Unknown, but lymphocytic infiltration of vessel	Necrotizing vasculitis, often at bifurcations leading to aneurysms	Renal-segmental necrotizing glomerulonephritis	1.8 per 100,000	40s and 50s
Kawasaki's disease	Medium muscular arteries but can affect all including **coronary arteries**	Direct antibody attack on vascular endothelium	Inflammation, endothelial proliferation and thrombosis	Mucous membranes, lymph nodes, cardiac	Rare	Children
Wegener's granulomatosis	Small arteries and veins	ANCA associated with likely abnormal proteinase 3 activity	Granulomatous inflammation and necrotizing vasculitis	Upper and lower respiratory tract (lung necrosis/ granulomas), renal—necrotizing glomerulonephritis	Rare	40s
Churg-Strauss syndrome	Small- and medium-sized arteries, veins	ANCA associated	Necrotizing vasculitis, eosinophil-rich and granulomatous inflammation	Lungs, viscera, cardiac, muscle and renal-focal segmental necrotizing glomerulonephritis	Rare *hx* of atopy	40s and 50s
Henoch-Schönlein purpura	Small arterioles and venules as well as capillaries	Immune complex mediated	Ig-A immune complex deposition, fibrinoid necrosis	Purpuric skin lesions, abdominal pain, arthralgias and renal-proliferative glomerulonephritis	14 per 100,000 *hx* x of atopy and recent URI	Children and teenagers
Thromboangiitis obliterans	Medium and small arteries and veins	Unknown	Acute or chronic inflammation with segmental thrombosis	Extremities	Primarily in heavy smokers	20s to 30s

Key Points

▸ Kawasaki's disease is a rare vasculitis that primarily affects children. Key features of the disease include inflammation of medium-sized vessels including coronary arteries associated with inflammation of the mucus membranes and lymph nodes.

▸ **Anti-neutrophil cytoplasmic antibodies (ANCA)** target myeloperoxidase located in the primary granules of neutrophils. **P-ANCA** is associated with polyarteritis nodosa and primary glomerular disease. **C-ANCA** is associated with Wegener's granulomatosis and microscopic polyangiitis.

▸ Blood vessels are composed of three layers: the innermost **tunica intima** composed of endothelium, basal lamina and connective tissue; **tunica media** made up of elastic fibers and smooth muscle; and the **tunica adventitia** composed of connective tissue and in large vessels, smooth muscle and the **vasa vasorum.**

Questions

1. Which part of the patient's blood vessels are *most likely* the primary target of the inflammation?

   A. Endothelium
   B. Intima
   C. Elastic fibers
   D. Tight junctions
   E. Epithelium

2. In a patient with Kawasaki's disease, the elevated ESR is best explained by the

   A. increased weight of individual erythrocytes.
   B. decreased impedance by fewer leukocytes.
   C. increased platelet aggregation.
   D. increased acute phase proteins.
   E. decreased rouleaux formation.

3. A 28-year-old Japanese woman presents to her doctor complaining of malaise, arthralgias, and double vision. She has no past medical history and is not taking any medications at this time. The patient smokes a pack of cigarettes a day. On physical examination the patient is noted to have mildly elevated blood pressure and her pulses are noted to be asymmetrically decreased. Which of the following is the best test to confirm her diagnosis?

   A. ESR
   B. P-ANCA
   C. EKG
   D. Arteriography
   E. Renal biopsy

4. A 45-year-old man with asthma presents to the emergency room for an acute asthma exacerbation. He has a long history of asthma which, until recently, has been relatively well controlled. On further questioning the patient reveals that he has also experienced fever, malaise, and weight loss over the past year. CBC shows a slightly increased WBC with increased numbers of eosinophils. A chest x-ray is obtained and reveals patchy, nodular infiltrates. What of the following is the *most likely* diagnosis?

   A. Pneumonia
   B. Churg-Strauss syndrome
   C. Goodpasture's disease
   D. Polyarteritis nodosa
   E. Winiwarter-Buerger's disease

HPI: LO, a 52-year-old male executive, presents to your office complaining of severe pain in his right big toe. He states that the pain is sharp and started abruptly overnight awakening him from sleep. The pain is excruciating and, on a scale of 1 to 10, LO rates the pain as a (10.) He has been unable to do anything but suffer from the pain. "Even having the sheet over my foot was torture," he exclaims. This is the first time LO has ever experienced anything like this. Despite Tylenol the pain has persisted and is making it difficult for LO to walk. He denies any trauma to the toe. Most of his time is spent behind his desk at the office or out at restaurants wining and dining clients. Aside from this pain LO has no other complaints. The patient's past medical history is significant for gastrointestinal (GI) reflux disease, hypertension, and a history of kidney stones. He is currently on omeprazole and atenolol. He has no drug allergies. The patient is a smoker and reports consuming approximately three to four drinks per day.

PE: BP 138/90; pulse 98; T 37.0°C; RR 19. Gen: obese man, + discomfort but not in acute distress. HEENT-PERRLA, EOMI, OP: clear, neck supple no LAN. CVR: RRR. Chest: CTA bilaterally. Abd: soft, NT, ND, + BS. Extremities: no edema, clubbing or cyanosis, first metatarsophalangeal joint on the right swollen, tender, warm, no lesions, ulcers.

Labs: WBC 14; Hct 44; Plts 250; ESR 70; uric acid 10.

Thought Questions

- What is the *most likely* cause of this patient's pain? How is the diagnosis made?

- What is the normal pathway for uric acid production? How is it eliminated?

- What is the pathophysiology of the arthritis?

- If untreated what would be the likely progression of this disease?

- What is the difference between gout and pseudogout?

Basic Science Review and Discussion

This patient has an acute attack of gout. Otherwise known as the "disease of kings," gout is the result of hyperuricemia. It is seen primarily in men age 40+. Most cases are due to an idiopathic increased production or decreased clearance of uric acid. Rarely, this disorder can be secondary to other diseases that cause overproduction or underexcretion of uric acid. Specific enzyme defects such as deficiency of **hypoxanthine-guanine phosphoribosyltransferase (HGPRT)** or overactivity of **PRPP synthetase** cause an overproduction of uric acid. Excessive dietary intake of purines, diseases with increased nucleotide turnover such as myeloproliferative and lymphoproliferative disorders as well as hemolytic diseases, hypoxemia and tissue underperfusion, severe muscle exertion, and ethanol abuse can also cause excess uric acid production. Diseases leading to impaired renal function can cause underexcretion of uric acid.

Purine Metabolism　Uric acid is an end product of purine metabolism. Purines are the building blocks of nucleic acids and DNA. These are synthesized via two pathways: a de novo pathway, and a salvage pathway. In the de novo pathway purines (guanylic acid, inosinic acid, and adenylic acid) are formed from nonpurine precursors. Through a series of reactions a ribose-5 phosphate sugar is transformed into inosinic acid (IMP). Key enzymes in this pathway include **PRPP synthetase,** which converts the initial ribose sugar into 5-phosphoribosyl-1-pyrophosphate (PRPP); and **amidophosphoribosyltransferase,** which subsequently turns PRPP into 5-phosphoribosyl 1-amine. Glycine and formate are next added and the result is IMP, which can then be interconverted to guanylic acid (GMP) or adenylic acid (AMP). In the salvage pathway purines are derived from the breakdown of nucleic acids of endogenous or exogenous origin. **HGPRT** is a key enzyme in this pathway turning guanine and hypoxanthine into GMP and IMP respectively. **Adenine phosphoribosyltransferase** and **5′-nucleotidase** salvage AMP from adenine and adenosine. Enzymes involved in the breakdown of purines include **5′-nucleotidase** which, in addition to salvaging AMP from adenosine, transforms IMP into inosine; **purine nucleoside phosphorylase,** which facilitates the breakdown of inosine to hypoxanthine as well as the reverse reaction of hypoxanthine to inosine; and **xanthine oxidase,** which completes the breakdown of purines to uric acid catalyzing the reactions changing hypoxanthine to xanthine and finally to uric acid.

Pathophysiology of Gout　Underexcretion or overproduction leads to increased uric acid in the blood. Deposition of **monosodium urate crystals** in the joint space in turn causes the arthritis by inciting an intense inflammatory reaction involving both neutrophils and monocytes. Monocytes phagocytose crystals and in turn release Il-1 and TNF-α, which in turn causes cells in the joint to release proteases leading to tissue injury. Neutrophil chemotaxis is also triggered by the presence of urate crystals as well as the presence of Il-1 and TNF-α. Neutrophils phagocytose crystals and, in the process, release prostaglandins and free radicals. Subsequent lysis of these neutrophils causes release of lysosomal enzymes, which results in further tissue injury and inflammation.

If left untreated, the initial attack may last hours to days but will eventually resolve. The patient then enters an asymptomatic period that may or may not be marked by further attacks. Over time, as the disease progresses, attacks will become more frequent and involve more joints. Urate crystal deposits (tophi) develop in the articular and periarticular spaces and chronic inflammation associated with this deposition leads to joint destruction and deformities.

Diagnosis Definitive diagnosis of gout is made by analysis of synovial fluid. Evidence of inflammation is noted with

turbid fluid containing numerous white blood cells the majority of which are neutrophils. Gram stain and culture will be negative. However examination under polarized light microscopy will reveal needle-shaped negatively birefringent monosodium urate. If positively birefringent rhomboid-shaped crystals are seen then the patient has chondrocalcinosis (pseudogout).

Pseudogout Pseudogout is the result of hypercalcemia, which leads to the deposition of **calcium-pyrophosphate** crystals in the joint space. The distribution of the arthritis is similar to that of gout, affecting single joints such as the knee and wrist. Unlike gout, pseudogout is seen equally in men and women. It tends to occur later in life—in the 60s. All races are affected equally. Diseases that predispose patients to this type of arthritis are hemochromatosis, diabetes, and thyroid disorders.

Case Conclusion Synovial fluid is removed from the first metatarsophalangeal joint on the right and inspected under polarized light microscopy. Negatively birefringent needle-shaped crystals are noted. The patient is started immediately on nonsteroidal anti-inflammatory drugs (NSAIDs) and colchicine and his pain resolves by the next day. He is scheduled to return for follow-up in one week.

Thumbnail: Gout versus Pseudogout

	Gout	Pseudogout/Chondrocalicinosis
Mechanism of disease	Hyperuricemia with deposition of monosodium urate crystals in joint space	Hypercalcemia with deposition of calcium pyrophosphate crystals in the joint space
Epidemiology	male > female, 9:1 Pacific Islanders Age > 40	Male/female ratio even All races equally affected Age > 60
Risk factors	Lesch-Nyhan syndrome, diuretic use, cyclosporin use, malignancies, chronic renal disease, lead poisoning	Hemochromatosis, diabetes, hyperparathyroidism, hypothyroidism
Joint involvement	Monoarticular, typically first metatarsophalangeal, less commonly midfoot, knees, ankles, and wrists	Monoarticular, typically knee and wrist
Synovial fluid aspirate	Needle-shaped, negatively birefringent crystals	Rhomboid-shaped, positively birefringent crystals

---

Key Points

- Purines—GMP, IMP, and AMP—are synthesized via two pathways: a de novo pathway and a salvage pathway.
- Deficiency of **HGPRT** or overactivity of **PRPP synthetase** can cause an overproduction of uric acid.
- Molecular pathophysiology of gout-hyperuricemia → deposition of monosodium urate crystals in

joint space → phagocytosis of crystals by PMNs triggers release of inflammatory mediators (leukotrienes, cytokines and chemotactins) → inflammatory reaction which—if prolonged and involves the release of lysosomal enzymes—causes joint destruction

Questions

1. Which of the following would *not* prevent further complications of gout in this patient?
   A. Reducing alcohol intake
   B. Weight loss
   C. Allopurinol
   D. Colchicine
   E. Probenecid

2. In a patient who has both gout and hypertension, which antihypertensive medication is *contraindicated*?
   A. Beta-blockers
   B. Calcium channel blockers
   C. Thiazide diuretics
   D. ACE inhibitors
   E. Alpha-blockers

3. Serum uric acid levels are noted to be elevated in a teenage boy with developmental delay and joint pain. Which of the following enzymes is *most likely* to be deficient?
   A. Adenine phosphoribosyltransferase
   B. Hypoxanthine-guanine phosphoribosyltransferase
   C. Xanthine oxidase
   D. Phosphoribosylpyrophosphate synthetase
   E. Amidophosphoribosyltransferase

4. You suspect a patient has gout. Because it can be a cause of hyperuricemia and gout, which disease is important to ask about, when obtaining a past medical history?
   A. Hepatitis
   B. Leukemia
   C. Hyperthyroidism
   D. Hypercholesterolemia
   E. Renal artery stenosis

HPI: TD, a 66-year-old woman, presents to your office complaining of right knee and hip pain. The patient states that the pain started shortly after she began a daily weight-loss exercise program 3 months ago. Initially, the pain was intermittent occurring once or twice a week. Since then the pain has become increasingly frequent. It worsens with activity and improves with rest. Ibuprofen has provided some relief but causes stomach discomfort. TD is quite distressed, and states, "it's hopeless; after years of trying to work up the motivation to improve my health through exercise, I get started on a program and am now forced to quit because of this pain." The patient denies any recent trauma. She has no other symptoms. Her past medical history is significant for asthma, gastroesophageal reflux disease, elevated cholesterol, and obesity. She has no drug allergies. Her current medications include albuterol, omeprazole, and simvastatin. Family history is significant for mother and grandmother with "rheumatism."

PE: TD is an obese woman weighing 230 pounds. She is in no acute distress. Lungs are clear to auscultation bilaterally. Extremity exam reveals a normal appearing right knee without swelling, erythema, tenderness, or warmth. There is slight limitation in the range of motion and crepitus on palpation. Other joints are unremarkable.

Thought Questions

- What are the characteristic features of osteoarthritis? Which joints are most commonly affected? What are the risk factors for the development of this kind of arthritis?

- How would you describe the structure and primary functions of cartilage?

- What is the pathophysiology of osteoarthritis?

- What changes are noted in the bones of joints affected by osteoarthritis?

- How would you describe the process of bone remodeling that underlies these changes?

Basic Science Review and Discussion

Clinical Features Osteoarthritis, a degenerative joint disease, is the most common form of arthritis. It is characterized by the slow progressive loss of articular cartilage, the formation of new bone at the appositional surfaces of the joint as well as the formation of ostephytes at the joint margins. There are no systemic manifestations of this type of arthritis. Disease is often asymmetric and localized to just a few joints. The most commonly affected joints are weight-bearing joints such as the hips, knees, and spine. However, small joints of the hands (first carpometacarpals, proximal and distal interphalangeals) and feet (metatarsophalangeals) may also be affected. Joint pain in osteoarthritis typically worsens with activity and relieved by rest. Stiffness is most pronounced after periods of immobility. The pain may initially be intermittent and mild but worsens as the disease progresses. With severe disease there is decreased range of motion in the affected joints as well as nocturnal pain.

Etiology Osteoarthritis is seen most commonly in older people (> 50–60) with more than 60% of the population having some degree of cartilage abnormality in their joints. Heredity and mechanical factors play a role in pathogenesis. There are two types of osteoarthritis. The most common is primary in which the joint degeneration occurs insidiously without any obvious initiating cause. Secondary osteoarthritis is less common and can be seen in younger individuals (< 40–50). It is usually associated with joint injury such as a fracture; chronic overuse of a joint due to sports or occupational activity; metabolic disease such as hyperparathyroidism, hemochromatosis, ochronosis; or increased mechanical stress on joints caused by obesity. Regardless of the initiating cause of the degenerative joint disease, the disease process is the same: progressive loss of cartilage and bony remodeling in the joint.

Molecular Pathogenesis Articular cartilage is connective tissue that serves two primary purposes: (1) as a shock absorber, and (2) as a wear-resistant smooth surface for joint movement. This type of cartilage lacks blood supply, innervation, or lymph drainage. Articular cartilage is made up of hyaline cartilage that is composed of cells (chondrocytes) and extracellular matrix (fibers and ground substance). Type II collagen fibers form the skeleton of hyaline cartilage. These fibers are arranged in arches providing resistance to tensile stresses and allowing for transmission of vertical loads. The ground substance of articular cartilage is made up of proteoglycan aggregates. **Proteoglycans** are molecules composed of numerous hydrophilic polysaccharide chains (chondroitin sulfate and keratan sulfate) that are covalently linked to a protein backbone. In hyaline cartilage, proteoglycans form aggregates with hyaluronic acid. The hydrophilic portions of the proteoglycans attract water giving this type of cartilage its elasticity and turgor. Chondrocytes are responsible for the maintenance of the extracellular matrix.

Chondrocytes play a key role in the cartilage destruction found in osteoarthritis. Early in the disease, they are noted to be actively dividing and producing increased quantities of collagen, proteoglycans, and hyaluronic acid. However, these new products do not aggregate well and are not adequately stabilized in the extracellular matrix. Next, proteolytic and collagenolytic enzymes are released from chondrocytes and the extracellular matrix is degraded. IL-1 is believed to be the mediator initiating this process. TNF-α, TGF-β, and prostaglandins are thought to perpetuate this process through induction of the release of lytic enzymes from chondrocytes and inhibition of matrix synthesis.

Over time, remodeling and hypertrophy of the bone occur, leading to appositional bone growth and sclerosis. At the margins of the joints there is further growth of bone and cartilage resulting in osteophytes or bone spurs. X-rays reveal narrowed joint spaces with sharp articular margins; osteophytes; and thickened, dense subchondral bone at the articular surfaces.

This remodeling and hypertrophy of the bone that occurs at affected joints is a direct result of osteoclast and osteoblast activity. **Osteoclasts** are multinucleated cells that contain lysosomal enzymes and acid phosphatase. Their primary role is bone resorption. This function is controlled by local **cytokines** such as IL-1, TNF-α and IL-6; as well as systemic hormones such as parathyroid hormone and 1,25-dihydroxyvitamin D. **Osteoblasts** originate from stromal cells and are responsible for the production of bone matrix proteins including type I collagen, as well as proteins and particles that lead to bone mineralization. Formation of new bone is regulated by systemic hormones such as 1,25-dihydroxyvitamin D, as well as growth factors including TGF-β, IGF I and II, and platelet-derived growth factor (PDGF), which are stored in bone and likely released during the process of osteoclastic resorption. The signal responsible for initiating this process is unknown; however, it is clear that increased stress on the bone is one trigger. Therefore, in osteoarthritis, increased repetitive stress on the articular surfaces of the bones of affected joints leads to the start of this remodeling process. The final result is thicker, denser bone that can better withstand the increased forces that occur once the cartilage has been lost.

Case Conclusion   Differential diagnosis: rheumatoid arthritis, systemic lupus erythematosus (SLE), seronegative spondylopathies (ankylosing spondylitis, Reiter's syndrome, psoriatic arthritis), gout, pseudogout, and septic arthritis.

Labs are done and TD is found to have a normal white blood cell count and erythrocyte sedimentation rate (ESR). She is rheumatoid factor negative and ANA negative. The patient is then referred to a physical therapist who designs a low-impact exercise and stretching program that focuses on strengthening muscles surrounding the affected joints and increasing flexibility and range of motion. TD is instructed to discontinue the ibuprofen and take acetaminophen and celecoxib as needed for pain.

Thumbnail: Comparison of Different Types of Arthritides

Type of Arthritis	Epidemiology	Joints Affected	Symptoms	Extra-articular Manifestations	Physical Findings
Osteoarthritis	**Increase with age, in those with obesity, repetitive joint injury/ stress**	**Asymmetric** hips, knees, spine, DIP, PIP	Joint pain worse after activity, better with rest	None	Crepitus, joint enlargement, osteophytes, Bouchard & Heberden nodes
Septic Arthritis	**Non GC:** prior trauma, IV drug users **GC:** young women	**Monoarticular**	**Non GC:** sudden onset joint pain, fever, chills **GC:** prodromal migratory polyarthralgias, pain of joint	**Non GC:** None **GC:** skin rash	Joint inflammation GC: skin rash, necrotic pustules palms and soles
Rheumatoid Arthritis	**Women > men** Age 30s–40s	**Symmetric** wrists, MCP, PIP, ankles, knees, shoulders, hips, elbows, spine	Joint pain & swelling worse after rest/ inactivity better with activity Fatigue, malaise, anorexia, weight loss	Subcutaneous nodules, vasculitis, eye, pleuritis, pericarditis	Early swelling, warmth, erythema, pain Late deformities: hammer toe, swan-neck, boutonniere
SLE	women ≥ men African American age 15–40	**Symmetric** Small joints of hands, wrists, and knees	Joint pain, anorexia, fever, weight loss, photosensitivity Oral ulcers	Skin rashes, oral ulcers, pleuritis, pericarditis, seizure, psychosis, anemia, leukopenia, lymphopenia, thrombocytopenia,	Malar rash, joint tenderness and inflammation Deformities rare
Seronegative Spondylopathies	Men > women Age 20s–30s	**Asymmetric Monoarticular** Sacroiliac, spine, shoulders, hips, and knees	Mid- and low-back stiffness, pain, enthesopathy	Urethritis, conjunctivitis, psoriasis, inflammatory bowel disease	Spondylitis, sacroiliitis, enthesopathy, conjunctivitis, uveitis, psoriatic rash
Gout/Pseudogout	Men ≥ women Pacific islanders Age 40–50	**Asymmetric Monoarticular** First metatarsophalangeal, midfoot, knees, ankles, wrist	Acute onset of severe pain, typically nocturnal ±fever	Tophi with chronic disease	Early swollen, tender, red joints Late deformities due to tophaceous invasion of joints

DIP, distal interphalangeal; PIP, proximal interphalangeal; MCP, metacarpophalangeal; GC, gonococcal.

Key Points

▶ Articular cartilage is made up of chondrocytes, type II collagen, and proteoglycans. Chondrocytes maintain the cartilage by producing the extracellular matrix as well as enzymes that digest it.

▶ The cytokines that stimulate chondrocyte dysfunction and increased breakdown of cartilage in osteoarthritis are IL-2, TNF-α, and TGF-β.

▶ Bone remodeling is a direct result of osteoblast and osteoclast activity. **Osteoclasts** are responsible for bone resorption, whereas **osteoblasts** produce proteins that lead to bone formation.

Questions

1. TD returns to your office 7 years later complaining of increasing difficulty using her hands, which has forced her to give up knitting. Examination of her hands reveals

   A. swelling, erythema, warmth, and tenderness over the distal metatarsophalangeal joints.
   B. swelling, erythema, warmth, and tenderness over the distal interphalangeal joints.
   C. bony enlargement of the proximal interphalangeal joints.
   D. rheumatoid nodules over the distal interphalangeal joints.
   E. hyperextension deformity of the proximal interphalangeal joints.

2. TD's 45-year-old daughter LM has accompanied her on this visit. LM has no joint symptoms at this time but is concerned about developing osteoarthritis. Which of the following contributes the most to the elastic nature of LM's healthy articular cartilage?

   A. Osteoclasts
   B. Type II collagen
   C. Chrondrocytes
   D. Proteoglycans
   E. Synovial fluid

3. In a patient with advanced osteoarthritis of the hip who is about to undergo hip replacement, which of the following cells is most active in the affected joint?

   A. Chondrocytes
   B. Neutrophils
   C. CD8 T-cells
   D. Osteophytes
   E. Osteoblasts

Septic Arthritis

HPI: JC, a 34-year-old female intravenous drug user, presents to the emergency department with a chief complaint of right knee pain. The pain is excruciating and makes it difficult for JC to walk. The patient states the pain started suddenly on the night prior to admission. She denies any past history of problems with her knees or joints. However, she does report falling 3 days ago. Thus far she has taken no medications for this pain. She does report fevers and chills. JC's past medical history is significant for pelvic inflammatory disease (PID) and multiple skin abscesses. She currently works as an exotic dancer. She does not smoke but does consume three to four drinks a day and uses IV heroin.

PE: T 38.4°C; BP 118/67; pulse 78. Gen: thin woman, mildly diaphoretic. Skin: old scars over arms and legs, no rashes or active lesions. Cardiac: regular rate and rhythm, no murmurs. Lungs: clear to auscultation. Extremities: + swelling, warmth, redness, and tenderness over right knee; other joints unremarkable.

Thought Questions

- What is the *most likely* etiology of JC's arthritis?
- Which tests would confirm your diagnosis.
- How would you describe the findings?
- How do the synovial fluid findings in septic arthritis differ from those of other arthritides?
- Which organisms can cause infectious arthritis? What are the differences in clinical presentation of these different infections?

Basic Science Review and Discussion

JC most likely has septic arthritis. This type of arthritis typically affects a single joint—usually the knee, although other sites (hip, wrist, shoulder, and ankle) may also be involved. The most common infectious agents include *Staphylococcus aureus,* group A streptococci (GAS) and group B streptococci. In IV drug users gram negative bacteria such as *E. coli* and *Pseudomonas aeruginosa* may also cause infection of the joints. In post surgical patients *Staphylococcus epidermidis* can cause septic arthritis. Symptoms of septic arthritis include the sudden onset of monoarticular joint pain and inflammation that may or may not be associated with fever and chills.

Disseminated *Neisseria gonorrhoeae* infections can also cause a septic arthritis. However, this type of septic arthritis is distinct in its presentation. It is more insidious in onset. The arthritis itself is often preceded by 1 to 4 days of migratory polyarthralgias, and is often associated with a characteristic skin rash of the extremities, which is pustular in nature—in particular the palms and soles (Table 40-1).

Infection of the joint may occur through five possible routes: hematogenous spread; dissemination and extension of osteomyelitis; spread from adjacent soft tissue infection; contamination during diagnostic or therapeutic procedures; or penetrating damage by puncture or cutting. Once the organisms enter the body, an inflammatory reaction is initiated with migration of polymorphonuclear leukocytes and release of inflammatory mediators. Inflammation and pain subsequently results.

The diagnosis of septic arthritis is made via analysis of synovial fluid from the affected joint. Fluid is aspirated from the joint and initially examined. In this type of arthritis, the fluid will be noted to be turbid and opaque due to high numbers of white blood cells. Cell counts of the fluid will confirm this finding with > 100,000 WBCs per microliter. The majority of these leukocytes will be neutrophils. Gram stain of the fluid will reveal infectious organisms in 75% of staphylococcal infections and 50% of gram-negative infections. For *N. gonorrhoeae* Gram stain is positive in 25% of cases. Glucose levels are often lower than that of the serum. These findings stand in stark contrast to those in other types of arthritis. Although inflammation plays a role in arthritides such as gout, pseudogout, rheumatoid arthritis, systemic lupus erythematosus (SLE), and the seronegative spondylopathies (Reiter's, ankylosing spondylitis, etc.) the number or white cells is not nearly as elevated. Moreover, the percentage of neutrophils is lower. Glucose measurements of fluid will be lower than serum but not as markedly as in septic arthritis. Finally, Gram stain and culture will be negative. In noninflammatory arthritides such as osteoarthritis, synovial fluid will be clear and contain only minimal numbers of white blood cells. Glucose levels will be essentially equal to that of serum and, once again, Gram stain and culture will be negative.

Case Conclusion Synovial fluid is removed from the right knee and noted to be turbid. Analysis of this fluid reveals a cell count with > 50,000 WBC per microliter with 80% polymorphonuclear (leukocytes) (PMNs), glucose < 25 mg/ml. Gram stain of the synovial fluid shows Gram-positive cocci. Blood cultures are drawn and return positive for *Staphylococcus aureus*. JC is immediately started on IV nafcillin.

Table 40-1. Septic Arthritis—Gonococcal versus Nongonococcal

	Gonococcal	Nongonococcal
Organisms	*N. gonorrhoeae*	*S. aureus*, group A strep., group B strep., *E. coli*, *P. aeruginosa*
Epidemiology	Young, sexually active adults	Small children, elderly, immunosuppressed, prior joint damage or IV drug use
Signs and Symptoms	• 1 to 4 days of migratory polyarthralgias followed by monoarticular purulent monoarthritis most often affecting the knee • asymptomatic skin rash—small necrotic pustules on extremities especially palms and soles	• Sudden onset acute joint pain and swelling most often the knee • Possible chills and fever
Treatment	• Systemic antibiotics • Joint aspiration rarely needed as often quick response to abx	• Systemic antibiotics based on organism • Joint aspiration if medical management fails

Thumbnail: Findings in Different Types of Arthritides

Type of Arthritis	Pathophysiology	Synovial Fluid	Lab Findings
Osteoarthritis	Degenerative Abnormal stresses on nl cartilage or nl stresses on abnormal cartilage	Clear, minimal WBCs, glucose normal, Gram stain and culture negative	None
Septic Arthritis	Infectious	Turbid, markedly elevated WBCs, mostly PMNs, decreased glucose, +Gram stain and culture	Positive blood cultures in 40% to 50%
Rheumatoid Arthritis	Autoimmune Progressive **synovitis** leading to pannus formation and eventual erosion of articular cartilage, bone, and tendon	Cloudy, elevated WBCs with a slight increase in percentage of PMNs, decreased glucose, negative Gram stain and culture	- Elevated rheumatoid factor - Elevated ESR
SLE	Autoimmune	Cloudy, elevated WBCs with a slight increase in percentage of PMNs, decreased glucose, negative Gram stain and culture	+ ANA + ds DNA
Seronegative Spondylopathies	Noninfectious, inflammatory	Cloudy, elevated WBCs with a slight increase in percentage of PMNs, decreased glucose, negative gram stain and culture	- Elevated ESR - HLA-B27
Gout/Pseudogout	Noninfectious, inflammatory	Cloudy, elevated WBCs with a slight increase in percentage of PMNs, decreased glucose, negative Gram stain and culture **Urate or calcium oxylate crystals**	Elevated uric acid level, increased ESR

Key Points

▶ Most common microbes in septic arthritis include *Staphylococcus aureus*, group A streptococci and group B streptococci.

▶ In IV drug users gram-negative bacteria such as *E. coli* and *Pseudomonas aeruginosa*

▶ In postsurgical patients *Staphylococcus epidermidis*

▶ *Neisseria gonorrhoeae* can also cause septic arthritis, which is distinct from the other infections with a characteristic rash on the palms and soles and more insidious onset.

Questions

1. You are working in the local ER and find an unlabeled tube of synovial fluid on the counter waiting to be sent off to the lab. The fluid is noted to be turbid. You place a drop under the microscope and note numerous PMNs. A Gram stain reveals numerous gram-positive organisms in clusters. To which of the following patients does this fluid *most likely* belong?

   A. A 67-year-old obese woman presenting with chronic right knee pain

   B. A 42-year-old male executive with severe big toe pain

   C. A 37-year-old woman with a lupus flare

   D. A 15-year-old boy who fell out a second-story window

   E. A 55-year-old man returning with knee pain following arthroscopic surgery

2. A 22-year-old woman who is a marathon runner is brought in to your office by her boyfriend for left knee pain. The patient states that all she needs is pain medication to control her symptoms so that she can continue to train for an upcoming competition. However, her boyfriend is concerned that it could be something more serious and would like her to get examined. Currently, the pain is tolerable but increases with activity so she is unable to run. She denies any recent or past trauma. Review of systems reveals a week of increased fatigue and body aches all of which the patient ascribes to an increasingly rigorous training schedule. On physical exam the woman is noted to have a markedly inflamed left knee that is tender and hot to the touch. A rash is noted on her palms. The remainder of the exam is within normal limits. Arthrocentesis is performed and Gram stain of the fluid reveals which of the following?

   A. Marked lymphocytosis

   B. Gram-negative rods

   C. Gram-positive diplococci

   D. Gram-positive cocci

   E. Negatively birefringent crystals

3. Which of the following should be the next step in your management of this patient?

   A. Advise the patient to stop running and take non-steroidal anti-inflammatory drugs (NSAIDs) until her symptoms resolve

   B. Give the patient and her boyfriend shots of ceftriaxone

   C. Check for antinuclear antibody (ANA) and rheumatoid factor

   D. Start colchicine

   E. Admit and administer IV antibiotics until symptoms improve

Case 32

1. E
2. D
3. D
4. A

Case 33

1. B
2. C
3. F
4. C

Case 34

1. C
2. B
3. D

Case 35

1. C
2. B

Case 36

1. C
2. D
3. E

Case 37

1. A
2. D
3. D
4. B

Case 38

1. D
2. C
3. B
4. B

Case 39

1. C
2. D
3. E

Case 40

1. E
2. C
3. E

Answers

Case 1

1. D. The internal intercostal muscles point backward as they are followed from the upper rib to lower rib, such that contraction pulls the rib cage down and inward. This acts to decrease thoracic volume and facilitate forced expiration. The external intercostal muscles point forward, and contraction pulls the rib cage up and outward. The diaphragm in contraction acts to compress the abdominal contents and pull up the lower ribs. Scalene and sternocleidomastoid muscles are attached to the first two ribs and sternum, thus contraction pulls up the anterior rib cage. Any upward force on the anterior rib cage allows the entire rib cage to pivot up and out on its posterior hinge points on the thoracic vertebrae. Muscles that perform this action are accessory muscles of inspiration, and include the diaphragm, external intercostals, scalenes, and sternocleidomastoids. Accessory muscles of expiration pull down on the anterior rib cage and include abdominal muscles and the internal intercostals.

2. D. Diffusion of oxygen across the alveolar-capillary membrane is a rapid process in the normal lung, taking approximately 0.25 seconds for oxygen partial pressures to equilibrate on both sides. The transit time of pulmonary blood through capillary beds is about 0.75 seconds at rest, which allows ample time for oxygen diffusion to take place. The equation that governs diffusion of a gas across a membrane is Fick's equation: $v = \{A/T\} \times D \times (Pa - Pc)$, where A = area, T = thickness, Pa = partial pressure of gas in the alveolus, and Pc = partial pressure of gas in the capillary. D is a diffusion constant proportional to $Sol/(MW)^{1/2}$.

3. D. It is important to have a general idea of vascular pressures and know the differences between the pulmonary and systemic systems (see Figure 1-2). The pulmonary circulation is a low-pressure system. The right ventricle is much smaller than the left ventricle and produces only about 25 mmHg of pressure during systole. Pulmonary arteries are very thin-walled and do not provide diastolic recoil or much resistance to flow before it reaches the pulmonary capillary beds. The mean pressure in the pulmonary arterial system is about 15 mmHg and about 12 mmHg at the origin of the capillary beds. The majority of flow resistance in the pulmonary system occurs at the level of the capillaries where the pressure drops from 12 mmHg to about 8 mmHg, and the pressure in the left atrium is about 5 mmHg. In contrast, the left ventricle produces a high pressure (120 mmHg) during systole. The systemic arterial system consists of thick-walled elastic vessels that recoil during diastole and act to maintain a higher diastolic pressure (80 mmHg) and a higher overall mean pressure (100 mmHg). The majority of flow resistance in the systemic vasculature occurs in the small arterioles that contract and expand to regulate flow to certain vascular capillary beds during different physiologic needs. On average, the mean pressure drops from 100 mmHg to about 30 mmHg across these arterioles. Pressure across the systemic capillary beds drops to about 10 mmHg, and pressure in the systemic venous system drops to about 2 mmHg by the time blood reaches the right atrium.

4. D. Inspired air pressure is equal to ambient air pressure when there is no flow through the airways. Ambient air pressure at sea level is 760 mmHg, and thus inspired air pressure is 760 mmHg during full inspiration. The fraction of air composed of oxygen is 0.21; therefore, the partial pressure of oxygen is 0.21×760 mmHg, or 160 mmHg. However, this assumes that inspired air is dry, when in fact it picks up water vapor as it is inhaled through the respiratory airways. Water vapor consists of about 47 mmHg in inspired air, which means that the total dry gas pressure is about 760 mmHg − 47 mmHg, or 713 mmHg. The ratio of oxygen to total dry gas remains 0.21, and the partial pressure of inspired oxygen is 0.21×713 mmHg, or 150 mmHg. Once inspired air reaches the alveoli, it is further diluted by the presence of CO_2, which is discussed in Case 2.

Case 2

1. A. Peripheral chemoreceptors in the carotid bodies respond to decreases in arterial PaO_2, decreases in pH, and increases in arterial $PaCO_2$. Their response to hypoxemia is profound below oxygen tension levels of 70 mmHg, although smaller responses are present at oxygen levels slightly below normal. Even though the peripheral chemoreceptors respond to changes in pH and $PaCO_2$, the central chemoreceptors play a larger role in regulating CO_2 levels.

2. C. At high altitude, hyperventilation is triggered by the peripheral chemoreceptors in the carotid bodies as a response to hypoxemia. In the alveoli, the partial pressure of CO_2 ($PaCO_2$) is governed by the alveolar ventilation equation: $PaCO_2 = VCO_2/V_A \times K$, where VCO_2 is the production of CO_2 by peripheral tissues, V_A is alveolar ventilation, and K is a constant. At rest, VCO_2 remains constant and $PaCO_2$ is inversely proportional to V_A. Therefore, doubling the respiratory rate decreases the $PaCO_2$ twofold, or from the normal 40 mmHg to 20 mmHg. This accommodates a greater alveolar PaO_2, which is important in order to maintain the PaO_2 as close to the normal 100 mmHg as possible.

3. B. The first step to analyzing a blood gas is to look at the pH. If the pH < 7.4, then the primary disturbance is acidosis; if the pH

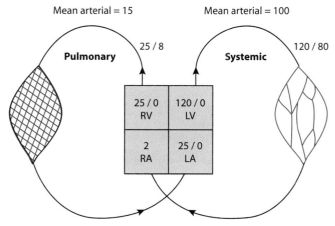

Figure 1-2. Vascular pressure found in the four heart chambers, and systemic and pulmonary circulation.

> 7.4, then the primary disturbance is alkalosis. Next look at the $Paco_2$ and $[HCO_3^-]$ to determine whether the process is respiratory or metabolic. If the primary disturbance is acidosis, then $Paco_2 >$ 40 means there is a respiratory acidosis (hypoventilation), and an $[HCO_3^-] < 24$ means there is a metabolic acidosis (excess organic acid). If the primary disturbance is alkalosis, then $Paco_2 < 40$ means there is a respiratory alkalosis (hyperventilation), and an $[HCO_3^-] > 24$ means there is a metabolic alkalosis (loss of organic acid). Once the primary disturbance is determined, the compensatory mechanism can be predicted by the ratio $[HCO_3^-]/[CO_2]$. In this instance, since the pH < 7.4 and the $[HCO_3^-] < 24$, the primary disturbance is metabolic acidosis. One can therefore predict that the compensation will be a decrease in $[CO_2]$. This is accomplished by hyperventilation, a common presenting symptom in patients with metabolic acidosis. In metabolic acidosis, Winter's equation predicts the level of $Paco_2$ when compensation is complete: $Paco_2 = 1.5 \times HCO_3^- + 8$, or in this case $1.5 \times (12) + 8 = 26$ mmHg, which is the measured value for $Paco_2$. This means that the compensatory respiratory alkalosis is complete. A quick rule of thumb for Winter's equation is that the measured $Paco_2$ should be equal to the last two digits of the pH for compensatory respiratory alkalosis to be complete (26 in this case).

4. A. Again, the pH < 7.4 indicates the primary disturbance is acidosis, and the $Paco_2 > 40$ mmHg indicates that it is a respiratory acidosis (e.g., effective hypoventilation or CO_2 retention that is typical of chronic obstructive pulmonary disease [COPD]). The ratio $[HCO_3^-]/[CO_2]$ dictates that the compensation will be an increase in $[HCO_3^-]$ that takes place at the level of the kidneys. This is a compensatory metabolic alkalosis and it takes at least 2 to 3 days to occur. Most patients with COPD have chronic respiratory acidosis and are referred to as CO_2 retainers because they have a chronically elevated arterial $Paco_2$. Their compensation is also therefore chronic, meaning that the serum $[HCO_3^-]$ is always elevated. As a rule of thumb, in chronic compensation for respiratory acidosis the $[HCO_3^-]$ is elevated 2 meq/L and the pH is decreased by 0.03 for every 10 mmHg elevation of $Paco_2$ above the normal 40 mmHg. In this patient, the $Paco_2$ of 60 mmHg is 20 mmHg above the normal value. Expected chronic compensation would be an increase in $[HCO_3^-]$ of 4 meq/L (or 28 meq/L) and a decrease in pH of 0.06 (or 7.34). This means that this patient's respiratory acidosis is fully compensated with a metabolic alkalosis.

Case 3

1. A. Henry's law dictates how much of a gas can be dissolved into a liquid depending on the partial pressure imparted on the liquid by the surrounding gas: $C_x = K \times P_x$, where C_x is gas concentration (mL/dL), K is a constant specific to the type of gas, and P_x is the partial pressure of the gas. For oxygen, K is 0.003 mL/dL/mmHg; therefore, the oxygen concentration of oxygenated blood is $C_x = 0.003 \times 100 = 0.3$ mL/dL. This is only about 1.5% of the total oxygen content of oxygenated blood (about 20 mL/dL). The remaining oxygen is bound to hemoglobin. Keep in mind that partial pressures (referred to as O_2 or CO_2 tension) are often used instead of actual concentrations when describing dissolved gas contents in blood. For example, the oxygen content of pulmonary venous blood is described as 100 mmHg, meaning that it contains the amount of

oxygen (both dissolved and bound to hemoglobin) that an equal volume of blood would if in contact with oxygen at a partial pressure of 100 mmHg. This number does not correlate with the actual pressure exerted on the fluid, which is only about 5–10 mmHg in the pulmonary venous system. Similarly, the CO_2 content of mixed venous blood ($Pvco_2$) is reported as 40 mmHg, which means that when venous blood comes in contact with the alveolar membranes it will result in an alveolar partial pressure of CO_2 ($Paco_2$) of 40 mmHg.

2. D. As explained in Case 1, diffusion across the alveolar membrane is governed by Fick's equation: $v = \{A/T\} \times D \times (Pa - Pc)$, where A = area, T = thickness, Pa = partial pressure of gas in the alveolus, and Pc = partial pressure of gas in the capillary. D is a diffusion constant proportional to $Sol/(MW)^{1/2}$. The solubility of carbon dioxide is about twentyfold greater than that of oxygen, which accounts for its more rapid diffusion across the alveolar-capillary membrane. Carbon dioxide therefore reaches equilibrium much quicker than oxygen.

3. D. The oxygen tension is the partial pressure of oxygen if the blood were placed in a closed container and allowed to equilibrate. Based on Henry's law, it is proportional to the amount of oxygen dissolved in the blood. Physiologically, the container represents the alveoli, and the partial pressure of oxygen is dictated by the partial pressure of oxygen in inspired air. At higher altitudes the barometric pressure (air pressure, 760 mmHg at sea level) decreases, yet the ratio of oxygen to total air molecules remains 0.21. Therefore, the partial pressure of oxygen decreases in the alveoli, which translates into a lower oxygen tension in arterial blood. Even though hemoglobin is the primary oxygen carrier in the blood, oxygen tension is independent of hemoglobin; therefore, anemia and CO poisoning have no effect on oxygen tension. They do, however, have a great effect on the oxygen-carrying capacity. Each gram of hemoglobin is capable of carrying 1.39 ml of oxygen. The normal hemoglobin concentration is about 15 g/dL; therefore, the normal carrying capacity of blood is about 20.8 mL/dL assuming a saturation of 100%. Again, compare this to the 0.3 mL/dL oxygen dissolved in blood that was calculated in question 1, Case 3. All of the factors listed in this question decrease oxygen delivery to peripheral tissues.

4. C. A shift to the right of the oxygen-hemoglobin dissociation curve occurs in conditions of increased temperature, acidity, Pco_2, and 2,3-DPG; all conditions that exist in exercising muscles. Shifting the curve to the right has the effect of decreasing the size of the plateau and moving the steep portion of the curve toward higher oxygen tensions. Therefore, for a given oxygen tension, the saturation of hemoglobin will be less. This means that hemoglobin binds less avidly to oxygen and off-loading is facilitated. In the pulmonary capillary beds the opposite conditions exist, shifting the curve back to the left and making the plateau larger. This represents the greater avidity of hemoglobin for oxygen in the pulmonary capillaries. CO poisoning causes hemoglobin to adhere strongly to oxygen molecules and prevents off-loading in peripheral tissues. This is represented by an extreme shift to the left of the oxygen-hemoglobin dissociation curve. The normal P_{50} (O_2 tension at which hemoglobin is 50% saturated) is about 27 mmHg. The P_{50} increases when the curve is shifted to the right. Of note, the oxygen tension of mixed venous blood is about 40 mmHg, corresponding to about 60% saturation, which is still above the P_{50} level.

Case 4

1. A. Emphysema is the result of alveolar wall destruction and its associated elastic properties. Alveolar wall destruction results in increased dead space where gas exchange cannot occur. Loss of elasticity results in greater lung compliance, or distensibility. This hinders the ability for normal passive exhalation to occur, resulting in increased functional vital capacity (FRC) and residual volume (RV). Without the normal recoil mechanism, the thoracic cage expands, which increases total lung capacity (TLC) and results in the characteristic barrel-chest. This results in decreased vital capacity.

2. B. In chronic obstructive pulmonary disease (COPD), air trapping occurs mostly at the bases, which results in shunting of ventilation to the apices where little perfusion occurs. This results in a ventilation-perfusion mismatch, which has a deleterious effect on gas exchange. The lung tissue is more "relaxed" at the bases due to the settling effect of gravity. This increased compliance at the bases, along with the loss of alveolar integrity, causes respiratory bronchioles to collapse when intrathoracic pressure is applied during exhalation.

3. C. Respiratory acidosis is the result of poor alveolar ventilation, which causes the inadequate elimination of carbon dioxide. It is the characteristic metabolic disorder in those who have lost their respiratory drive due to central nervous system lesions, sedative overdose, or muscular disorders (e.g., kyphoscoliosis, rib fractures). It is also the primary metabolic disorder seen in obstructive lung disease. Acute CO_2 retention results in an increase in $PaCO_2$ and a decrease in pH. As a rule of thumb, the pH decreases by 0.08 for every increase of 10 mmHg in $PaCO_2$. Over the course of several days renal compensation occurs with retention of HCO_3^- and an increase in the pH. However, the pH will not fully return to 7.40 until serum $PaCO$ has normalized. The rule of thumb for chronic CO_2 retention is that for every 10 mmHg increase in $PaCO_2$ over 40, the pH will be decreased by 0.03 and the $[HCO_3^-]$ increased by 2 meq.

4. B. Increasing lung volume results in stretching of alveoli and interstitial elastin, causing greater stiffness and recoil; therefore, compliance diminishes as lung volume increases. As mentioned previously, lung volumes are increased in those with COPD, which means that they function at a point on the pressure-volume curve where compliance is significantly lower. Thus, more work is required to generate a sufficient amount of negative intrapleural pressure to draw in the same volume of air.

Case 5

1. B. Laminar flow in a tube is governed by Poiseuille's law, which states that flow resistance is proportional to the tube length and gas viscosity and inversely proportional to the radius of the tube to the fourth power ($R = 8nl/\pi r^4$). This means that resistance increases exponentially as the diameter of the tube decreases. This is the reason why flow resistance in asthma increases dramatically in bronchioles where the resistance is typically low due to its laminar flow characteristics, short length, and large total cross-sectional area. Bronchiolar constriction causes a significant decrease in the total cross-sectional area and therefore a significant increase in overall resistance. In general, the greatest resistance to flow is encountered in the medium-sized bronchi; however, the larger proportion of smooth muscle in the bronchioles accounts for the increased airway resistance seen in asthma.

2. C. Trapping occurs in asthma as a result of closing of bronchioles during exhalation. During exhalation, the tethering effect on the bronchiolar walls of the expanded elastic lung tissue decreases causing their diameter to decrease. As a result of smooth muscle contraction, bronchiolar wall edema, and lumen secretions, some bronchioles close off and prevent air from escaping. Although increased lung compliance, or decreased elasticity, is seen in asthma, it does not contribute significantly to airway collapse as it does in chronic obstructive pulmonary disease (COPD). Similar to COPD, air trapping occurs preferentially in the bases due to the weight of the lungs causing a more positive intrapleural pressure and therefore greater pressure exerted inward on the bronchiolar walls. This results in increased ventilation to the upper lung fields and the creation of a ventilation/perfusion (V/Q) mismatch. Obstruction during inhalation is not a problem because decreased intrapleural pressure and increased lung volume both act to increase the diameter of bronchioles.

3. D. Mild to moderate asthma results in a V/Q mismatch, relative hypoxia, and a compensatory increase in minute volume. Exchange of CO_2 at the alveolar membrane occurs readily, resulting in the net transfer of pulmonary capillary CO_2 into the alveolar space. Therefore, arterial $PaCO_2$ is decreased and, subsequently, the pH is increased. Arterial HCO_3^- will also decrease slightly in order to maintain equilibrium of the Henderson-Hasselbach equation ($H_2CO_3 \leftrightarrows H^+ + HCO_3^-$). This is referred to as respiratory alkalosis. As asthma becomes more severe and the patient is unable to ventilate adequately, CO_2 is no longer eliminated and its alveolar accumulation results in an increased arterial $PaCO_2$ and subsequent acidosis. This is referred to as *respiratory acidosis*.

4. C. Flow can be defined at its extremes as either laminar or turbulent. Transitional flow is considered in between these two states. Laminar flow is more efficient because it results in greater forward velocity with much smaller resistance. For a patient with asthma this translates into better ventilation requiring less work of breathing. Flow is laminar or turbulent depending on the conduit, flow rates, and characteristics of the fluid. These factors are summarized by the Reynold's equation (Re = 2rvd/n). For a gaseous fluid (i.e., air), viscosity (n) plays little role. Therefore, the Reynold's number is determined by the radius of the conduit, the velocity of the flow, and the density of the gas. At higher Reynold's numbers (typically > 2000), the flow's transition is from laminar to turbulent. Flow in the trachea is typically turbulent given the large conduit diameter and high flow velocity. In the terminal bronchioles, the conduit diameter and flow rates have decreased dramatically, and the resulting flow is laminar. Heliox is often used in acute asthma exacerbations in order to optimize laminar flow and reduce the work of breathing. Heliox is a mixture of 80% helium and 20% oxygen, where helium has one-eighth the density of nitrogen. This mixture therefore decreases the Reynold's number and promotes laminar flow in the bronchi and larger bronchioles.

Case 6

1. E. Restrictive lung disease is characterized by decreased lung volumes measured by pulmonary function testing, including total lung capacity (TLC), functional vital capacity (FVC), forced expiratory volume in 1 second (FEV$_1$), functional residual volume (FRV), and residual volume (RV). Decreased FEV$_1$ is characteristic of obstructive lung disease; however, a better measurement of pure obstructive pathology is the ratio of gas expired during the first second (FEV$_1$) over the total volume of gas expired to residual volume (FVC). This ratio is FEV$_1$/FVC, and it is universally decreased in obstructive lung disease. In restrictive disease, FEV$_1$ may be decreased only because the total expired capacity is decreased, as opposed to an actual obstructive pattern. Therefore, in purely restrictive disease, the ratio FEV$_1$/FVC is often normal or increased.

2. B. Pulmonary fibrosis is the common final pathway for a number of disease processes. The initial insult may be a result of direct toxicity (e.g., drug- or radiation-induced fibrosis), an inflammatory response (e.g., pneumoconioses, hypersensitivity pneumonitis), or through an immunologically mediated reaction (e.g., collagen vascular disease, pulmonary vasculitides). Regardless of inciting injury, the subsequent influx of inflammatory cells into the pulmonary interstitia results in deposition of collagen and fibrotic tissue. This fibrosis leads to contraction of the interstitial space, decreased lung volume, decreased lung compliance, and increased alveolar-capillary diffusion distances with resulting decreased diffusion capacity (DLCO). The numerous diseases that can result in pulmonary fibrosis are detailed in Table 6-2.

3. E. Asbestos is used generically to refer to several different types of mineral silicates that form fibrous dust particles possessing excellent thermal and electric insulating properties. Therefore, asbestos had previous widespread use in construction materials, pipe fittings, tile and roofing material, and brake lining. Onset of asbestosis is typically delayed by decades from the exposure. The presence of pleural plaques implies only past exposure and does not necessarily mean that pulmonary disease exists. Asbestosis significantly increases the risk for squamous cell and adenocarcinoma of the lung. This risk is multiplied by the additional risk of ciga-

rette smoking. Mesotheliomas are also associated with asbestos exposure, although this risk is neither augmented by cigarette smoking nor asbestos-dose related. Silicosis is the result of exposure to free silica, or crystalline quartz, in the form of rock dust. Exposure occurs primarily in mining, stone cutting, granite quarrying, sandblasting, tunneling through rock rich in quartz. Classic radiographic findings include rounded, small opacities in the upper lobes with calcified hilar adenopathy that create an "eggshell" pattern. For reasons unknown, silicosis has a high association with tuberculosis. Byssinosis, or hypersensitivity to cotton dust, is often referred to as "Monday's disease." Cotton dust exposure occurs in cotton mills before the cotton is spun; it causes bronchoconstriction and obstructive pulmonary function tests. Symptoms tend to improve on the weekends when workers are away from the mill and recur on Monday when they return. Coal workers' pneumoconiosis, like asbestosis and silicosis, is a fibrotic infiltrative disease in response to inhaling inorganic coal dust.

4. D. Sarcoidosis is a disease characterized by the formation of noncaseating granulomas that consist of T-lymphocytes and phagocytic monocytes. It is an exaggerated cellular immune response, either acquired or inherited, to an unknown antigen or self antigens. The lung is most often affected, although skin, eyes, and lymph nodes are also commonly affected. In the United States the disease occurs more frequently in African Americans, although this does not necessarily hold true for other regions of the world (e.g., higher prevalence in whites in Europe). In the lung, sarcoidosis typically causes hilar adenopathy, and up to 15% of diagnosed persons develop progressive interstitial fibrosis. Erythema nodosum is a common skin finding and consists of erythematous painful nodules located on the anterior shin. Eye, lymph node, and liver involvement are also common. Any other organ system may be involved as well, including bone marrow, spleen, nervous system, kidneys, musculoskeletal system, heart, endocrine, and reproductive organs.

Table 6-2. Etiologies of Pulmonary Fibrosis

Idiopathic pulmonary fibrosis
Pneumoconioses —Asbestosis, silicosis, coal workers' pneumoconiosis
Hypersensitivity pneumonitis —Bacteria (especially *Actinomyces* in Farmer's lung), fungi (molds), animal proteins (bird droppings, animal dander), amoeba (humidifier lung), drugs (especially nitrofurantoin)
Collagen vascular disease —Rheumatoid arthritis, SLE, scleroderma
Drug-induced fibrosis —Amiodarone, bleomycin, chlorambucil, chronic sulfonamides
Pulmonary vasculitis (e.g., Wegener's granulomatosis)
Radiation pneumonitis

Case 7

1. E. Risk factors for pulmonary embolism (PE) include a recent surgical procedure or orthopedic injury, postpartum, heart failure with low cardiac output, cancer, oral estrogen replacement or contraceptive pills, smoking, or a familial history of clotting disorders. The strongest risk factor for PE is history of a prior deep venous thrombosis.

2. C. Acute mitral or aortic valvular stenosis causes a sharp rise in pulmonary venous pressure which, by back-pressure, results in recruitment of collapsed vessels and dilatation of open vessels. This increases the total effective cross-sectional diameter of the pulmonary vasculature and results in a decrease in pulmonary vascular resistance. Both positive pressure ventilation and forced exhalation result in increased intrathoracic pressure, which causes constriction of pulmonary capillaries and increased resistance. Breathing gas with a Fio$_2$ of 0.10 (i.e., hypoxic mixture) results in hypoxic vasoconstriction and thus increased pulmonary vascular resistance. A pneumonectomy, or the removal of lung tissue and related pulmonary vasculature, effectively decreases the total cross-sectional area of the pulmonary vasculature and thus increases total vascular resistance.

3. C. Acute pulmonary embolism causes local vasoconstriction as a result of a local decrease in PaO_2. Increased flow resistance locally, and an overall increase in pulmonary artery pressure, results in vasodilation of unaffected capillary beds via recruitment and dilatation. Despite the relative decrease in vascular resistance as a result of this vasodilation, the overall effect of a pulmonary embolism is to increase pulmonary vascular resistance. As a result of the V/Q mismatch, the PaO_2 of arterial blood is decreased, which translates to an increased A-a gradient.

4. C. It is important to understand the physiologic differences between lung regions in order to understand the pathophysiology of many pulmonary diseases. Zone 1 (lung apices) is a region where the alveoli are hyperexpanded due to the effect of gravity pulling the tissues down. As a result of the increased volume and stretching of interstitial tissues, this region "lives" higher on the pressure volume curve, meaning that it takes larger increments of pressure to effect a change in volume. This is by definition *lower compliance.* The difference between intrathoracic and alveolar pressure is equal throughout all regions of the lung during inspiration. Therefore, because zone 3 (lung bases) has a higher compliance, the increase in volume of the alveoli in zone 3 is greater, resulting in greater ventilation to zone 3 and less ventilation to zone 1. Perfusion is also greater in zone 3 due to the higher pulmonary capillary pressure as a result of gravity. Perfusion (Q) is reduced in zone 1 to a greater degree than ventilation (V); and as a result, the V/Q ratio in zone 1 is much greater than that in zone 3.

Case 8

1. B. Increased pulmonary vessel hydrostatic pressure results in the flow of edema fluid into the interstitium that separates the capillaries from the alveoli. Increased interstitial fluid both increases interstitial hydrostatic pressure and decreases interstitial oncotic pressure. Both of these effects promote the flow of fluid back out of the interstitium and into the capillaries, thus providing negative feedback to the development of pulmonary edema. However, when the pulmonary vessel hydrostatic pressure is so great as to counteract these effects, the interstitial hydrostatic pressure builds to a degree where alveolar membrane damage occurs. This results in an increased membrane permeability coefficient and the influx of water, ions, proteins, and cells into the alveoli.

2. A. Alveolar edema washes away pulmonary surfactant and negates its effect of lowering alveolar wall surface tension. This increased surface tension promotes alveolar collapse, thus decreasing overall alveolar ventilation. The decreased ventilation with relatively unaffected perfusion results in an overall decrease in the V/Q ratio. Unventilated alveoli can also be thought of as a physiologic shunt that provides unventilated mixed venous blood into the arterial circulation, which results in low blood oxygen content and hypoxemia. As a result of gravity and thus increased pulmonary hydrostatic pressures in zone 3, pulmonary edema effects the lung bases greater than the apices. During inspiration, recruitment and opening of apical alveoli occurs causing increased ventilation

to this region. Similarly, hypoxic vasoconstriction in the bases leads to recruitment and dilatation of apical vessels and perfusion to the apices is increased as well.

3. C. Early pulmonary edema is manifested by filling of basilar alveoli and the development of a V/Q mismatch and physiologic shunting. This results in arterial hypoxemia and the physiologic response of increased minute ventilation. This translates to increased ventilation to apical alveoli whose V/Q ratio is greater than 1.0. Because of the already saturated oxygen-hemoglobin curve in these regions, arterial oxygen content increases little. However, by nature of the more linear CO_2-hemoglobin curve the off-gassing of carbon dioxide is facilitated. The decrease in $PaCO_2$ leads to a primary respiratory alkalosis as seen in choice c. Choice a represents a mixed respiratory acidosis (high $PaCO_2$) and metabolic acidosis (low $[HCO_3^-]$). Both choices b and e represent a metabolic acidosis (low $[HCO_3^-]$) with a small compensatory decrease in PCO_2. Choice d represents a metabolic alkalosis (high $[HCO_3^-]$) with a small compensatory increase in $PaCO_2$.

4. E. Pulmonary edema is a disorder of fluid transudate into peripheral alveoli. Sometimes the edema is such that peripheral bronchioles become fluid-filled as well, and clinical findings of expiratory wheezes are not uncommon. This finding is referred to as *cardiac wheeze.* Unlike reactive airways disease, this wheeze is not a result of bronchoconstriction; and therefore, the use of beta-agonist nebulizers is not helpful.

Case 9

1. D. This patient presents with symptoms and signs of classical pneumonia, which is typically caused by bacterial pathogens such as *S. pneumoniae, H. influenzae, M. catarrhalis,* or *S. aureus. Mycoplasma pneumoniae* is the most common causative organism for atypical pneumonia in young, healthy adults.

2. C. The illness described is Legionella pneumonia, caused by the organism *Legionella pneumophila.* This organism is ubiquitous in moist environments. Outbreaks have been linked to a variety of sources including cooling towers, air-conditioning systems, whirlpools, respiratory nebulizers, and other man-made water-containing units. *Legionella* is thought to consist of 10% of both community- and hospital-acquired pneumonias. *Legionella* pneumonia is usually preceded by a prodrome of malaise, headache, myalgia, and weakness. Later, the onset of high fevers and rigors is not uncommon. Patients usually have a nonproductive cough and may have pleuritic chest pain. The radiographic findings include a patchy, diffuse infiltrate, but they may also include focal consolidation. Gastrointestinal symptoms are a hallmark of *Legionella* infection and include diarrhea, vomiting, and abdominal pain. Relative bradycardia is also common. The treatment of choice for *Legionella* is erythromycin, a macrolide. Other macrolides (e.g., azithromycin, clarithromycin), sulfamethoxazole/trimethoprim (Bactrim), and fluoroquinolones are effective as well.

3. A. This patient most likely has *Mycoplasma pneumonia,* which is the most common bacterial atypical pneumonia. Other likely etiologies for a young healthy patient would be *Chlamydia pneu-*

moniae or a viral pneumonia. First-line treatment would be a macrolide (e.g., azithromycin, clarithromycin, erythromycin). A fluoroquinolone is a good alternative. Amoxicillin/clavulanate and cephalosporins are not active against *Mycoplasma* because of its lack of a true cell wall.

4. B. This patient presents with a syndrome typical for *Pneumocystis carinii* pneumonia. Common presenting symptoms include fever, dyspnea, and nonproductive cough. Physical exam usually reveals tachypnea, tachycardia, hypoxia, and ill-appearance. Pulmonary exam is often unrevealing. The chest x-ray findings show bilateral, diffuse, interstitial infiltrates that tend to be perihilar. Lab abnormalities often include an elevated serum lactate dehydrogenase (LDH), which likely reflects parenchymal lung damage. The two mainstays of therapy for *Pneumocystis* include trimethoprim-sulfamethoxazole and pentamidine, both of which are administered intravenously. Other drugs used include dapsone, clindamycin, and primaquine. Studies have shown that administration of glucocorticoids is beneficial for patients with a $PaO_2 < 70$ mmHg or an A-a gradient > 35 mmHg. *Pneumocystis* prophylaxis is indicated for AIDS patients with a CD_4 count < 200 because these patients are at high risk for contracting *Pneumocystis.* Prophylaxis consists of either trimethoprim-sulfamethoxazole one double-strength tablet daily or aerosolized pentamidine administered in an inhaler.

Case 10

1. D. Primary infection with tuberculosis occurs by inhaling bacilli into the lungs where these are phagocytized by alveolar macrophages and carried to regional lymph nodes. During the first few weeks after primary infection, the bacilli replicate locally and T-cell-mediated cellular immunity develops. Lymphocytes and monocytes migrate to the area of infection and form histiocytic cells that organize into a granuloma. These granulomas most often contain the infection and eventually become calcified. Tuberculosis bacilli remain viable within macrophages in the granuloma for years and often never reactivate. Primary infection is usually asymptomatic; however, a small percentage of patients develop active tuberculosis after primary infection. Once infected, patients develop life-long immunity to reinfection as is manifested by a positive response to PPD antigen. Patients with primary infection are not contagious as long as the infection is contained within a granuloma.

2. C. Secondary tuberculosis, or reactivation tuberculosis, usually occurs many years after the primary infection. Reactivation is more prevalent in the elderly, debilitated, and immunocompromised. It occurs when contained bacilli begin to multiply and proliferate. As pulmonary lesions progress, they necrotize and become caseating granulomas. These can necrotize into adjacent bronchi and become cavitary lesions. Secondary tuberculosis can also manifest as lobar infiltrates. It is during this phase that patients are contagious. The PPD typically remains *positive* during secondary tuberculosis. Anergy, or a false-negative PPD test, often occurs in end-stage AIDS and in miliary tuberculosis, which is a widespread hematogenous spread of bacilli.

3. B. The size of the PPD reaction considered positive depends on the likelihood of disease in that particular patient. This is done because there is some degree of cross-reactivity with other antigens and subsequent false-positive reactions in some patients. Therefore, the threshold of positivity is set higher for patients with relatively low risk to avoid overtreating false-positive reactions. For immunocompromised patients, any reaction is considered positive because of the high prevalence of anergy. Persons who are exposed to active tuberculosis are considered positive with reactions of 5 mm or greater. For individuals at elevated risk for TB (e.g., homeless, urban-dwellers, highly endemic region) reactions of 10 mm or greater are considered positive.

4. A. The most common side effect of treatment for tuberculosis is hepatitis. Isoniazid, rifampin, and pyrazinamide can all cause hepatitis. Isoniazid is also known to cause peripheral neuropathy. Rifampin causes orange urine and flu-like symptoms; it can also cause thrombocytopenia. Pyrazinamide can cause hyperuricemia. Patients who are started on isoniazid or rifampin must have liver function tests done at 2 weeks and followed up every several months thereafter.

Case 11

1. D. Acute respiratory distress syndrome (ARDS) is most commonly caused by bacterial sepsis as a result of endotoxin-mediated damage to pulmonary capillary endothelium. Etiologies for ARDS are many and include direct pulmonary alveolar damage from infection, aspiration, toxic inhalation, or blunt trauma. Indirect damage can occur with narcotics overdose, host immunologic reactions to disease, and other systemic disease processes that cause hypotension. The latter include acute necrotizing pancreatitis, severe burn injuries, and multisystem trauma with prolonged hypotension. ARDS is also a known complication of major surgery involving cardiopulmonary bypass.

2. C. ARDS is characterized by damage to pulmonary capillary endothelium resulting in destruction capillary-alveolar barrier and increased permeability to water, ions, proteins, and cells. This is reflected in the Starling equation by an increase in the filtration coefficient (K_f). As a result of increased permeability, interstitial hydrostatic and oncotic pressures will also increase, approaching those pressures present in pulmonary capillaries. Local lymphatics can increase their flow fifteenfold in response to increased interstitial hydrostatic pressure. Once this outlet is overwhelmed, increased interstitial hydrostatic pressure causes damage to alveolar epithelium, which results in alveolar exudates.

3. A. ARDS results in alveolar hypoventilation in the face of relatively normal perfusion (i.e., decreased V/Q ratio). This in effect creates physiologic shunting of mixed venous blood past unventilated alveoli into pulmonary venous return to the heart, creating a large A-a gradient and arterial hypoxemia. Early in the course of ARDS, increased minute ventilation will result in off-loading of CO_2 and respiratory alkalosis (choice c) as discussed with other disease processes. However, alveolar flooding occurs rapidly in ARDS, and increased minute ventilation is not able to compensate for the degree of hypoxemia that develops, and respiratory failure ensues. This is heralded by CO_2 retention (i.e., increased $PaCO_2 > 40$ mmHg) and acidemia (i.e., respiratory acidosis). At the same time, peripheral hypoxemia results in anaerobic metabolism and the formation of lactic acid that causes a simultaneous metabolic acidosis (i.e., decreased [HCO_3^-]). Choice a reflects this mixed acid-base disorder. The other options include primary metabolic acidosis (choices B and E), respiratory alkalosis (choice C), and metabolic alkalosis (choice D).

4. B. Increased positive end-expiratory pressure (PEEP) (10–15 mmHg) is beneficial for patients with ARDS. Alveolar filling washes away surfactant, which maintains low alveolar surface tension and thus alveolar patency. As a result, alveolar collapse occurs in the face of increased interstitial hydrostatic pressure. PEEP counteracts this tendency for alveoli to collapse, and it is especially important during the expiratory phase when airway pressures are low. Increasing the number of patent alveoli has the effect of decreasing peak inspiratory pressures required to provide a given tidal volume (i.e., increased lung compliance). As a result, a larger tidal volume can be given and thus an increased minute volume (tidal volume $\times$ respiratory rate). This allows more effective oxygen delivery to a greater surface area of alveolar membrane. PEEP applies pressure to the intrathoracic cavity, which results in decreased venous return to the right atrium and increased pulmonary vascular resistance. This in turn leads to decreased blood return to the left atrium (i.e., decreased preload). As depicted by the Frank-Starling curve, decreased preload results in decreased cardiac output. For this reason, arterial blood pressure must be closely monitored while increasing PEEP.

Case 12

1. A. Squamous cell carcinoma, which accounts for about 40% of bronchogenic carcinomas, tends to occur more centrally. It is locally invasive and has a tendency to cavitate into surrounding bronchi, which leads to hemoptysis. Massive hemoptysis results from tumor invasion through the wall of a bronchiolar vessel. Because of its undifferentiated and invasive nature large-cell carcinoma also tends to cavitate; however, the tumors tend to be more peripherally located and thus hemoptysis is less common. Adenocarcinoma is also a peripheral tumor with less likelihood to cavitate. Small-cell carcinoma is centrally located but not locally invasive and does not cavitate. It does, however, metastasize rapidly by hematogenous spread.

2. B. Adenocarcinoma, which also accounts for about 40% of bronchogenic carcinomas, has a variation referred to as *bronchioloalveolar* carcinoma because of its more diffuse involvement of bronchioles and alveoli. This type of carcinoma can appear on chest x-ray as diffuse, peripheral, multinodular or fluffy infiltrates. Diagnosis is usually made via cytologic examination of bronchoalveolar lavage fluid. Adenocarcinoma and squamous cell carcinoma metastasize slower than large- or small-cell carcinomas; therefore, lesions are often amenable to surgical resection. The 5-year survival for solitary tumors less than 4 cm in diameter are 40% and 30% for squamous cell carcinoma and adenocarcinoma, respectively. In general, adenocarcinoma tends to be more common in women and in nonsmokers. About 90% of patients who develop bronchogenic carcinoma have a strong history of tobacco use. Tobacco is very strongly associated with both squamous cell and small-cell carcinoma.

3. C. This patient likely has a postobstructive pneumonia as a result of a bronchial tumor. This must be suspected in patients with pneumonia that does not resolve with appropriate therapy, especially in elderly patients with risk factors for bronchogenic carcinoma. In some hospitals, the next step in the work-up for this patient would be further imaging of the chest in an attempt to identify an obstructing mass and to identify mediastinal metastases. CT scan is the quickest and most cost-effective imaging study that will provide enough detail regarding pulmonary parenchyma and mediastinal structures. Whether or not a mass is identified by CT scan, this patient would likely undergo bronchoscopy to directly visualize the bronchi and obtain washings for culture and cytology. This test has the highest likelihood of arriving at a specific diagnosis.

4. E. Bronchogenic carcinoma can lead to a number of physical exam findings that are both related to tumor invasion of local thoracic structures and to systemic neuroendocrine effects of factors released by the tumor. Eyelid drooping is one feature of Horner's syndrome (ptosis, myosis, anhydrosis) that can occur as result of tumor invasion of the cervical sympathetic chain that originates anterior to the thoracic vertebrae in the posterior mediastinum. Hoarseness can result from invasion of the recurrent laryngeal nerve near the lung apices. Facial swelling can be the result of superior vena cava syndrome, which is caused most frequently by small-cell carcinomas that obstruct the thoracic outlet and compress the superior vena cava. This results in decreased venous return from the head and upper extremities. Leg swelling is an indication of a lower extremity deep venous thrombosis, which occurs frequently in patients with cancer. The specific etiology of cancer-related hypercoagulability is not understood, although it is thought to be an alteration of normal clotting factor function.

Case 13

1. D. Cystic fibrosis (CF) results from a mutation at position 508 on the long arm of chromosome 7. This region codes for a protein that functions as a cAMP-mediated chloride channel on normal epithelial cells. This chloride channel performs different functions depending on the location of the epithelial cells. In respiratory epithelia, this channel functions to secrete chloride into respiratory mucus and, as a result, sodium and water will follow. This keeps secretions well hydrated and fluid. In CF, chloride secretion is diminished; therefore, sodium and water is reabsorbed into the cells, resulting in dehydrated, thick, tenacious mucus. In skin, the CFTR chloride channel functions to reabsorb chloride back into epithelial cells. Therefore, dysfunction of these channels results in abnormally elevated NaCl secretion from sweat ducts.

2. A. In addition to the lungs, CF causes profound dysfunction and morbidity related to the gastrointestinal tract. In the pancreas, absence of the cystic fibrosis transmembrane regulator (CFTR) chloride channel results in dysfunction of the chloride-bicarbonate exchanger, resulting in decreased secretion of sodium bicarbonate from the exocrine pancreas. This inhibits the secretion of exocrine pancreatic enzymes and results in destruction of the exocrine pancreas. Lack of pancreatic enzymes results in malabsorption of fat and vitamins, leading to steatorrhea. Pancreatic beta cells are often spared, and therefore hyperglycemia and insulin requirement is a late finding in a small percentage of patients. Lack of chloride and water secretion from the intestinal crypts results in obstruction that can manifest as meconium ileus in infants. Distal intestinal obstruction occurs in adolescence and adulthood as well. In the hepatobiliary system, decreased secretion of chloride and water results in sludging of secretions, hepatobiliary cirrhosis, chronic cholecystitis, and bile duct proliferation.

3. D. Respiratory manifestations of CF start early in life, typically as chronic cough and rhinorrhea as an infant. Chronic sinusitis and nasal polyps are common in childhood. Although airway colonization with *Streptococcus* is a likely occurrence, the classic pathogens related to CF early in life are *S. aureus* and *H. influenzae*. Thereafter, *Pseudomonas* becomes the prevalent pathogen and emergence of the highly-resistant mucoid form is common. Other typical pathogens found in CF patients include gram-negative rods such as *Klebsiella, Proteus,* and *E. coli.* The fungus *Aspergillus fumigatus* is also a common pathogen. Chronic infection and inflammation leads to necrosis of the bronchial walls and result in chronic bronchiectasis. Thick mucus causes chronic bronchial plugging and a resultant obstructive pattern on pulmonary function tests. This airway obstruction is initially reversible with clearance of thick mucus from small airways but, as the disease progresses to chronic bronchiectasis, airway obstruction persists. Common complications of CF include atelectasis and pneumothoraces, the former as a result of mucus plugging and the latter as a result of obstruction and hyperinflation. Bronchial wall destruction and bronchiectasis typically results in hemoptysis.

4. F. Antibiotic therapy for pneumonia in CF patients should be tailored to the specific pathogens cultured and antibiotic sensitivities. However, one must know which antibiotic classes are most effective against *Pseudomonas*. Due to the high resistance of most *Pseudomonas* species and to ensure adequate antimicrobial activity, it is common practice to double-cover, or give two antibiotics from differing classes. Antipseudomonal penicillins include piperacillin, mezlocillin, and ticarcillin. Fluoroquinolones have variable effectiveness against *Pseudomonas* only variably, and resistance is increasing; however, levofloxacin and ciprofloxacin are often effective. Antipseudomonal cephalosporins include cefepime, ceftazidime, and cefoperazone. Other third-generation agents (e.g., ceftriaxone, cefotaxime) have variable effectiveness. Aminoglycosides (e.g., gentamicin, tobramycin, amikacin) are mainstays of therapy against *Pseudomonas*. A typical regimen against *Pseudomonas* includes antipseudomonal penicillin combined with an aminoglycoside.

Case 14

1. B. Gastroesophageal reflux disease (GERD) develops when acidic gastric contents splash into the distal portion of the esophagus irritating the tissues. It is true that GERD can be associated with lower esophageal sphincter (LES) atrophy and scleroderma but the LES would be open in GERD, whereas in achalasia it would be closed. Remember, the question asks which is *less likely* to occur with acha-

lasia. In achalasia, the LES does not relax and has increased resting tone resulting in diminution of the possibility of developing GERD. Scleroderma is associated with achalasia. Answer choices C, D, and E may or may not occur in this patient, but are unrelated to the increased resting tone often observed in achalasia.

2. C. Hirschsprung's (congenital megacolon) and achalasia both lack ganglion cells. In achalasia the cells are missing from the myenteric plexus; in Hirschsprung's they are missing from the Meissner's and myenteric plexus. In both instances, patients have dilation of the respective portion of the GI tract: the colon in Hirschsprung's (resulting in loss of bowel function and inability to pass stool) and the esophagus in achalasia. Collagen vascular disease and squamous cell carcinoma rates are increased in patients with achalasia.

3. A. Answers B, C, D, and E are all possible sequelae of achalasia. Collagen vascular disease is associated with achalasia but does not result from the disorder.

4. C. Congenital megacolon is not a component of CREST syndrome, which is characterized by *c*alcinosis, *R*aynaud's phenomenon, *e*sophageal dysfunction *s*clerodactyly, and *t*elangiectasia.

Case 15

1. A. Corrosive esophagitis from ingestion of a strong alkaline agent such as lye results in liquefactive necrosis. Coagulative necrosis is produced by ingestion of acids. Gangrenous necrosis occurs when the tissue or bone has severely limited or absent blood flow (e.g., diabetic, *Clostridium p.*). Fat necrosis occurs when areas of fat are traumatized and devoid of blood flow. Radiation necrosis is caused by large doses of radiation

2. D. Long-standing gastroesophageal reflux disease (GERD) can lead to metaplastic columnar cells and Barrett's esophagus with subsequent increases risk for adenocarcinoma of the distal esophagus. Transitional cell types are common in the bladder. Metaplastic squamous cells can occur in precancerous conditions in many types of tissues (e.g., breast, prostate, uterus, cervix, lung). Microvilli and squamous cells are not pathologic.

3. E. This patient offers several clues that he may in fact have AIDS. Although the other blood tests may impact the treatment of his illnesses, his long-term health will be most benefited by treatment with antiretrovirals if he is in fact HIV positive. ELISA is the screening test of choice for HIV infection. CBC with diff, chest x-ray, and sputum culture can indicate infection (e.g., pneumonia, tuberculosis) with an elevated white blood cell count, a density or growth of acid fast bacilli, respectively. TSH is a screening tool for thyroid dysfunction.

Case 16

1. D. Neutrophils above the basement membrane only is the classic pathophysiology of acute gastritis. Answer A with absent epithelium, a purulent exudate, and bleeding would indicate an erosion that is a more severe form of gastritis. Answer B—thinned and flattened rugae and mucosa—is a gross observation of gastritis rather than a histological description. Answer C is the classic description of *H. pylori* gastritis. Finally, the specimen should contain no pre-malignant features in acute gastritis.

2. E. Disorders of the thyroid and adrenal glands are associated with pernicious anemia; the other disorders listed are not. HIV should be screened only for those individuals at increased risk.

3. B. Gastrin levels are elevated in chronic gastritis. The other gastric hormone levels are unchanged.

4. A. The increased risk of gastric carcinoma is 2% to 4%. The other answers (C, D, and E) are, fortunately, too high.

Case 17

1. C. Cimetidine, although effective, has various side effects listed in the question stem as well as gynecomastia, which is an enlargement of the breast tissue in the male or other anti-androgenic effects. Stevens-Johnson syndrome (skin rash, fever, and multiple lesions of the oral conjunctival and vaginal mucous membranes) is often caused by sulfa-based drugs or ethosuximide. Agranulocytosis is a reaction to the antipsychotic clozapine or the anti-epileptic carbamazepine. Microcytic anemia is a type of anemia with a low mean corpuscular volume (MCV). Depression is an adverse effect of some β_2 blockers like propranalol.

2. B. Nonsteroidal anti-inflammatory drugs (NSAIDs) are theorized to promote ulceration formation by suppression of mucosal prostaglandins. Ischemia may also impair mucosal defense; however, this is common in the setting of hypovolemic shock. Answers C and D are theorized as mechanisms for ulceration of the carcinoid tumor Zollinger-Ellison syndrome or other conditions of hyperacidity. Increased gastric emptying occurs in dumping syndrome.

3. E. Gastric ulcers and chronic gastritis increase the patient's risk of gastric carcinoma. Duodenal ulceration is not known to increase a patient's risk of duodenal carcinoma. Answers A, B, and D are not known complications of ulcers.

4. D. This patient has evidence of gastric ulcer perforation as indicated by the free air shown on the KUB. Commonly performed ulcers are repaired with an omental patch (Graham patch). This patient is not a candidate for outpatient pharmacologic management (answers B and C). Barium swallow is contraindicated in a patient with a perforated ulcer. Admission with serial abdominal examinations is employed in a patient with an acute (surgical) abdomen of unknown etiology but does not offer definitive treatment in this patient.

Case 18

1. D. This patient has a history that indicates chronic Chagas' disease. In acute Chagas' disease, parasites from *Trypanosoma cruzi* invade myocardium and rarely result in progressive cardiac dilation and failure. In chronic Chagas' disease, 5 to 15 years after initial infection, an autoimmune response results in an inflamma-

tory infiltration of the myocardium causing dilated cardiomyopathy and cardiac arrhythmias. Gummas are a finding in tertiary syphilis. Endocarditis and interstitial fibrosis are not sequelae of Chagas' disease. The bite marks—from the bites of the reduviid bug—indicate the manner in which patients acquire Chagas' disease. Scabies are not associated with Chagas' disease.

2. A. Hypokalemia is most likely the cause of this infant's condition. Hypokalemia may result from Hirschsprung's and is manifest as hyporeflexia, flaccid paralysis, muscular weakness, and EKG changes. The abnormal state of feeding in Hirschsprung's often results in low albumin levels. Hyperkalemia may result in weakness but is commonly asymptomatic. Decreased caloric and water intake cannot describe all of the infant's findings.

3. E. Although the skin derives from the ectoderm—the precursor of the neural crest—it does not become skin. The other choices originate in the neural crest.

Case 19

1. A. This child most likely has rotavirus. Norwalk and adenovirus both cause nonbloody diarrhea in children; however, rotavirus is more common in infants and toddlers. Salmonella is often transmitted via the oral fecal route and causes typhoid fever with diarrhea and bradycardia, absolute neutropenia, and hepatosplenomegaly. Necrotizing enterocolitis is more common in infants and neonates born prematurely but commonly presents with fever and dysentery.

2. E. *Campylobacter* usually has multiple superficial ulcers from the small intestine to the colon with crypt abscesses on pathologic specimen. Other causes of bloody diarrhea are represented in this question. *Shigella* characteristically results in purulent exudate and erosions in the distal colon, whereas *Yersinia* results in mucosal hemorrhage and ulceration. *Salmonella* destroys enterocytes and results in linear ulcers in the ileum and colon. Shortened villi and lymphocytic infiltration of the lamina propria is a common finding for viral enterocolitis.

3. B. The most likely agent is *Vibrio cholerae* and the patient may be describing "rice water stools" from the severe secretory diarrhea. The mechanism of action for *Vibrio* is stimulation of adenylate cyclase. Enterotoxigenic strains of *E. coli* produce heat labile and heat stable toxins that stimulate guanylate cyclase. Endocytosis and transcytosis are used by *Salmonella* and *Yersinia*. Viruses such as Norwalk and rotavirus destroy enterocytes.

Case 20

1. D. A deficiency of vitamin K results in a prolonged PT and aPTT that can result in increased bleeding (anticoagulation). Vitamin A deficiency causes night blindness and dermatitis, whereas an excess may result in the listed symptoms. Vitamin D deficiency leads to rickets in children and osteopenia in adults, whereas excess results in elevated calcium levels and anorexia. Vitamin E deficiency causes increased fragility of erythrocytes, not dermatitis.

Finally, folic acid deficiency leads to anemia but it is a water-soluble vitamin, not a fat-soluble one.

2. A. This patient exhibits several physical signs of not absorbing enough vitamin K and is consequently bleeding. A PT and aPTT should be checked and if abnormal vitamin K should be administered in an intramuscular injection. Small intestinal biopsy is important in making the diagnosis of celiac sprue and in determining if a gluten-free diet will be effective. Because this patient is not adhering to her diet, a biopsy would not yield additional information. Likewise, a stool specimen for fecal fat is commonly used to make an initial diagnosis but not to guide treatment. Screening other family members is warranted because there is an increased familial incidence.

Case 21

1. C. T-cell lymphoma is associated with one of the common causes of malabsorption: celiac sprue. The other listed cancers are not known to increase in patients with sprue.

2. E. Streptomycin is an aminoglycoside and that class of drugs may cause nephrotoxicity and ototoxicity; the nephrotoxicity observed more commonly in patients is concurrently treated with a cephalosporin. Metformin is known to cause lactic acidosis; the statin drugs cause myositis. Gastrointestinal distress is a common reaction to many antibiotics including penicillin. Chloramphenicol causes gray-baby syndrome.

3. B. Giardiasis is a result of consuming water from a contaminated water. Giardia commonly contaminates water not filtered by sand and results in nutrient malabsorption. Shigella is less likely because it commonly causes a bloody diarrhea. Amebiasis is another common cause of bloody diarrhea and liver abscesses. Cholera does not exhibit a malabsorption syndrome but rather presents as rice water stools and profound dehydration. Viral syndromes are not known to cause malabsorptive diarrhea.

Case 22

1. E. In alcoholic liver hepatitis, you would expect an increase in aspartate aminotransferase (AST) and alanine aminotransferase (ALT) but usually the AST is approximately twice as high. The conjugated bilirubin is usually increased by 50% of the total.

2. C. Palmar erythema, gynecomastia, skin telangiectasias, and hypogonadism result from the altered metabolism of estrogens and resultant hyperestrinism. Patients with alcoholic cirrhosis have coagulopathy secondary to poor production of clotting factors. Hematemesis and hemorrhoids are a result of increased pressure in the portal venous system.

Case 23

1. D. Dubin-Johnson and Rotor's are both types of conjugated hyperbilirubinemias. The defect in Dubin-Johnson is in the bile canalicular membrane, affecting transport of the conjugated

bilirubin. Rotor's, also a type of conjugated jaundice, is differentiated from Dubin-Johnson pathologically in that it has no black pigment in the liver. Gilbert's, ABO incompatibility, Crigler-Najjar, breast milk, and physiologic jaundice are all unconjugated types. Severe hemolytic disease and Crigler-Najjar type I often cause kernicterus.

2. E. Reviewing the production and breakdown of bilirubin is the key to answering this question correctly. An excess of heme resulting in too much bilirubin, decreased hepatic uptake of bilirubin, and decreased conjugation all give predominantly unconjugated bilirubinemia. If the conjugated bilirubin is not excreted or bile flow is decreased secondary to obstruction then a conjugated hyperbilirubinemia exists.

3. B. In Crigler-Najjar type I, the gene that codes for the enzyme—UDP glucuronyl transferase—is absent, which results in an unconjugated hyperbilirubinemia. Gilbert's also gives an unconjugated hyperbilirubinemia secondary to decreased bilirubin UGT. Dubin-Johnson syndrome is an autosomal recessive disorder of conjugated hyperbilirubinemia with a canalicular membrane defect that results in a pigmented liver. Rotor's is a conjugated type with defective uptake by the hepatocyte.

Case 24

1. D. Patients who have been exposed to hepatitis B virus (HBV) and have immunity possess both anti-HBs and antiHB$_c$IgG. The patients in choice E are actively immunized and have anti-HBs antibodies but no antibodies to the core antigen as the vaccine immunizes against only surface antigen protein. Anti HB$_c$IgM may indicate current viral replication or acute infection. The patient in choice A is neither immune nor infected. The patient described in choice B most likely has an acute infection. Patient C most likely has a chronic infection.

2. E. Pruritis results from increased bile acids deposited in the skin. Hyperbilirubinemia leads to jaundice. Hyperbilirubinuria leads to dark urine. The CD8 T-lymphocytes lead to injury of hepatocytes. Ground-glass cytoplasm is present in hepatocytes filled with HB$_s$Ag. Hepatitis D is able to infect hepatocytes only in the presence of hepatitis B. Both hepatitis A and D are transmitted via the fecal-oral route.

Case 25

1. D. Primary sclerosing cholangitis results in a lymphocytic inflammatory infiltrate that leads to obliterative fibrosis and dilatation of the bile ducts. Antimitochondrial antibodies are associated with primary biliary cirrhosis, whereas alcoholic liver disease results in terminal venule fibrosis. Ballooning degeneration and apoptosis is observed in liver specimens from patients with active infectious hepatitis, whereas right heart failure leads to "nutmeg" liver or chronic hepatic congestion.

2. C. Patients with primary sclerosing cholangitis (PSC) are likely to have inflammatory bowel disease. Patients with primary biliary cirrhosis (PBC) are more commonly asymptomatic females with insidious onset of pruritis, jaundice, and fatigue. Pathologically, livers with PBC reveal granulomatous destruction of interlobular bile ducts with fibrosis and nodular regeneration, whereas those with PSC have a patchy lymphocytic infiltrate in the ducts that leads to obliteration.

Case 26

1. A. Risk factors for stone formation are decreased bile acids or bile salts with or without increased cholesterol solubilized in bile. Simply stated, solubilizing bile acids and lecithin are overwhelmed by an increase in the levels of cholesterol. The stone itself is not enough to cause disease because over 80% of gallstones do not cause pain or other complications. In approximately 90% of cases, acute cholecystitis is precipitated by an obstruction of the gallbladder neck or proximal cystic duct. Bacterial infection may follow these events; however, it is not an inciting event. Enzyme degradation and shistosomes are not known to cause cholecystitis.

2. C. Both C and E are correct but C is the current treatment of choice. The extended spectrum penicillins cover relevant bacteria. Also, third-generation cephalosporins plus metronidazole or clindamycin to kill anaerobe (*Clostridium* and *Bacteroides*).

3. D. The likely diagnosis based on the information provided is gallstone ileus. Rarely can a large stone erode through the wall of the gallbladder and into an adjacent loop of small intestine. Please see Key Points in Case 26 for differentiation of acute cholecystitis and gallstone pancreatitis. Ascending cholangitis is an infection of the bile ducts secondary to obstruction and is characterized by fever, right upper quadrant pain, jaundice, shock, and neurologic symptoms known as Reynold's pentad. Cytstic fibrosis is an autosomal recessive disorder characterized by respiratory, pancreatic, and urogenital disease.

4. B. Unlike the rest of the gastrointestinal tract, the gallbladder does not contain a submucosal or muscularis mucosa. It does contain the other layers listed in this question's choices.

Case 27

1. D. A prolonged QT interval is common in a patient with hypocalcemia. A short QT interval is observed in a patient with hypercalcemia. ST segment depression is an EKG change associated with ischemia, whereas diffuse ST segment elevation is common in pericarditis. Peaked T-waves are common in hypercalcemia.

2. E. In acute pancreatitis, elastase is partially responsible for the destruction of vessel walls. Cholecystokinin (CCK) stimulates the pancreas to release zymogens, whereas colipase requires bile acids to split fats. Trypsin does cleave pro-enzymes but α-amylase is secreted in active form. Enterokinase cleaves chymotrypsin to create the activator trypsin.

Case 28

1. B. All of the listed illnesses are in the differential diagnosis and laboratory evaluation is necessary to prioritize this list. Pelvic inflammatory disease (PID) is likely based on the patient's risk factors—3 days of pain, nausea, vomiting, multiple sexual partners—and physical examination. Although an ectopic pregnancy is also possible, it is unlikely based on her last period. A urine or blood pregnancy test would help. Gastroenteritis is usually a diagnosis of exclusion. This patient denies urinary symptoms and has normal bowel movements, thus renal stones or Crohn's disease is unlikely.

2. E. Diverticulitis and acute appendicitis are similar in that they both involve obstruction, often by a fecalith. Lymphoid hyperplasia as an obstructive source for appendicitis is a factor only in adolescents and young adults. The Western diet is proposed as the reason for diverticula to form and it is due to *decreased* not increased fiber in the diet. Bacterial invasion takes part in both appendicitis and diverticulitis; however, this is secondary not primary.

Case 29

1. D. Pseudopolyps are a common finding in areas where the mucosa is regenerating and bulges. This is uncommon in Crohn's disease. However, skip lesions, transmural involvement of the bowel wall, entire alimentary tract involvement, and fistula formation are common features or complications of Crohn's disease.

2. A. Patients with Crohn's disease are at risk for general or specific malabsorption including protein losing enteropathy (low albumin) as well as electrolyte abnormalities. Low calcium levels result in tetany, whereas decreased absorption of vitamin D results in osteopenia. A low hematocrit and microcytosis results from iron deficiency anemia, among other sequelae. This question describes a pernicious anemia of malabsorption that is so severe that the patient has neurologic sequelae; namely, a B_{12} deficiency.

3. C. Toxic megacolon is more common in patients who suffer from ulcerative colitis (UC) secondary to chronic cases of active disease that heal and attenuate the bowel wall leading to a thinned and weakened structure. The other choices—fistulas, aphthous ulcers, granulomas, and malabsorption—are characteristics or complications of Crohn's.

Case 30

1. A. In an elderly patient with an acute lower gastrointestinal bleed, the most likely cause is diverticulosis. Angiodysplasia can also result in an acute bleed in patients in their 60s; however, angiodysplasia is less common. Diverticulitis rarely causes brisk bleeding. Adenocarcinoma often causes persistent bleeding with microcytic, iron deficient anemia; these patients often have heme (+) stools. Appendicitis does not cause rectal bleeding.

2. D. The most clinically important bacterium not covered by the aminoglycoside you chose is *Bacteroides fragilis,* which is an anaerobic gram-negative rod that can be treated with clindamycin or metronidazole. The other categories of bacteria and protozoa are not applicable to common diverticulitis

3. E. A diet high in fiber (20–35 grams of fiber a day) increases stool bulk that decreases transit time, lowers pressures, and decreases muscle hypertrophy. A high-fiber diet is *not* theorized to strengthen the mucosa.

Case 31

1. A. This patient has evidence of ischemic bowel and likely necrotic bowel. While all of the choices are important and may help, this patient needs surgical intervention to remove the inciting event (if possible) and restore vascular supply to the bowel. Fluid management is important with evidence of acute renal failure and dehydration. Nasogastric (NG) decompression will alleviate her symptoms but will not add blood supply to the dying bowel. Although imaging may or may not add helpful information, it will only delay definitive treatment. Admission and observation is not an option.

2. C. In intussusception there must be a nidus for the telescoping to occur.

Case 32

1. E. It is possible that this patient has systemic lupus erythematosus (SLE) like her sister. Familial occurrence of SLE has been documented and it is known that family members have an increased risk of developing the disorder. Moreover, it has been shown that unaffected first-degree relatives have higher levels of auto-antibodies and immunoregulatory abnormalities. However, an important part of the patient's sister's history that cannot be overlooked is the fact that she has been taking hydralazine for her elevated blood pressure. A lupus-like syndrome can be caused by this drug as well as by the drugs procainamide, isoniazid, chlorpromazine, quinidine, and methyldopa. The clinical features of this drug-induced syndrome are similar to those of SLE and include positive antinuclear antibody (ANA) titers. However, important differences do exist. First, the gender prevalence of this disorder is equal as opposed to predominantly female. Second, renal and central nervous system (CNS) involvement is not typical. Third, although these patients are positive for ANA, they are neither usually positive for antidouble-stranded DNA antibodies nor are their complement levels markedly decreased. Finally, the symptoms of the drug-induced, lupus-like syndrome are milder and resolve once the drug is discontinued. Discoid lupus is characterized primarily by characteristic skin lesions that begin as erythematous papules or plaques with scaling that may become thick and adherent with a hypopigmented central area. Other symptoms, such as arthritis, are usually absent in this disorder.

2. D. Unfortunately, at this point in time, a perfect diagnostic test for SLE does not exist. All of the answer choices can be positive in patients with this disease. The most sensitive test for screening is antinuclear antibodies. Nearly all patients with SLE have these antibodies. However, this test is not specific and is elevated in a number of other disorders: systemic sclerosis, scleroderma, Sjögren's syndrome, rheumatoid arthritis, polymyositis/dermatomyositis, mixed connective tissue disorder, Wegener's granulomatosis, leprosy, infectious mononucleosis, liver disease, primary pulmonary fibrosis, and vasculitis. Moreover, approximately 5% to 15% of normal individuals have low titers of these antibodies. In contrast, antibodies to double-stranded DNA are found in only 50% of patients with SLE, but are rarely found in any other disorders. Erythrocyte sedimentation rate (ESR) is typically elevated in SLE, but is seen in a wide variety of inflammatory processes. Rheumatoid factor is observed in only 20% of patients with lupus. Lupus anticoagulant is an antiphospholipid antibody seen in 7% of lupus patients which, contrary to its name, is actually associated with venous and arterial thrombosis as well as to placental infarction. Unlike the other antibodies that are tested for by actually measuring the amount of antibody present in serum through titers, lupus anticoagulant is identified by looking at coagulation tests like prolongation of the activated PTT and Russel viper venom test.

3. D. This patient most likely has SLE—an autoimmune disorder characterized by the production of auto-antibodies. The loss of tolerance leading to this immune dysfunction is likely due to abnormalities in clonal anergy. Clonal anergy is the process that occurs in the peripheral blood circulation whereby lymphocytes that react with self antigens are inactivated. Clonal deletion occurs in the thymus and bone marrow as lymphocytes mature. In this process self reactive T-cells and B-cells are eliminated and self tolerance results. Release of sequestered antigens and molecular mimicry are two other mechanisms postulated to be involved in the development of autoimmune phenomenon. However, these are not believed to play a role in SLE. Enzyme deficiency can play a role in other arthritides such as gout, but has no role in this lupus.

4. A. Systemic lupus erythematosus is by definition a multiorgan system disorder. Systemic manifestations include fever, anorexia, weight loss, fatigue, and malaise. Skin and mucocutaneous features include a malar rash, discoid rash, alopecia and oral ulcers. The eyes can also be affected with conjunctivitis, photophobia, transient blindness, and blurring of vision. Pulmonary involvement can be seen as pleurisy, pleural effusion, bronchopneumonia, and pneumonitis. Pericarditis, cardiac arrhythmias, and cardiac failure secondary to myocarditis and hypertension are all possible heart manifestations. Also, Libman-Sacs endocarditis characterized by small single or multiple irregular verrucous lesions on any valve of the heart, on either surface of the valve leaflets can be seen. Neurologic symptoms include psychosis, organic brain syndrome, seizures, neuropathies, and depression. Glomerulonephritis is the main renal manifestation. Hematologic abnormalities seen in SLE include hemolytic anemia, thrombocytopenia, lymphopenia, and leukopenia. Finally, arterial and venous thrombosis as well as vasculitis characterized by "onion skin lesions" of the central arteries of the spleen can complicate the disease. Although joint involvement is a key feature of SLE, the arthritis seen rarely leads to joint destruction and deformities.

Case 33

1. B. Synovial fluid in early rheumatoid arthritis reveals evidence of the severe noninfectious inflammatory process occurring in the joints. It is typically turbid with elevated levels of WBCs the majority of which are neutrophils. This type of fluid can also be seen in gout and pseudogout, both of which are also characterized by noninfectious inflammation of the joints. In septic/infectious arthritis synovial fluid is also turbid, but levels of WBCs are even greater than that seen with noninfectious arthritis. Fragments of *Chlamydia trachomatis* can be found in the synovial fluid of patients with Reiter's syndrome (reactive arthritis). Bloody fluid can be seen whenever the arthrocentesis is traumatic, regardless of the type of joint pathology. Birefringent crystals seen under polarized light microscopy are characteristic of gout. Although levels of rheumatoid factor can be elevated in rheumatoid arthritis, these antibodies are tested for primarily in the blood.

2. C. The patient was most likely started on methotrexate, which is commonly used in patients with severe rheumatoid arthritis unresponsive to nonsteroidal anti-inflammatory drugs (NSAIDs) and other slow-acting agents such as gold salts, chloroquine, and D-penicillamine. Methotrexate is an immunosuppressant medication that is often used in the treatment of cancer. This chemotherapeutic agent is structurally similar to folic acid and acts by inhibiting dihydrofolate reductase, leading to decreased DNA and RNA production, and eventually decreased protein synthesis and cell death. The doses given for patients with rheumatoid arthritis are significantly lower than those given for chemotherapy. However, the side effects of oral ulcers and nausea are still commonly seen. More important, methotrexate can lead to decreased WBC production and subsequent immunosuppression, which places these patients at increased risk for infection. Aplastic anemia is not typically seen with methotrexate but can be associated with use of gold salts and penicillamine. Renal damage can be seen with methotrexate but usually occurs only with high-dose therapy. Hepatic function can also be impaired, but this occurs only with long-term use. Decreased rheumatoid factor is seen with the use of penicillamine.

3. F. Severe, long-standing rheumatoid arthritis with chronic inflammation of the joint space leads to destruction of the cartilage and underlying bone. On radiographs this is seen as joint space narrowing and bony erosions. Joint space narrowing is initially observed at the juxta-articular margin, which is not protected by cartilage. However, with continued inflammation and destruction of the cartilage, erosions can be seen in the remainder of the bony articular surfaces of the joint. Demineralization of bone and decreased bone density is seen with osteoporosis. Increased bony cortex of increased density is seen in Paget's disease and is characterized by excessive bone turnover. Joint space narrowing, osteophytes, and dense subchondral bone are seen in osteoarthritis. A "bamboo spine," characterized by calcification of the anterior and lateral spinal ligaments with squaring and demineralization of the vertebral bodies, is seen in late-stage ankylosing spondylitis. "Punched out" osteolytic lesions of the skull and long bones are characteristic of multiple myeloma.

4. C. This patient's reaction is an example of a type I hypersensitivity reaction. This immediate/anaphylactic hypersensitivity occurs when an antigen—in this case something in the shellfish—binds to and cross-links IgE on the surface of mast cells causing mast cell degranulation. Mediators such as histamine, eosinophil chemotactic factor of anaphylaxis, leukotrienes, prostaglandins, and thromboxanes are thus released. This release leads to swelling, vasodilation, and increased capillary permeability, which in turn can manifest as urticaria, angioedema, allergic rhinitis and bronchospasm. IgA is found mostly in the mucus membranes and serves *primarily* to prevent attachment of bacteria and viruses. It is not involved with mast cell degranulation and release of histamine. IgG-mediated immune complexes deposited in the skin is an example of type III hypersensitivity that occurs when immune complexes are deposited in tissues and subsequently activate complement. The onset of this type of reaction is delayed and usually occurs from a few days to a couple of weeks following exposure to the antigen. Serum sickness is an example of such a reaction. IgG-mediated complement lysis is an example of type II hypersensitivity that occurs when IgG antibodies directed at antigens of the cell membrane activate complement and lead to cell membrane destruction through the membrane-attack complex. Rh hemolytic disease is an example of this kind of hypersensitivity reaction.

Case 34

1. C. Reiter's syndrome is characterized by arthritis, conjunctivitis, and urethritis. It often follows chlamydial urethritis or dysentery caused by *Salmonella, Shigella, Yersinia* or *Campylobacter*. Skin manifestations are not typically a part of this syndrome. Psoriatic arthritis is, however, characterized by arthritis conjunctivitis and a psoriatic rash that is usually macular papular in nature with scaling.

2. B. Reiter's syndrome is associated with HLA-B27 and often follows chlamydial, not gonococcal, infection. Urethral cultures are therefore often positive for *Chlamydia*. This infection is believed to cause inflammatory symptoms through molecular mimicry whereby portions of the infectious agent are homologous to self proteins and thus—when infected—the resulting immune response leads not just to resolution of the infection but also to inflammation of self tissues. The infection itself is not responsible for the arthritis. Examination of synovial fluid reveals presence of chlamydial peptides but cultures are negative for the organism. HLA-D4 is associated with rheumatoid arthritis and Type 1 diabetes

3. D. Class I MHC molecules are found on all cells and present antigen to CD8 cells leading to cytotoxic T-cell destruction by the CD8 cells. Class II MHC molecules are found only on B-cells and macrophages and present antigen to CD4 cells, which in turn can lead to a T-cell mediated humoral response that triggers the complement cascade. HLA-DR3 and HLA-DR4 are examples of class II MHC molecules. HLA-B27 is a class I HLA molecule.

Case 35

1. C. In the first 24 hours of wound healing the most important process that occurs is the formation of new blood vessels, angiogenesis. Vascular endothelial growth factor (VEGF) is the most important growth factor in angiogenesis. It promotes angiogenesis by increasing vascular permeability, stimulating endothelial cell migration and proliferation, and up-regulating the expression of enzymes crucial for remodeling the extracellular matrix. Interferon gamma (IFN-gamma) is a cytokine, which is a major stimulator of monocytes and macrophages and thereby plays a role in the inflammatory response. Platelet-derived growth factor plays an important role in wound healing through recruiting monocytes, stimulating fibroblast migration and proliferation, increasing collagen synthesis, and collagenase secretion. However, it has no role in angiogenesis. Interleukin-1 (IL-1) is a cytokine produced by macrophages that activates, T- and B-lymphocytes, neutrophils, epithelial cells, and fibroblasts. It also plays a role in wound healing and inflammation. However, it has no role in angiogenesis. Tumor necrosis factor beta (TNF-β) is another inflammatory mediator released primarily by activated T-lymphocytes. It increases the synthesis of adhesion molecules by endothelial cells thereby allowing neutrophils to adhere to blood vessel walls at the site of infection. This mediator also activates the respiratory burst in neutrophils enhancing their killing power.

2. B. This infant most likely has osteogenesis imperfecta, a genetic disease caused by defects in the synthesis of type I collagen. These defects usually result from mutations in the genes coding for the α-1 and α-2 chains of the collagen molecule. Severe cases like the one described here likely involve mutations in the molecules that prevent normal formation of the triple helix of collagen. Type I collagen is the most common type of collagen found. It makes up skin, bone tendon, and the cornea. Defects in this form of collagen would therefore lead to skeletal abnormalities, "brittle bones," and blue sclera. Elastin is one of the fibrillar proteins that make up elastic fibers. These fibers form branching, irregular networks in connective tissue found in large arteries, trachea, and skin. Type II collagen is found primarily in cartilage, and the vitreous body. Type III collagen is made up of thin fibrils arranged in reticular networks found in lymphoid organs, blood vessels, and skin. Type IV collagen is arranged in sheets and makes up the basil lamina.

Case 36

1. C. Salivary gland biopsy is crucial in making the diagnosis of Sjögren's syndrome. In this disease, lymphocytic infiltrates are noted in the major and minor salivary glands. Elevated levels of SS A (Ro) antibodies are another criteria used in diagnosing Sjögren's; however, their presence is ascertained by checking titers in serum. These antibodies are not visualized in salivary gland biopsies. Collagen deposition and fibrosis of the salivary glands are more typical of scleroderma, not Sjögren's syndrome. Glandular proliferation with resulting loss of normal salivary gland architecture is characteristic of salivary gland tumors. Neutrophils are inflammatory cells that can be seen in bacterial infections of the salivary glands. They are typically seen in Sjögren's.

2. D. The predominant cell type seen in the salivary gland biopsy in a patient with Sjögren's syndrome is the helper T-lymphocyte. The primary immune function of this cell is to enhance the immune response through (a) the production of cytokines, which in turn activate B-cells and stimulate their maturation into antibody-producing plasma cells; and (b) activate macrophages and cytotoxic T-cells. B-cells—not T-cells—are responsible for antibody production. Cells of the B lineage also have memory that allows them to respond rapidly when reexposure to antigens occurs. Opsonization is the process by which foreign bacteria are coated with antibodies or complement protein C3b, which facilitate phagocytosis by macrophages and polymorphonuclear cells. The complement cascade leads to lysis of cells such as bacteria, allografts, and tumor cells. This system also generates mediators that contribute to the inflammatory response and attract phagocytes. Finally, this system contributes C3b that opsonizes foreign bacteria. The cascade is activated via two pathways: the classic pathway that is initiated by antigen-antibody complexes, and the alternative pathway that is triggered by cell surface substances such as bacterial lipopolysaccharides, fungal cell walls, and viral envelopes.

3. E. Rheumatoid arthritis often improves during pregnancy. While there are no clear adverse pregnancy outcomes associated with rheumatoid arthritis, women with this disorder often possess a number of different auto-antibodies including anti-SS A (Ro,) which has been associated with neonatal systemic lupus erythematosus (SLE) and congenital heart block. Therefore it is often advisable to check titers in pregnant women with autoimmune diseases such as SLE, rheumatoid arthritis, and Sjögren's syndrome. Both antinuclear antibody (ANA) and rheumatoid factor may be present in women with rheumatoid arthritis; however, neither correlates well with disease severity and activity, nor do levels of either correlate with pregnancy outcome. Although both an amniocentesis as well as serum or amniotic fluid AFP (alphafetal protein) would provide information on the potential for chromosomal or structural defects in this child, neither would be obtained at 7 weeks' gestation. Serum AFP is usually checked at 14 to 20 weeks' gestation. Elevated levels are correlated with midline structural defects as well as neural tube defects. Decreased levels are associated with chromosomal anomalies. Amniocentesis is not usually performed until at least 15 to 18 weeks' of gestation.

Case 37

1. A. Blood vessels are composed of an outer adventitia layer, inner media, and innermost intima. The intima is composed of endothelium, basal lamina, and subendothelial connective tissue. Arteries contain an internal elastic lamina separating the intima from the media. Muscular arteries also have an external elastic lamina to facilitate diameter changes. As the innermost layer with maximal exposure to foreign antigens and immunosurveillance the endothelium is the most affected in Kawasaki's disease.

2. D. The erythrocyte sedimentation rate (ESR) has been the most widely used and studied index of the acute-phase response of inflammatory disease. Elevations in the speed of sedimentation in anticoagulated blood was known to ancient Greeks. Increased acute-phase proteins—particularly fibrinogen and immunoglobulins—causes increased aggregation of erythrocytes (rouleaux formation or stacking). This is facilitated by the decreased natural tendency of erythrocytes to repel each other with negatively charged polysaccharide surface molecules.

3. D. This patient most likely has Takayasu's arteritis—a chronic vasculitis of the aorta and its branches—most commonly seen in young women of Asian descent. Initial symptoms include malaise and arthralgias. As the disease progresses and there is increasing fibrosis and narrowing of the aorta, headaches, visual changes, and angina pectoris may develop. On examination, peripheral pulses are noted to be asymmetrically decreased and hypertension can be seen. Patients with this disorder are noted to have an elevated ESR. However, this is not specific for the disease and is seen in numerous other systemic inflammatory disorders. An EKG may reveal ischemic disease if the aortitis affects the coronary artery ostia. Renal disease is rare in this disease and is usually related to ischemia or hypertensive changes. Thus, a renal biopsy is not useful in diagnosis. Arteriography is the best test for confirming the diagnosis. An aortogram usually reveals the narrowing of the great vessels. P-ANCA is associated with polyarteritis nodosa, not Takayasu's arteritis.

4. B. Pneumonia can cause an acute asthma exacerbation. However, it is an unlikely diagnosis in this patient who has chronic symptoms and evidence of systemic inflammatory disease. In pneumonia, one would most likely see an elevated WBC count with increased neutrophils and a left shift, and chest x-ray would reveal focal consolidation as opposed to patchy or nodular infiltrates. Churg-Strauss syndrome, polyarteritis nodosa, and Goodpasture's disease are all systemic vasculitides that can affect the respiratory tract. In polyarteritis nodosa, patients have constitutional symptoms such as fever and malaise. Joint pains and skin manifestations are also common. Lungs may be affected but this occurs only rarely. Goodpasture's disease is characterized by a necrotizing hemorrhagic interstitial pneumonitis with concomitant proliferative glomerulonephritis. The primary pulmonary symptom is not an asthma exacerbation but hemoptysis. Chest x-ray in these patients usually reveals focal pulmonary consolidation. Churg-Strauss syndrome is often seen in people who have a history of asthma or allergic disease. Patients have symptoms of systemic inflammatory disease, fever, arthralgias, myalgias, and weight loss. Asthma exacerbation is often the initial pulmonary symptom. Eosinophilia is characteristic of this disease. Diagnosis is confirmed by biopsy of involved vascular or renal tissue, which would reveal inflammation and necrotizing microgranulomas with eosinophilic infiltrates. Buerger's disease is seen in heavy smokers and is characterized by acute and chronic inflammation of medium and small arteries of the extremities in conjunction with segmental thrombosis. It does not usually affect the vessels of the lungs.

Case 38

1. D. Colchicine is effective only for relieving the pain of acute gouty attack, and reducing the frequency of attacks. It works by binding tubulin a microtubular protein important in cellular movement thereby disrupting the mobility of granulocytes decreasing the number of these cells that migrate to the affected joint. This medication also inhibits the synthesis and release of leukotrienes. However, it does *not* prevent progression of the disease. The other two medications are useful in the prevention of complications and recurrent acute episodes. Allopurinol decreases the production of uric acid by inhibiting xanthine oxidase—the enzyme that catalyzes oxidation of hypoxanthine to xanthine as well as that of xanthine to uric acid. Probenecid enhances the renal excretion of uric acid. Because obesity and excess alcohol intake are associated with gout, weight reduction as well as decreased alcohol intake are also recommended for prevention of complications.

2. C. Thiazide diuretics have actually been associated with acute gouty attacks. These inhibit renal excretion of uric acid and are therefore not recommended for the treatment of hypertension in patients with gout.

3. B. Hypoxanthine-guanine phosphoribosyltransferase is an enzyme involved in the salvage pathway for synthesis of purines. It transforms guanine to guanylic acid (GMP) and hypoxanthine to inosinic acid (IMP). Deficiency of this enzyme leads to increased synthesis of purines via the de novo pathway thereby leading to increased uric acid production. The degree of deficiency of this enzyme can vary. A complete absence of this enzyme results in Lesch-Nyhan syndrome, which is an x-linked disorder seen only in males. Patients with this syndrome have severe neurologic deficits, hyperuricemia, gouty arthritis, and are noted to exhibit self-mutilation. Minimal deficiencies in this enzyme, on the other hand, can cause only hyperuricemia and gouty arthritis with only mild neurological deficits. This patient likely has only a partial deficiency. Adenine phosphoribosyltransferase is another enzyme involved in the salvage pathway of purine synthesis. It catalyzes the transformation of adenine into adenylic acid (AMP). Deficiency of this enzyme would lead to a build-up of adenine. AMP could still be salvaged from adenosine or be created from IMP. Xanthine oxidase is involved in the de novo pathway transforming hypoxanthine into xanthine. Deficiency of this enzyme would lead to build-up of hypoxanthine and inosine, and a decrease in the amount of uric acid produced. Phosphoribosylpyrophosphate synthetase is an enzyme involved in the de novo pathway. Overactivity—not deficiency—of this enzyme can lead to increased uric acid. Amidophosphoribosyltransferase is another enzyme involved in the de novo pathway. Like phosphoribosylpyrophosphate synthetase, overactivity rather than deficiency would lead to increased uric acid.

4. B. Gout can be seen in medical conditions that cause hyperuricemia by increasing the production of uric acid or by decreasing its elimination. Conditions that involve an increase in the breakdown and turnover of purines include myeloproliferative disorders, lymphoproliferative disorders, carcinoma and sarcomas, chronic hemolytic anemias, cytotoxic drugs, psoriasis. Conditions that cause decreased renal clearance of uric acid include kidney disease and disorders in which renal tubular transport is impaired such as lactic acidosis and ketoacidosis. Hepatitis, hyperthyroidism, hypercholesterolemia and renal artery stenosis have no effect on uric acid production or elimination and are not therefore likely to be a cause for gout. However, leukemia with its increased production of granulocytes and increased purine metabolism *can* lead to hyperuricemia and gout.

Case 39

1. C. This patient has had progressive joint destruction and most likely has developed osteophytes, or bone spurs in the joints of her hands that are limiting the range of motion in these joints and causing increased pain. When these bony enlargements are found in the proximal interphalangeal joints they are called Bouchard's nodes. When they affect the distal interphalangeal joints they are called Heberden's nodes. Acute inflammation characterized by swelling, erythema, warmth, and tenderness is not commonly seen in osteoarthritis; it is more characteristic of the inflammatory arthritides such as rheumatoid arthritis, gout, and septic arthritis. The metatarsophalangeal joints are found in the feet, not in the hands. Rheumatoid nodules are subcutaneous nodules seen in rheumatoid arthritis. Hyperextension of the proximal interphalangeal joints, otherwise known as "swan neck" deformities, are seen in advanced rheumatoid arthritis.

2. D. Articular cartilage is composed primarily of hyaline cartilage that is formed by a framework of type II collagen, proteoglycans aggregates that make up most of the extracellular matrix, and chondrocytes. It is the hydrophilic proteoglycan aggregates that bind to water and give this type of cartilage its elasticity. The collagen provides tensile strength and resilience. Chondrocytes produce the extracellular matrix and collagen, but do not themselves contribute to any supportive properties of cartilage. Osteoclasts are found in bone and involved primarily with bone reabsorption and remodeling. Synovial fluid is found in the joint space and acts as a lubricant as well as providing nutrition for the cartilage.

3. E. In advanced osteoarthritis such as this patient has, there has been destruction of the cartilage and extensive bony remodeling. Osteoblasts are likely to be the most active cells in the joint at this point because these are involved in laying down more bone in response to the increased stress on the joint with the loss of the articular cartilage. In advanced disease, chondrocyte activity is likely low because most of the cartilage has been destroyed. Neutrophils are involved in acute bacterial infection of the joint and unlikely to be seen in osteoarthritis. CD 8 T cells play a key role in cell mediated immunity. These are not likely to be found in osteoarthritis, which is a degenerative—not autoimmune-mediated—arthritis. Osteophytes are not cells but the bony spurs formed late in the disease as a result of bony remodeling.

Case 40

1. E. This fluid is characteristic of septic arthritis. Although other inflammatory arthritides—rheumatoid arthritis and gout—can cause an inflammation in the joint space, the degree is not as marked as in an infection of the joint. A 55-year-old man who recently underwent knee surgery is at risk for infection, particu-

larly with *Staphylococcus epidermidis.* The older woman with chronic knee pain (choice a) most likely suffers from osteoarthritis, which is a degenerative disease that does not require synovial fluid aspiration because the fluid would be normal in appearance. In a 42-year-old man with severe, sudden onset of big toe pain, the most likely diagnosis is gout. Examination of the fluid of the affected joint in this patient would reveal cloudy fluid with some polymorphonuclear (PMN) leukocytes present. The characteristic finding in this patient would be needle-shaped, negatively birefringent crystals seen with polarized light microscopy. A 37-year-old woman with a lupus flare would most likely present with polyarthritis as well as other symptoms. There would not likely be a single affected joint to tap. If a tap was done on an affected joint it would reveal evidence of moderate inflammation but not severe inflammation with turbid fluid and numerous PMNs. In a 15-year-old boy who experiences a traumatic injury to a joint, arthrocentesis would reveal grossly bloody fluid.

2. C. Although this patient is at high risk for traumatic or degenerative joint changes due to her running, her signs and symptoms indicate an infectious arthritis due to *Neisseria gonorrhoeae.* This type of arthritis is seen most commonly in young, sexually active individuals. It is characterized by an insidious onset in which the monoarticular joint pain is preceded by polyarthralgias. These patients typically develop a pustular rash on their palms and soles and have affected joints that are extremely tender, swollen, and warm to the touch. Synovial fluid analysis of this patient's affected joint would reveal marked leukocytosis with a predominance of neutrophils, not lymphocytes. Gram stain would show gram-positive diplococci. Gram-positive cocci would be seen in infections with *Streptococcus* or *Staphylococcus* infections. Gram-negative rods would be seen in *E. coli* or *Pseudomonas* infections, which are most commonly seen in IV drug users. Negatively birefringent crystals are observed in gout when polarized light microscopy is used; these are not visualized with Gram stain.

3. E. Gonococcal arthritis usually responds well to antibiotic treatment. The patient should be admitted and IV antibiotics given until her symptoms resolve. Although this type of infection has been treated with outpatient antibiotics in the past, increasing antibiotic resistance has led to current recommendations for hospitalized IV therapy until improvement in symptoms. Third-generation cephalosporins are usually effective. Once patients show improvement, they may be switched to an oral third-generation cephalosporin or ciprofloxacin to complete a 7- to 10-day course. Usually, antibiotic therapy alone is enough and therapeutic arthrocentesis is rarely needed. This patient's boyfriend should also be treated for gonorrhea; however, a single injection of ceftriaxone would be inadequate to treat this patient's problem. NSAIDs and rest alone is inadequate treatment for infectious arthritis. The patient is not likely to have rheumatoid arthritis or systemic lupus erythematosus so tests for rheumatoid factor and antinuclear antibody are unwarranted. Colchicine is a treatment option for an acute attack of gout, not for infectious arthritis.

Index

Index note: page references with *b, f,* or *t* indicate a box, figure, or table.